$\mathcal{N}$OURISHING DESTINY

NOURISHING DESTINY

THE INNER TRADITION OF CHINESE MEDICINE

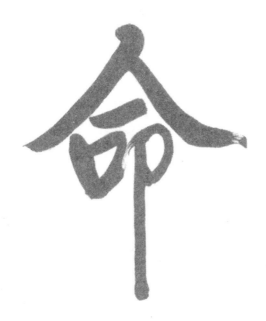

Lonny S. Jarrett

Help create the future of Chinese medicine online at Nourishingdestiny.com
http://www.spiritpathpress.com
Email: spiritpathpress@aol.com

Copyright 1998, 2000, 2001, 2004, 2009 Spirit Path Press
Published by Spirit Path Press,
PO Box 1093, Stockbridge, Massachusetts, 01262

Library of Congress Catalog Card Number: 98-91097
ISBN Number: 0-9669916-0-5

Book Design by Ruth Kolbert
Composition by Toni Kenny,
Elements of Design: elementsofdesign@adelphia.net

DISCLAIMER

This book is designed to provide information on the covered subject
matter. It is sold with the understanding that the material herein is schol-
arly in nature and that any clinical application is the sole responsibilty
of the practitioner. Readers should consult a licensed herbalist before
making use of any plant for medical purposes.

Every effort has been made to make this text as accurate as possible.
However, there may be errors in content or that are typographical in nature.
The author and Spirit Path Press have neither liability nor responsibility
to any entity or any person with respect to any loss, injury, or damage
caused, directly or indirectly, by the information contained in this book.

If you do not agree to the above, you may return this book to the
publisher for a full refund.

This work
is dedicated to my grandmother
Betty Dobkin
whose love and kindness touch all who I have touched.

CONTENTS

FOREWORD

Sitting here, pen in hand, stranded beside the information superhighway. Why another book about Chinese medicine? This one neither an easy read nor a compendium of treatment formulae (the two most successful strategies for budding authors in this field).

From the moment I first met Lonny Jarrett, I felt that he had in him a touch of genius akin to that of his inspirator, J.R. Worsley. Both seem to meet the criteria for spirits and sages in the *Nan Jing:* "One who looks and knows it is to be called a spirit. One who listens and knows it is to be called a sage." I had seen this uncanny ability in Lonny, and numerous examples can be found in *Nourishing Destiny,* confirming the author's gift for diagnosis at a glance, whether in person or even by a telephone answering machine! After more than two decades at practicing these skills myself, I believe it fair to conclude that heaven bestows these gifts with the same frequency and scatter as with all other remarkable facilities, be they perfect pitch in musicians or the ability to make automatic calculations in mathematicians. As a corollary, I suspect we each have our own special treasure hidden within us, only awaiting self-discovery. This premise is explicitly developed as a major theme of the book in hand: How each of us begins life with a unique destiny, granted by heaven (or nature or the *Dao*—take your pick) and it is up to each of us, with the help of our fellows, to fulfill that destiny otherwise known as our life's purpose. Of course, first we must find out what that purpose is . . .

It is high time someone address the relationship between Chinese medicine and an understanding of life's purpose. *Nourishing Destiny* presents many novel and intriguing thoughts on this matter, ultimately based on the classics. Like Worsley before him, Jarrett has synthesized material from a wealth of different traditions. His work is the first in English that seriously attempts to integrate in a clinical context the essential teachings of philosophical Daoism, Daoist alchemy, traditional acupuncture in its various incarnations, and Chinese herbal medicine. It is really a work in progress, and though it may be difficult to fathom all that is offered, there is much here to inspire both the lay reader and the practitioner. I hope this work reaches the wide audience who might benefit from its wisdom.

Peter Eckman M.D., Ph.D, M.Ac.(U.K)

Peter Eckman

PREFACE

―――――

A View of the Labyrinth from Above

A scholar of the Chinese language once commented to me that in order to read and comprehend a passage written in Chinese one has to already have read it. This is because the meaning of Chinese characters is purely contextual. We do not possess a context for understanding the meaning of characters that appear at the beginning of a passage until we have already read the entire piece. A corollary of this principle when teaching Chinese medicine is that one cannot present any topic without constantly referring to other topics which have, by necessity, not yet been presented. Similarly, the information that appears throughout this book only emerges in context once the entire book has been read. Readers accustomed to a more linear presentation of information may find this approach confusing at times. Therefore, I offer here an overview of the text to help orient you before embarking on your journey.

This book is divided into three sections corresponding to the divisions of heaven, human, and earth. Part I, Chapters 1 through 7, corresponds to heaven. This material represents the theoretical foundations and language of the inner tradition. Part II (Chapters 8–11) corresponds to humanity. I discuss the notion of five-element constitutional type as it provides insight into the human condition. I also examine the physiology of blood and *qi* from the perspective of the inner tradition. Part III, Chapters 12 through 15, corresponds to earth. These chapters provide grounding for the theoretical considerations of the first two parts by applying them to the process of diagnosis and treatment.

Heaven

All models of medicine are based on scientific systems which, in turn, are predicated on a culture's assumptions about the fundamental nature of existence. In Chapter 1 I focus on Chinese creation mythology as it lays the foundational assumptions held by the ancient Chinese about the nature of life and the human condition. I examine the Daoist enumeration of being as it describes the generation of the material universe and establishes the theme of heaven and earth being blended back into a primordial unity by a whirling vortex of *qi*. As nonbeing evolves into being, humans emerge to blend heaven and earth through the fulfillment of personal destiny. The myth of Emperor Yu controlling the floods exemplifies the importance of channeling *dao* and fulfilling destiny as a way of restoring original nature.

Chapter 2 examines the importance of destiny, which serves as the foundation for the inner tradition. Fulfillment of destiny involves actualizing the potential virtues present in our constitutional endowment of *jing, qi,* and *shen*. The human who fulfills destiny is able to acknowledge original nature, initiate actions consistent with manifesting his or her innate purpose, and utilize every situation encountered in life as an opportunity for self-cultivation.

The first sentences of the *Dao De Jing* suggest that language creates reality. The ways in which many of the characters that are foundational in Chinese medicine have been defined in modern texts often reflects both a materialistic ideology and causal quality of thought. In Chapter 3 I redefine some of the fundamental terms of Chinese medicine in order to reflect more accurately the worldview and theoretical assumptions of the inner tradition. This discussion focuses on defining the relative contribution of innate and acquired influences to human nature.

Although heaven may will a destiny for each of us, it cannot force us to manifest the seed it has planted within. Chapter 4 examines the importance of human will *(zhi)* in acting as a conduit between the activating impulse *(shen)* from our hearts and our innate potential *(jing)* to manifest in the world. I also examine the role of will in mediating the interaction of the inherited and acquired constitution.

Chapter 5 discusses the fulfillment of human destiny as it is predicated on the integrated functioning of our primordial endowment of *yin* and *yang*, *jing* and *shen*, and the innate and acquired constitutions. These three dualities are blended into one totality within the fires of *mingmen*, the gate of destiny. The integrity of these processes largely depends on the fidelity with which each human is able to perceive life uncolored by the interpretations of his or her own mind. Acquired belief systems that do not conform to true self dampen the flames of *mingmen* and suppress the expression of one's innate purpose.

The infant possesses original nature that may be returned to by the sage through the cultivation of virtue. It is destiny that each of us loses original nature, but it is not certain it will be regained in our lifetime. Chapter 6 enumerates seven stages of distancing from original nature organized according to the theories of Daoist scholar Liu Yiming. Here we examine the separation of *yin* and *yang* and the emergence of our five-element constitutional type. The human journey from conception to death is explored in terms of its clinical significance for the inner tradition.

In the Daoist enumeration of being, the number seven corresponds to the loss and return of original nature. Chapter 7 discusses the clinical significance of the separation of *yin* and *yang* in the context of Chinese pulse diagnoses and the husband/wife imbalance. Here we view the mechanism that determines whether an individual awakes to original nature in his or her lifetime or dies estranged from true self. I discuss the physiological consequences of becoming estranged from one's destiny.

Humanity

Part II is concerned with the process of diagnosing the functional dynamics that lead to the loss and return of original nature.

Chapter 8 introduces the five-element system as a method of assessing the human being's functional relationship to nature. The theoretical foundations of the five-element system are presented in relationship to the holographic paradigm. Diagnosis by color, sound, odor, emotion, and pulse is presented as a method for assessing the specific quality of a patient's constitutional endowment.

Chapter 9 elaborates the notion of constitutional type. The path of healing for each individual is defined as the transformation of a disordered emotion back into its corresponding virtue. A case study illustrates how an individual's interpretation of his life experience may ultimately be embodied as pathology. The role of constitutional diagnosis and treatment is presented as it empowers his healing and reconnection to true self. Emphasis is placed on the interaction of the practitioner with the patient as a potential source of healing.

Chapter 10 presents the twelve officials of Chinese medicine as they comprise the window through which we may view each of the constitutional types. The *yin* and *yang* officials associated with each element are discussed as they comprise, respectively, the functions of heart and mind. The importance of the heart/kidney axis in maintaining functional integrity of the heart and mind is presented. Several case studies illustrate the constitutional attributes of each official.

In Chapter 11 the physiology of *qi* and blood is discussed as it empowers the fulfillment of destiny. *Qi* is defined as that which enables one to act virtuously and blood is defined as that which empowers us to be virtuous. The difference between blood and *qi* is described as the difference between being and doing.

Earth

Part III emphasizes the principles of treatment in aiding the return to original nature and the nourishment of destiny.

Chapter 12 presents the notions of illness, health, and healing as they are inherent in the inner tradition. The healing crisis is discussed as it pertains to the turning point in a patient's process of treatment. The mechanism by which Chinese medicine promotes health and empowers the fulfillment of destiny is elaborated. The virtue of the sage, as exemplified in Daoist writings, is discussed as a role model for the practitioner who aspires to be a healer.

Chapter 13 reiterates the themes found throughout the text as they occur in the names and functions of specific acupuncture points. Acupuncture points are described as foci at which multiple aspects of being overlap and may be simultaneously influenced.

Chapter 14 presents the role of the intake in gathering all relevant diagnostic information necessary to perform a constitutional diagnosis. All interactions with patients from the moment of hearing their voice on the answering machine through watching them walk away from the intake are analyzed for their potential value in diagnosis. I discuss the role of diagnosis in initiating the patient's movement toward healing.

Chapter 15 presents the theoretical principles discussed throughout the book within the context of two case studies. The entire intake and its interpretation is presented along with a detailed pulse and tongue analysis. I describe the results of the first eight to ten treatment sessions including the reasoning behind each acupuncture point needled and herb prescribed. The outcome of treatment is discussed in both cases.

Appendix

Western science involves the quantitative analysis of structure, and traditional Chinese science involves the qualitative assessment of function. The appendix examines the complementary natures of Chinese and Western medicine as they flow from the foundational assumptions inherent in the worldviews on which they are based.

ACKNOWLEDGMENTS

Words truly fail to express the heartfelt gratitude I feel toward so many for having taken the time to teach and encourage me over the years. First, I must express thanks to my family for their care and nurturance throughout this lifetime. My parents have always encouraged me to pursue my interests and follow my heart. My wife Devajyoti and my children Anjelica Li and Zev Elijah are shining stars and I am truly blessed for their presence in my life. I love you all.

I feel fortunate to have had several excellent teachers early in life including Stuart Feinstein, Hilda Robbins, and Al Tartaglia. I am also proud to have attended Hampshire College where the school motto is, "To know is not enough." The behavior genetics course I took there with teachers Lynn Miller and Ray Coppinger helped form the foundation for my ability to write and to think critically. A heartfelt thanks to Pat Model at the Albert Einstein College of Medicine, who taught me the virtue of taking pride in my work.

I would like to thank my teachers in the martial arts who taught me discipline and helped empower me to embody my beliefs as virtues—with a deep bow to Masters Marion Taylor, Ron Dephino, Danny Chang, Master James B.C. Yu, and James Holloway. In the field of

Chinese medicine I owe special thanks to two of my early teachers, Paul Gallagher and Jonathan Klate, who have remained encouraging to this day. Lots of love to my first practitioner Letha Hadady and thanks for her generosity and care. I also am thankful to Leon Hammer for his shared knowledge and friendship. I thank Ted Kaptchuk with whom I studied herbal medicine. His approach to Chinese medicine is profound and he has done something beautiful with this art. I would also like to acknowledge Dianne Connelly, who taught me the power of proper intention in speaking and Professor J.R. Worsley for having worked tirelessly to preserve the spirit of something beautiful in this world.

Thanks to those who have supported my teaching over the years, both as students and workshop organizers, including Bobbi Aqua, Carl Dahlgren, Michael Gaeta, Tom Gentile, Nancy Hokenson, Chris Hudson, and Deborah V. Smith. I would also like to thank Bob Duggan, Barbara Ellrich, and Barbara Ely at the Traditional Acupuncture Institute, Laura Mignosa at the Connecticut Institute of Herbal Studies, and Dan Seitz at the New England School of Acupuncture.

I am indebted to Mary Ellen Zorbaugh and Volker Scheid for publishing my first articles. A special thanks to the entire staff at the *American Journal of Acupuncture,* especially Alison Shafer and W.G. Grace for their diligence in helping me refine my early work. Sandy Camper was quite helpful in editing the initial stages of this text. A heartfelt thanks to Anne Lesser, who through masterful editing helped complete and polish this book to final form. I appreciate the help of Ruth Kolbert for designing the text and cover and of Toni Kenny for page-setting the book. Special thanks to Subhuti Dharmananda, Iona Marsaa Teegaurden, and Jeffrey C. Yuen for taking much time to read and comment on my book. Special thanks as well to Marlow Brooks for her beautiful calligraphy throughout the text and to Jin Huai Wang for his calligraphy on the front cover. I am also indebted to Peter Eckman for his foreword and for taking the time to read several revisions of this text as it was in preparation. Thanks to my friends Peter Kadar and Will and Bobbie Morris for providing input on the project at different stages of completion.

I would also like to thank my special friends Chandrakant, Dick, Kurt, Lori, Patrick, and Robin who have shared the journey and lightened the path. There is not enough that I can say to thank my dear friends Thea Elijah and Will Wadsworth for the years of encouragement they gave me while I was writing this text. Many of the concepts in this book transitioned from vague impressions to formed ideas during endless hours of passionate discussion with Thea who "steers by the torch of chaos and doubt." She is inspiration itself.

The upper class of medicines . . . govern the nourishment of destiny and correspond to heaven. . . . If one wishes to prolong the years of life without aging, one should [use these].

The middle class of medicines govern the nourishment of one's nature and correspond to man. . . . If one wishes to prevent illness and to supplement depletions and emaciations, one should [use these].

The lower [class of] medicines . . . govern the treatment of illness and correspond to earth. If one wishes to remove cold, heat and [other] evil influences [from the body], to break accumulations, and to cure illnesses, one should base [one's efforts] on [drugs listed in] the lower [class of this] manual.
– SHEN NONG BEN CAO

Clearly, for the author of the *Shen Nong Ben Cao*, China's oldest herbal text, the highest aspect of healing involves helping the patient fulfill destiny in order to live out the years as allotted by heaven. Below that level of healing is the nourishment of humans' inborn nature *(xing:*性*)*. The lowest class of medicine treats only physical illness. As early as the third century C.E., the alchemist Ge Hong laments that these words "come from the highest sages," yet the people of his age have lost their belief in the efficacy of the highest forms of medicine.

In this book I examine the tradition of Chinese medicine, whose primary therapeutic focus is to help patients fulfill their personal destiny. I call this the "inner tradition of Chinese medicine," hereafter referred to as the "inner tradition." As suggested by Ge Hong, even in his time the practice of this inner tradition represented only a small part of the practice of Chinese medicine. Today, the quality of thought inherent in this tradition has been all but lost in the materialistic ideology of the modern era.

At the outset, it is important to comprehend precisely my use of the term "inner tradition." Ge Hong's texts, the *Wai Bian* and the *Nei Bian,* exemplify the distinction between the inner and outer traditions. The *Wai Bian* is an external *(wai:*外*)* text belonging to the Confucian school that addresses public affairs. The *Nei Bian* is an internal *(nei:*內*)* text of alchemy that focuses on spiritual transformation and the fulfillment of destiny.

All endeavors in life may be divided into both inner and outer aspects. For example, the practice of martial arts ranges along a broad continuum from relatively "soft" internal styles, such as Taiji, which focus on self-cultivation, promotion of health, and obtaining longevity, to relatively "hard" external styles, such as Tae Kwon Do, which focus predominantly on cultivating physical strength and self-defense. Despite this distinction, note that even a slow meditative style such as Taiji has self-defense applications and, likewise, a fast, hard style such as Tae Kwon Do may help cultivate inner virtues such as self-esteem and personal integrity. The inner and outer aspects of a discipline thus are not mutually exclusive. However, the particular point occupied by a given tradition of practice along the continuum from relatively internal (dealing with spirit) to relatively external (dealing with the body) tends to define the limits of practitioners in their ability to address the root of illness and imbalance.

The master practitioner must be able to take the therapeutic action most appropriate in the moment for the individual patient. This entails being able to access patients on many levels, ranging from their depth of spirit to the most superficial aspects of their physical being. Too often, the deeper aspects of treatment are neglected in modern traditions of Chinese medicine, thus depriving the practitioner of tools that could otherwise help to assimilate and apply the wealth of information continually emerging from the patient's depth of being. Were he present to observe modern practice, Ge Hong might be frustrated by the prevalent lack of belief in "the highest forms of medicine." However, in my travels as a teacher, I have noticed an increasing interest by practitioners of all traditions in the inner aspects of their art that might enable them to address more explicitly matters of emotion, mind, and spirit.

Historically, in China, practitioners of the numerous diverse family traditions of medicine were likely aware of, influenced by, and perhaps took for granted the writings that contain the quality of thought delineated in this text. In the West, contemporary practitioners of relatively external acupuncture and herbal traditions may be aware to one degree or another that their treatments affect their patients at deep levels of emotional and spiritual function and expression. However, in these traditions, no generally available framework explicates either diagnosis or treatment at this level. My work in this text represents an attempt to meet this need.

The term "inner tradition" refers to the practice of Chinese medicine in a way that places primary emphasis on the use of medicine as a tool to aid spiritual evolution. Most notably, a patient's progress in treatment is assessed primarily by indicators of conscious awareness and balanced emotional functioning rather than, as is done in more external traditions of practice, assessing response to treatment with primary emphasis on the relative presence or absence of pain or other physical symptomatology. Of course, inherent in the inner tradition is the expectation that as the constitutional basis of illness becomes balanced at a deep level, physical symptoms will improve. Similarly, practitioners of external traditions might expect a patient to show a deeper balance of mind and spirit as physical symptoms abate. The distinguishing factor between the inner and outer levels of practice is the level of being, be it physical, emotional, or spiritual, which figures most explicitly in diagnosis, directing treatment, and assessing improvement in the patient.

The inner tradition is most explicitly concerned with the psychospiritual basis of illness and views physical symptoms and signs as relatively superficial manifestations that are compensations for underlying constitutional issues. This view is expressed in the *Shen Nong Ben Cao*, which designates the treatment of physical illness as corresponding to the lowest class of medicine. In this regard the Daoist Liu Cao states,

If the basic energy is not stabilized, the spirit is insecure. Let insects eat away at the root of a tree, and the leaves dry up. Stop talking about mucus, saliva, semen, and blood—when you get to the basis and find out the original source, they are all the same. When has this thing ever had a fixed location? It changes according to the time, according to mind and ideas.[1]

Another hallmark of the inner tradition is that it explicitly serves as an extension of the practitioner's own spiritual quest and path. A foundational principle of this tradition is that a practitioner may only engender a virtue in a patient to the degree that he or she is able to access that virtue within. The diagnostics inherent in the inner tradition require the practitioner to listen with all senses and with increasingly deeper sensitivity to the cues that spontaneously emerge from the patient. This method of honing the senses may, in time, clear away the accretions of experience and interpretation that color the practitioner's own experience of reality. Hence, through discipline and attentive practice, the functions of the heart and mind of the practitioner may once again be reunited.

The core efficacy of the tradition of Chinese medicine that I delineate in this text does not stem from the collection of techniques which it embraces or even its philosophical orientation. Rather the efficacy stems from the embodiment of the tradition within the life of the practitioner. I consider the regular practice of an embodied discipline such as a martial art or pulse diagnosis to be essential in this regard. One's efficacy as a healer lies, in large part, in having become one's art.

A major factor that initially inspired me to research and write this text was my inquiry into how Chinese physiology reflects the emphasis on spirit found in early Daoist texts such as the *Dao De Jing (Tao Te Ching)* and the *Zhuangzi (Chuang Tzu)*. Further, I suspected truths arrived at in my clinical practice had been addressed in the literature of Chinese medicine. In part, this text is an elaboration of my inquiry into the theoretical and spiritual foundations of my own clinical insights. My training in the neurosciences led me to understand that models of medicine are based on assumptions about the nature of being that are inherent in the scientific models on which they are based. These assumptions define the relative strengths and weaknesses of any medical paradigm based on them. All too often, practitioners of medicine remain ignorant of the fundamental assumptions of the medicine they practice. My goal here is to present the thread I have discovered at the heart of my own practice of Chinese medicine.

In elucidating the inner tradition, I have drawn heavily on the teachings of Chinese spiritual alchemy. Alchemy as a branch of medicine constitutes the meeting ground between disciplines such as acupuncture, herbalism, pure philosophy, and religion. That this is so is well reflected in the alchemist Ge Hong's citation of the *Shen Nong Ben Cao* in his own text of inner alchemy, the *Bao Bu Zi*. The language used to describe Chinese spirituality, alchemy, and medicine is remarkably similar, and these authors, working in overlapping disciplines, were likely to have been well aware of the other contexts in which important characters such as *shen, ling, jing,* and *qi* were also used. My own exposition of the language of Chinese medicine is informed equally by my research into the etymology and usage of characters and the role these concepts play in my daily clinical practice.

In ancient China, cosmologists sought a unified theory of the universe. They believed that, if their theoretical models were correct, they would be able to build pitch pipes that would resonate to the vibrational changes at each solstice and equinox, causing music to spontaneously emerge from them. They further reasoned that if the cosmological models were correct, they would be able to produce an accurate calendar. However, their calendar required continual readjustment, and the pitch pipes never sounded. Eventually, Europeans came to China bearing a telescope and an accurate calendar, demonstrating that a precise calendar could be formulated, but through measurement rather than cosmological and spiritual considerations. The impact on China of this quantitative and materialistic science was impressive. No longer were pitch pipes made and no longer were cosmological maps drawn from inner knowing. Thus it has been winter in Chinese medicine since that time. As its practice has spread throughout the world to other cultures, however, a new diversity is emerging and it appears to be springtime once again for this ancient and precious art and science.

Perhaps it is not that the pitch pipes never sounded, but rather that the pitching of the pipes was not listened for with inner hearing. Perhaps the ancient calendar was never correct because the cosmologists were mapping a realm where no time exists. Perhaps it is time once again to build pitch pipes and to draw maps of life based on the heart's wisdom as well as the mind's capacity to analyze data. It is time once again to listen to life with our hearts rather than just to "objectively" dissect life with our minds.

By ascribing the term "inner tradition" to five-element constitutional medicine, I do not mean to imply an elevated status over other traditions of practice. A great virtue of Chinese medicine is the diversity

of practice and theory it embraces. The spiritual path defined in this
text involves removing all constructs creating separation between the
functioning of one's own heart and mind and the hearts and minds of
others. Therefore, it is imperative that practitioners of all traditions
hold dearly that aspect of their own practice which is closest to their
own hearts without diminishing the value of the practice of others.

Diversity emerges as the natural expression of a balanced relationship between human will and the will of heaven. The will of heaven is
continuous, creative, evolutionary change. Humans formulate ways of
knowing that consist of models and systems. Newtonian physics,
quantum mechanics, and the five-element system are examples. These
models represent the human attempt to understand the earth and the
nature of our lives upon it. It is human nature to cling to these models
and the momentary stability that they appear to afford amid continuous change. Our models remain static, and as we build them into
towering monolithic structures whose foundations consist of assumptions and meanings we create, the true nature of life continues to
evolve and outgrow them. The edge of this creative change is always
just beyond the grasp of our deepest intuition. The momentary stability afforded by such models is an illusion because the essential nature
of life remains chaotic and unknowable. Models are tools, elaborate
stories, and we must recognize them as such. Diversity is what emerges
when individuals are each able to embrace the freedom to create their
own mythology while simultaneously allowing others that same freedom. For the sage, all stories are created equal inasmuch as they
empower the creative flow of life.

In conclusion, to the degree that my thesis conforms to the beliefs
and practices of those who have come before me, I am happy to cred-
it them. To the degree that this work challenges those who attach
importance to historical antecedents as a requisite condition for defining what is "true" Chinese medicine, I am happy to admit that "I made
this work up" and to let a self-aware inner tradition begin with this
text. This inquiry is offered to practitioners of relatively more external
traditions of practice who seek a deeper access to diagnostic and therapeutic skills focused on emotional and spiritual levels of human
experience. Further, it is my hope that this text may provide practitioners of internal traditions with a better grounding in the theoretical
basis of their practice and the historical sources of input to their art. It
is my hope that this text may provide a window for the inquisitive
mind to follow more deeply into the universe that is Chinese medicine.

Structure and Conventions of the Text

Structure

In writing this text I examine the lineage of thought regarding destiny that is present throughout the writings of many authors in the related disciplines of Chinese medicine, philosophy, alchemy, and religion. In essence, I have attempted to perform a constitutional diagnosis on Chinese medicine itself, seeking out what represents its deepest spirit. One purpose in writing this book is to provide a vision of Chinese medicine that extends from its primordial roots all the way to the realities of daily clinical practice in the modern era. We begin by examining Chinese creation mythology and the Daoist enumeration of being as they are present in the *Dao De Jing* and the *Zhuangzi*. This represents the primordial aspect of being out of which all of life arises and ultimately returns.

I then discuss the principles inherent in this worldview as they exist in the language of Chinese medicine and physiology. The nature of human consciousness, health, illness, healing, and the human journey through life is presented with an eye toward always relating the discussion back to the foundational notions present in myth. After establishing the human path from conception to death, I introduce the five-element system as a method that allows the practitioner to comprehend the qualitative nature of a patient's destiny and the way that failure to fulfill destiny is being embodied as illness. Finally, case studies are presented that elaborate the notions expressed in this text as they occur clinically.

In a sense, this book is comprised of two broad components. The foundational component consists of a lineage of thought regarding the nature of health, illness, and healing as it lies thematically at the heart of Chinese medicine. I then extend this quality of thought into the clinical component of the book, which is predicated on the five-element system. The basic theory and foundational concepts presented are grounded in the classics, but the extension of these principles into clinical practice represents only my own interpretations, insights, and experience. It is my hope that you readers will consider how the words and thoughts of China's great thinkers speak to your own tradition of practice.

A notion often repeated to me by my genetics professor in college was that the caliber of a scientist is defined by the quality of the questions that he or she asks. At the end of each chapter I pose several questions meant to help focus the spirit of inquiry contained in each chapter. It is my hope that they will serve the reader as they continue to serve me.

The organization of this book may be compared to the structure of a collapsing telescope. A telescope's basic function is to focus attention on and illuminate or enlarge a particular object, just as this book's purpose is to focus attention on and examine a particular concept: how Chinese medicine can impact the fulfillment of individual destiny. A collapsing telescope is basically an arrangement of overlapping cylindrical sections, starting with a small section, with each overlapping section becoming increasingly larger as necessary to encompass the whole. Hence many concepts are repeated from chapter to chapter, but expanded on with each new chapter adding more detail. The perspective on each topic becomes more embodied as the book moves from Chinese creation mythology to the realities of clinical practice. In a sense, the organization of this book may be likened to a hologram in which each chapter serves its own discrete function yet, through reference to the same foundational principles, always contains an implicit image of the whole.

Conventions

All transliterations of Chinese in this text are written in pinyin, a system for romanizing Chinese ideograms. For the sake of consistency, I have changed all source material, including direct quotes, to pinyin. For readers who may be more familiar with the names of Chinese philosophers as they appear in the Wade-Giles system of transliteration, see parenthetical reference after first mention.

This is essentially a work on human nature and therefore I have written the text to be as gender neutral as possible. For ease of reading, certain chapters make either the practitioner or patient male or female throughout, which is noted at the outset of the chapter.

———

NOTES

1. Liu Cao is presumed to be the teacher of Zhong Boduan (983–1082) and Wang Zhe (1113–1171), founders of the southern and northern schools of complete reality Daoism, respectively. See Cleary, 1989, p. xxvi.

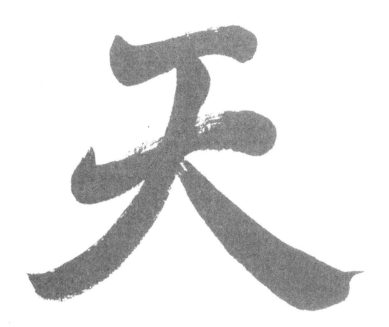

I

COSMOGONY

I am the wilderness before the dawn.
– *Dao De Jing* [1]

ALL MODELS OF MEDICINE ARE BASED ON WORLDVIEWS THAT reflect the underlying beliefs and assumptions about life inherent in their host culture. To appreciate the inner nature of Chinese medicine, we must first understand how the early Chinese thought about their world. The ways of knowing in ancient China focused on understanding the movements of the *dao*—the ultimate principle, the creative influence—as they are manifested externally in the universe and internally in humans. The *Dao De Jing* and the *Zhuangzi* are the earliest documents extant associated with the naturalistic philosophy of the Daode school.[2] They establish the fundamental assumptions about the nature of existence, inherent in the inner tradition of healing in Chinese medicine.

Human life must ultimately follow the ontogeny of the *dao*, for the implicit nature of the *dao* forms the foundation of our journey from birth to death. The developmental stages of the *dao*, as being emerges from nonbeing, are enumerated in the early Daoist texts. Enumeration is essential to understanding the functioning of the *dao* in the evolution of being. Reference to numbers also allows an understanding of the implicit movement of the *dao*, which lies at the heart of all observed phenomena in life. Think of it as the Daoists' attempt to order the different qualitative stages in the *dao's* evolution as they are inherent in phenomenological existence.

Daoist enumeration can be found in the domains of both mythology and science. Certainly, the use of numbers found in Daoist texts constitutes an essential part of early Chinese creation mythology. This enumeration was also used by the early Chinese to organize their perceptions of the world and the important functional relationships inherent in life. In this way, enumeration came to constitute a theoretical and scientific basis of the inductive synthetic worldview that lies at the heart of the inner tradition of Chinese medicine.[3]

It is important to note the emphasis here on the Daoists *qualitative* use of numbers as opposed to the *quantitative* use of numbers found in mathematics. The Daoists employed numbers to label nodal points at which different aspects of being were found to have similar functional qualities. For example, both heaven and *yuanqi* may be assigned the number "one" because they denote the influence of primal *yang* in the macro- and microcosm, respectively.

In this chapter, I explore some of the fundamental assumptions about the nature of life presented in the foundational texts of the inner tradition. I review Daoist enumeration relating to the evolution of the universe, as "being" *(wei:*為*)* emerges from "nonbeing" *(wuwei:*無為*)*. This presentation serves as the basis for a later discussion of humanity's gain, loss, and return to original nature.

The Ontogeny of the Dao: *Early and Later Heaven*

Chapter 42 of the *Dao De Jing* describes the basic numerical sequence of the creation of the material universe. It enumerates four stages, moving from the unity of nonbeing (the *dao*) to being (the ten thousand things):

> Dao *gives birth to one,*
> One *gives birth to two,*
> Two *gives birth to three,*
> Three *gives birth to the ten thousand things.*
> — *DAO DE JING* [4]

This enumeration describes the functional dynamics of being at increasing levels of complexity. The first three stages of evolution describe the paradise condition associated with the primal *dao*. Here the *dao* is like a cosmic womb from which being has not yet emerged. This stage of evolution is referred to as "early heaven" *(xiantian:先天)*. In Chinese physiology, early heaven corresponds to one's primordial endowment of *jing, qi,* and *shen* that are granted to each human at conception. This endowment is the physiological foundation of human evolution and individual purpose. It represents the seed of heaven's intent to provide an internal standard that may guide us through life.

The fourth stage of evolution at which the ten thousand things are born from the womb of the *dao* into material existence is referred to as "later heaven" *(houtian:後天)*. In Chinese physiology, the influence of later heaven corresponds to the essential *qi* acquired during life from food, air, and the positive interpretation of experience. As stages of human development, early heaven corresponds to the period of time from conception to the infant's first breath and later heaven corresponds to the period of time from the first breath to death. The interface of early and later heaven is the central axis along which the theme of each human life unfolds. Next I examine the essential characteristics of these domains according to Chinese enumeration and myth.

Early Heaven: The Womb of the Dao

> Let us go back to the Beginning: Before the Beginning was the *dao*. Let us call the *dao* zero, neither negative nor positive: pure potential *(ling)*. Then, the primordial energy will be one; it will be a kind of treasure *(bao)*, and that is exactly what the Chinese call it, comparing it to a single pearl in the midst of a boundless ocean.[5]

To begin at the beginning, we must discuss the fundamental nature of "no-thingness" itself, the *dao*. The qualitative nature of the *dao* is present throughout all creation and lies eternally in the depth of each being to which it gives birth. The *dao* is that all-embracing principle whose properties are inherently present throughout all of human existence. The inner path of healing in Chinese medicine consists in finding this kernel of truth that lies deep within each heart and assisting in its cultivation. To arrive at an understanding of the essential nature of the *dao* is of utmost importance, but an inherent pitfall awaits anyone who tries. Laozi (Lao Tzu), referring to the ultimate principle, says, "I do not know its proper name, but will call it *dao*."[6]

Dao is not the proper name of the ultimate principle, for what Laozi terms the *dao* is fundamentally unknowable by the human mind and, therefore, can have no proper name. In the very act of its naming, the "eternal" *dao* changes to the *dao* of transient existence, and the process of creation begins. Whatever we may say about the fundamental nature of the *dao*, eternal truth always lies beyond the reach of words, residing only in the realms of feeling and intuition. Laozi acknowledges that the name given by the character *dao* simply serves as a means to carry on a discourse on the subject of life's essential nature. With this caveat firmly in mind, we are now equipped to begin the inquiry into the fundamental nature of life itself.

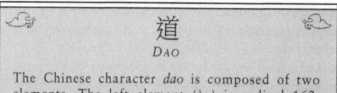

道

DAO

The Chinese character *dao* is composed of two elements. The left element (辶) is radical 162, which in its complete form (*zu*: 足) pictures a foot, signifying walking. The element on the right is the character *shou* (首), or radical 185, which signifies the head. Wieger tells us that the character denotes a road, a principle, or a doctrine.[7] The meaning conveyed by the character *dao* is the continuous progression and unfolding of nature along its evolutionary path. The character *dao* can also be constructed from the phrase *mu zi tou shou chuo* (目自頁首辶), which is comprised of characters meaning "to see," "self," "head," "understand," and "way," respectively. Thus we may comprehend *dao* as "the way one comes to see and understand oneself."[8]

The Dao *as One*

There was something chaotic yet complete,
Which existed before the creation of heaven and earth.
Without sound and formless,
It stands alone and does not change.
It pervades all and is free from danger;
It can be regarded as the mother of the world.

– DAO DE JING[9]

The *dao* is the state that exists before the creation of duality in the world and, as such, it precedes the creation of the ultimate duality, heaven and earth. It is the eternal, unnamed *dao* that gives rise to the one—the eternal principle named. The *dao* as one is the ground of all being, characterized in the *Dao De Jing* as "chaotic yet complete." Chaos *(hun:*混*)* and completion *(cheng:*成*)* are ultimate principles of life.

The *dao* is the complete totality that encompasses and harmonizes all opposites. In this primal state of *dao* all things are "formless," existing only as potential *(ling:*靈*)*. The potentiality of all things is interpenetrating, as the *dao* is implicit in all things and all things are implicit in one another. This state in which the *dao* "pervades all," and every "thing" contains an implicit image of every other "thing," is the basis of the holistic model that is foundational in the quality of thought contained in the inner tradition.

The undifferentiated oneness that is the eternal *dao* exists as chaos and is the source of randomness in the universe. Wang Bi defines chaos as "that which one cannot succeed in understanding."[10] The human mind is incapable of knowing the *dao* intellectually as unity because, as soon as it is known and named, it is no longer the one but the two: that which knows and that which is known. Recognizing that chaos is the foundation of existence, Zhuangzi states, "it is impossible to establish any constant rule."[11] Thus the essential nature of the *dao* as the ultimate principle is that of a unity embracing all of being and yet lying eternally just beyond the reach of human comprehension.

The inability of the human mind to comprehend the *dao* is emphasized again in Chapter 14 of the *Dao De Jing*:

> *What is looked at but not seen,*
> *Is named the extremely dim.*
> *What is listened to but not heard,*
> *Is named the extremely faint.*
> *What is grabbed but not caught,*
> *Is named the extremely small.*
> *These three things cannot be comprehended,*
> *Thus they blend* [hun] *into one.*[12]

The *dao*, the vast sea of potentiality, gives birth to the two, heaven and earth, the active and quiescent poles of the cosmos. Heaven rises out of the primordial chaos *(huntun:*混屯*)*, like a single star cast out over a boundless ocean. Radiating down *(shenming:*神明*)* upon the silent sea from which it rose, heaven extends *(shen:*神*)* its influence toward earth. The qualities of the two universal poles, heaven and earth, are perfectly blended *(chong: 沖)* by the *chongqi (沖氣)*. Sung dynasty scholar Wang An Shi (C.E. 1021–1086) described the *chongqi* as the empty whirling vortex revolving between heaven and earth. "The *dao* is *chong* and the *chongqi* is the original dynamism of the world."[13]

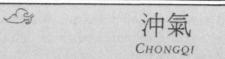

沖氣
CHONGQI

The character *chong* is composed of the water radical on the left and the phonetic component *zhong*, meaning "middle," "within," or "between," on the right. *Chong* has other meanings, including "to blend," "to infuse," and "to soar to." The character *chong*, when paired with the character *xu (虛)*, refers to the void between heaven and earth.[14] Hence the character pair *chongqi* may be taken to denote the quality of *qi* that lies at the center of all things, which, like a giant whirlpool, perfectly harmonizes all dualities and extremes back into the unity that is the essential nature of each being. This quality of *qi* holding steady at the center allows us to continually return to balance in life through the act of "centering" our self. This attribute of the *chongqi*, the harmonization of apparent opposites, is a central concept of the inner tradition of Chinese medicine. Chapter 42 of the *Dao De Jing* teaches us that all things carry *yin*, embrace *yang*, and achieve harmony by the mixing of *qi* *(chongqi)*.[15] Note that *chongmai (衝脈)*, one of the eight extra meridians, possesses the function of blending the influences of heaven and earth, and *yin* and *yang*, as they are mediated by the conception and governor vessels, respectively.

These three—heaven, earth, and *qi*—exist in what Girardot calls a state of "ordered chaos," a "paradise condition" that "returns to and duplicates the harmony of absolute unity."[16] During this paradise time, the one, although eternally engendering the stages of the two and the three, reverts naturally and spontaneously to its original nature as the unnamed *dao* (see Figure 1.1). Hence the *Dao De Jing* teaches us,

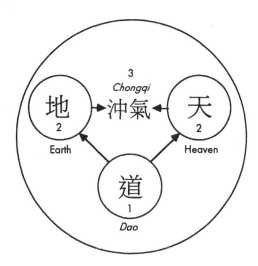

Figure 1.1
EARLY HEAVEN

Heaven, earth, and qi *compose the fundamental unity of the primordial* dao. *These three, remaining forever in a state of undivided totality, constitute "early heaven," or reality before the evolution of material existence.*

"These three things cannot be comprehended, thus they blend *(hun)* into one."[17] That which cannot be comprehended is *hun,* the primal chaotic nature of the *dao.*[18]

Humans are incapable of understanding the *dao* as unity, because as soon as it is known and named, the *dao* is no longer the one but transforms into the two: that which knows and that which is known. This duality exists in all "things" that can be comprehended by the human mind and is represented at the most primal level by division of the *dao* into the complementary poles of heaven and earth.

In fact, it is the human attempt to understand that splits apart the primal unity of heaven, earth, and *qi* to generate the material universe of the "ten thousand things." The human heart may "know" or understand unity through intuition and feeling, but the mind may never "know" unity, for its evaluative process equips it only to understand the pieces and parts of material existence. The Chinese character *de* (virtue) implies bypassing the mind to know truth with the heart. Chinese medicine, as a science, does not study "things," but rather the "functional relationships" that exist between "things." For it is in the empty space between things—not in the things themselves—that the eternal *dao* is to be found.

The Movement of the Dao

Although the eternal *dao* is unchanging, it does have an implicit movement:

> *I do not know its proper name but will call it* Dao.
> *If forced to give it a name, I shall call it great.*
> *Great means "moving away."*
> *"Moving away" means "far away"* (yuan),
> *And "far away" means [ultimately] to return.*
>   – DAO DE JING[19]

Laozi characterizes the movement of the *dao* as an eternal "self-becoming" *(ziran:*自然*).*[20] The expression *ziran* means that, at every moment, the *dao* spontaneously becomes itself, forever cleaving from and then spontaneously reverting to its original nature. The virtue of *ziran* empowers the spontaneous return to original nature once it has been lost and represents the Daoist ideal of health.

In its movement away from and return to itself, the *dao* centers on an axis or "pole of emptiness" *(xuji:*虛極*).*[21] This central axis is thought to unify heaven and earth and may be identified with the function of the *chongqi.* In the *dao*'s primordial journey, the fourth stage is always a returning to itself, showing that the movement of the *dao* mimics its ontogeny. These four stages and central axis may be thought of as constituting the cosmological basis of the five elements. In addition to its eternal cycling, the *dao* also exhibits a rising and falling motion similar to breathing. This action is like a bellows and may be thought of as the breath of the *dao.* The various "stages" of the *dao* are correlated with its movement, as shown in Figure 1.2.

Chapter 4 of the *Dao De Jing* characterizes the movement of the *dao* as a "whirling emptiness."[22] The use of the character *chong* for "whirling" indicates that the cyclical movement of the *dao* is synonymous with its motivating force of harmony and evolution. By calling the *dao* "fathomless" *(yuan:*淵*),* the *Dao De Jing* likens this dynamic movement to a deep, dark *(xuan:*玄*)* whirlpool. As our cosmic ancestor, this implicit movement of the *dao* is present in all things to which it gives birth.

Later Heaven: The Fall

> *We have just already become one, so how can I say any-thing? But I have just said that we are one, so how can I*

not be saying something? The one and what I said about it
make two, and the two and the original one make three.
– ZHUANGZI[23]

At the most primal level of enumeration, the fourth stage of the *dao* is the spontaneous return, or fall, of the three back to the original nature of the one. In the infancy of the *dao* (the "great"), there is no movement toward generating material reality. It is simply destiny that paradise is lost, and the unity of the *dao* eventually breaks down to "flood" the universe with the ten thousand things. Hence, as the egg of primordial *dao* hatches to yield material existence, the fourth stage of *dao* may also represent a fall from the primordial state of

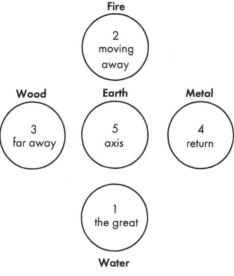

Figure 1.2
STAGES OF *DAO*

The stages of the dao *correlate with qualities of its movement. The fifth stage is the central axis around which the* dao's *whirling movement occurs. The movements of* dao *are the cosmological basis of the five elements. The first stage of* dao *corresponds to the element water which, like* dao, *represents the potential basis for all manifestation in life. As the North Star rises out of the ocean to create the two poles of heaven and earth, so too does the generation of the fire elements correspond to the second stage of* dao. *The generation of fire from water signifies that the* dao *has "moved away" from its original nature. The creation of these two poles engenders the third stage which corresponds to the wood element. The function of wood is to blend water and fire back into one by harmonizing qi. The fourth stage signifies a return from the duality of water and fire back into the original nature of* dao *as unity. These four transitions occur around a center that corresponds to the earth element and yields the fifth stage of* dao.

unity. This fall from original nature plays itself out eternally in the microcosm of both humankind and society.

The different levels of enumeration describe simultaneously occurring processes, with each successive level representing a further distancing from the primal *dao*. Hence, at the next higher level of existence, it is humans who take the place of the *chongqi* to mediate between heaven and earth. Humans who assume this role must, like the *chongqi*, perfectly blend the qualities of these two cosmic poles. This interaction must occur unhampered by the human tendency to interpret life if we are to maintain both the unity of the *dao* and our unity with the *dao*.

Only the infant and the sage are capable of moving effortlessly through the transitions of life unencumbered by the fetters of the mind's interpretations. As Zhuangzi points out, once the ultimate principle is named, there are two things: the unnamed *dao* and the named *dao*.

The *Dao De Jing*'s view of later heaven and the fall begins:

> The dao *that can be spoken of,*
> *Is not the Everlasting* (chang) dao.
> *Name* (ming) *that can be named,*
> *Is not the Everlasting name.*
> *Nameless* (wuming), *the origin* (shi) *of heaven and earth;*
> *Named* (youming), *the mother* (mu) *of ten thousand things.*
>
> – *DAO DE JING* [24]

The act of naming changes early heaven into later heaven and the everlasting *dao* into the ephemeral *dao*, the transitory basis of material "reality." To give a thing a personal name is synonymous to granting it a destiny and life. By naming, the ten thousand things become illuminated and thus are drawn out from the dark obscurity of chaos. This is an interesting example of characters sounding alike (termed homophones) and having similar shades of meaning. The Chinese characters for the words "destiny," "name," and "illumination" are all pronounced *ming*. The three concepts are philosophically and spiritually related.

The very act of talking about "things" causes the *dao* to become self-conscious, for humans are the *dao*, and thus humans talking are the *dao* talking to itself, about itself. In other words, the process of humans speaking about the nature of existence may be thought of as the *dao* judging itself and therefore losing spontaneity. That only humans name things suggests a direct role of human consciousness in the generation of material existence.

The *Dao De Jing* offers this human-centered and, more important-ly, consciousness-centered view of material reality.[25] Humans are vessels through whom the eternal *dao* detaches from and returns to itself while evolving in the process. Laozi gives his advice for maintaining connection with the primordial *dao*: "Reduce your sense of self and limit your desires,"[26] for it is our hopes and desires that draw the soul into the body and move us from nonbeing to being.[27]

Summary

The enumeration of existence found in the Chinese creation myths form the theoretical basis of the inner tradition of Chinese medicine. The concept of the two being harmonized and blended back into the one by a third factor is fundamental to all aspects of traditional practice. Even the physical sensation of *deqi*, experienced by both patient and practitioner when an acupuncture point is needled, is a manifestation of the *chongqi* in the microcosm as it harmonizes the unbalanced excess and deficient aspects of the patient's being from the two back into the one.

The Daoist enumeration of being describes a succession of levels of existence, but the different stages are not to be thought of as occurring at different times. The "paradise time" associated with the primordial *dao* did not happen in the distant past, with the present representing paradise lost and the ten thousand things. All stages must be understood to exist fully present in each moment and to occur simultaneously. For each moment holds the opportunity to focus our attention in a way that corresponds to either a return to, or a separation from, our original nature, the primal *dao*.

The essential qualities of the *dao* permeate every aspect of the reality that constitutes human existence. The fundamental unknowability of life is well illustrated in this quotation from Albert Einstein:

> Physical concepts are free creations of the human mind, and are not, however it may seem, uniquely determined by the external world. In our endeavor to understand reality, we are somewhat like a man trying to understand the mechanism of a closed watch. He sees the face and the moving hands, even hears it ticking, but he has no way of opening the case. If he is ingenious, he may form some picture of a mechanism which could be responsible for all the things he observes, but he may never be quite sure his picture is the only one which could explain his observations. He will never be able to compare his picture with the real mechanism and he cannot even imagine the possibility of the meaning of such a comparison.[28]

In sum, humans believe that the meaning they attribute to events in life constitutes reality. But by naming our experience, we cause the *dao* to separate from itself and, in so doing, we lose sight of its original nature. Having lost touch with the fundamental unity of life we also lose touch with our own original nature. The ultimate truth at the foundation of human existence is essentially unknowable and always lies just beyond the grasp of the human mind. Human life follows the basic movement of the *dao*, as individuals move away from and ultimately return to their original nature.

Having examined the basic assumptions about the nature of existence outlined in the early texts, we now turn our attention to these themes in Chinese myth and allegory.

Myth and Meaning

The early Chinese conception of the universe is reflected in Chinese creation mythology. It is through the mythology contained in early Daoist texts that the spirit of Chinese medicine emerges to speak to us directly. Hence the Chinese characters for the English word "myth" are *shenhua* (神話), which means, literally, "spirit talk." Next I explore some of the fundamental myths from Chinese culture about the cosmological origins of the universe and human life.

Self-consciousness kills the original chaotic nature of the *dao*, a principle exemplified in the story of the death of Emperor Huntun:

> The emperor of the South Sea was called Shu [Brief], the emperor of the North Sea was called Hu [Sudden], and the emperor of the central region was called Huntun [Chaos]. Shu and Hu from time to time came together for a meeting in the territory of Huntun, and Huntun treated them very generously. Shu and Hu discussed how they could repay his kindness. "All men," they said, "have seven openings so they can see, hear, eat, and breathe. But Huntun alone doesn't have any. Let's try boring him some!" Every day they bored another hole, and on the seventh day, Huntun died.[29]

Huntun takes the role here of the *chongqi*, as mediator between heaven (the South Sea) and earth (the North Sea).[30] True to his name, he had "no understanding" until given the "gift" of the senses, at which time he died. Human beings, in their attempt to control chaos and thereby "civilize" the world, kill the spontaneous nature of both the *dao* and themselves in the process. This begins the generative cycle that gives birth and brings death to material existence.

Interestingly, the combined names of the other two emperors, *shu* and *hu*, mean, literally, "lightning."[31] The concept of lightning striking the primordial chaos to produce life is remarkably similar to modern evolutionary theory.

After the death of Huntun (chaos), it was the giant Pangu, the ancestor of the human race, who took the place of the *chongqi* as mediator between heaven and earth. The earliest extant version of this myth dates from the third century C.E.:

> Heaven and earth were in the chaos condition *[huntun]*, like a chicken's egg, within which was born Pangu. After 18,000 years, when heaven and earth were separated, the pure *yang* formed the heaven and the murky *yin* formed the earth. Pangu stood between them. His body transformed nine times daily, while his head supported the heaven and his feet stabilized the earth.[32]

Pangu here represents the pivot of equilibrium between heaven and earth and denotes the perfectly balanced duration of the "three," the duration of cosmic incubation. In the Daoist enumeration of being, nine is the number of completion, and Pangu, by transforming nine times, completes the formation of the material universe. The theme of the number nine representing completion is reiterated in the *Nei Jing Su Wen* which states, "According to the final calculations nature begins as one and ends as nine. The first is heaven, the second is earth, and the third is man. These are the three. Three times three is nine and corresponds to the nine wild regions upon earth. Thus man is composed of three parts, and each part has three subdivisions which decide upon life or death."[33]

The myth of Pangu also explains the macro- and microcosmic relationship of the human body to the universe:

> After the death of Pangu, his breath became the wind and clouds, his voice the thunder, his left and right eyes the sun and moon, his four limbs and five "bodies" (fingers) the four quarters of the earth and five great mountains, his blood the rivers, his muscles and veins the strata of the earth, his flesh the soil, his hair and beard the constellations, his skin and body-hair the plants and trees, his teeth and bone the metals and stone, his marrow gold and precious stones, and his sweat the rain. The parasites on his body, impregnated by the wind, became human beings.[34]

Chinese medicine is based on the science of understanding the functional process of nature as it exists within the human being. Processes are seen as permeating both nature (the macrocosm) and the human being (the microcosm) and extending from one to the other in an unbroken chain. For example, in the macrocosm the polestar and the sun may be considered life-giving centers that control and orient the movements of the other stars and planets. In the microcosm of human society the emperor may be viewed as the life-giving center who utilizes the special function of each minister in the kingdom. In the microcosm of the human being, the heart may be said to fulfill the function of controlling the other officials (organs) in one's inner kingdom. The polestar, sun, emperor, and heart are all different physical manifestations that are functionally related and are therefore thought to be empowered by the same fundamental aspect of being, in this case heaven.

The death of Pangu gave rise to the phenomenal universe as we know it. As the universe is modeled on our "ancestor of the center," so, too, our bodies and lives are microcosmic representations of the fundamental process of the *dao*. Humankind mirrors the fundamental order of the universe as human lives follow the movements of the *dao*.

Chaos and the Floods

> *The great* dao *floods over.*
> – DAO DE JING[35]

After separating into the complementary poles of heaven and earth, the unity of the primal *dao* is maintained by the *chongqi*. This huge whirling abyss blends perfectly all qualities of the earthly *yin* and heavenly *yang*, so that these three—heaven, earth, and *qi*—return to and replicate the pristine quality of the primal *dao*. But the human disrupts this natural harmony and destroys the natural spontaneity of the *dao* by naming it. In early Daoism, humankind's attempt to create civilization and control nature reflects its own loss of self.

However, it is impossible to permanently block the will of heaven, whose force exerts itself like the flow of a mighty river. Controlling floods was a continual problem for the early Chinese, whose livelihood as farmers depended on both the irrigation and transportation provided by China's great rivers. In early myth, the imagery of the floods represents the *dao's* efforts to assert its original, spontaneous nature in human society, where it had been "civilized."

The *Dao De Jing* characterizes the *dao* as a vast whirlpool continually "moving away" from and "returning" to its source in the process of its own "self-becoming" and tells us that the fundamental nature of *dao* is chaotic.[36] Zhuangzi informs that the sage, in aligning himself with the *dao*, "steers by the torch of chaos and doubt."[37] In the words of Lagerwey,

> If chaos is eternal, the order introduced into chaos of the universe has an end, as it has a beginning. This is because slowly names given cease to fit; political systems invented in simpler times cease to function; old irrigation ditches get choked up with new vegetation; the waters of chaos begin to mount.[38]

The *dao* is like a river whose waters are continually rising, and the *Dao De Jing* is our survival manual, informing us that by cultivating virtue (*de:*德), we may channel the flood and avoid being inundated. Zhuangzi states that even though floodwaters pile up high to reach the sky, the sage will not drown.[39]

Controlling the floods was a daunting problem for the early Chinese, and early mythology is permeated with the imagery and theme of a brother and sister who float in a giant gourd to survive a great flood and land on Kunlun Mountain, procreate incestuously, then give birth to the human race.[40] The flood itself signifies the *dao*'s efforts to assert its original, spontaneous nature in human society, where it has been "civilized," and to wipe the slate clean for a new beginning. This drama is played out eternally as humans lose their original nature and try in vain to control the ensuing chaos. The theme of the flood in the myth of Gun and Yu lays the foundation for understanding the inner tradition of healing in Chinese medicine. It elaborates the virtue of fulfilling destiny by aligning one's will with the will of heaven and the futility of attempting to prevent heaven from expressing its own will.

The Myth of Gun and Yu

There are two Chinese histories: that history verifiable by archeological and written evidence and that history of legend which cannot be verified. The Shang dynasty is considered to be the first Chinese dynasty, dating to 1766 B.C.E. All previous dynasties referred to in the text comprise the legendary period, meaning they are not substantiated and exist only in myth. Still, these myths provide us with the fundamental archetypes inherent in the ancient Chinese view of their world.

During the time of Yao (c. 2356 B.C.E.), the overflowing waters reached up to the sky, so Yao enlisted Gun, the great-grandson of Emperor Huang Di, to control the flooding.[41] Gun set about building dams out of magic earth which he stole from Huang Di. But the dams collapsed again and again under the weight of the flood despite his efforts. For failing to control the floods and thereby neglecting his destiny, Gun was executed by Huang Di's heavenly executioner Zhurong, the spirit of fire, on Feather Mountain.[42] In the end, Gun was condemned to the bottom of an abyss becoming its spirit in the form of a tortoise. The image of Gun as a tortoise appears on the Ma Huang Dui funerary banner, excavated from a tomb in Hunan province in 1973 and belonging to the son of Li Zang, a minister in early Han times (206 B.C.E.–5 C.E.). On the banner Gun is portrayed as holding the world up and out of the primordial chaos.

Following Gun's failure, his son Yu was assigned the task of controlling the floods in place of his father. Yu worked devotedly for thirteen years, cutting ditches and tunneling through mountains to provide a way (dao) for the water from the rivers to be channeled to the sea. Here, the imagery of the sea represents that great abyss, which, like the dao, can receive all things without being filled up, yet is never depleted even though tapped continuously. The Zuo Chuan warns that he who ignores his own destiny (ming:命) "probably will not return home again."[43] Gun, who ignored his destiny, fell into the abyss, never to return home. But Yu, the embodiment of commitment, although he passed by his own doorway three times in thirteen years, returned home only after the floods were under control, thereby fulfilling his contract with heaven—his destiny.

Yu, in passing his doorway three times without entering, demonstrated his commitment to fulfilling his destiny. The number three signifies the primordial unity of heaven, earth, and qi, which was restored when Yu quelled the floods. The name of Emperor Yu (禹) is a homophone for the character yu (愈), meaning "to heal." It pictures a boat (俞) over a heart (心). This yields an image of the heart being carried safely from one shore to another. A related character also pronounced "yu" (俞) denotes a class of acupuncture points. This association suggests a functional connection between Emperor Yu's method of channeling the floods and the acupuncturist's role in guiding the flow of qi. Another homophone for the name of Emperor Yu is found in the word yu (遇), meaning "to meet."

During the time Yu was busy channeling the waters, he became intimately familiar with the people, places, animals, and plants that he met on his journey. Whenever he came to a famous mountain or a big swamp, he would summon its spirit and ask it about the deep structure of the mountains and rivers, and about the kinds of precious stones, birds, beasts, and reptiles found there. He queried the spirits about the

customs of the people in all eight directions and the boundaries, soil
quality, and size of the various states. He wrote all this down and
called it the *Shan Hai Jing* (The Scripture of the Mountains and Seas).[44]

After taming the floods, Yu founded the mythic Xia dynasty
(2205–1766 B.C.E.), becoming China's first emperor. With his mission
fulfilled, he ascended Mount Mao in order to receive in audience the
hundred spirits from the four directions and to inspect the feudal lords.
All of Yu's loyal subjects arrived on time except for one named
"Oppose-the-Wind" who attempted to disrupt the meeting and prevent Yu from ascending the throne. Yu beheaded his enemy and
displayed his head to the multitudes in order to make clear that all
under heaven belonged to him. He then held a great assembly to decide
how to rule the state. Having fulfilled his contract with heaven by
quelling the floods and ascending the throne, Yu then changed the
name of Mount Mao to the Mountain of the Assembly of Accounts.[45]

Having lost original nature, ancient China was inundated with the
floodwaters of chaos. Gun failed in his attempt to suppress the floods
and so died prematurely. Yu, by channeling the excess waters to the
sea, was able to heal his nation and restore its spiritual unity. In
ascending Mount Mao, Yu aligned himself with the polestar, the "heart
of heaven," and thereby unified heaven and earth, fulfilling his own
destiny and forging the destiny of his nation.

The Flood, Kunlun Mountain, and the Queen Mother

The mission of the flood is to return original nature to humankind
and to fulfill heaven's promise of an eternity filled with new beginnings. Humankind is not destroyed by the flood, but rather, at this
critical turning point, is given the opportunity to start again and to live
in conformance with the laws of nature. The "civilized" human is
inundated by the *yin*—mundane—influences acquired during life that
dampen the internal flame corresponding to *yang* and to heaven's
intent. If original nature is not restored, then the individual eventually
dies, just as life is swept by the flood back to the ocean of eternity that
is the *dao*.

In early Chinese mythology, the brother and sister, who represent the
primordial *yin* and *yang (yuanqi)*, land on Kunlun Mountain and cop-
ulate, rekindling the life of the human race.[46] In ancient China, Kunlun
Mountain was conceived of as the pillar that joined heaven and earth,
representing the axis of all creation.[47] As the root of heaven and earth,
Kunlun was thought to balance the primordial *yin* and *yang* and to

radiate this power through the expression of the five elements on earth—water, wood, fire, earth, and metal.[48] Kunlun Mountain is located in the West, and there Xi Wang Mu, the "queen mother of the West," resides.

In religious Daoism, Xi Wang Mu is considered to be the first woman to attain the *dao* and thus the queen of Daoist immortals. The oldest mythological representations depict her as a tiger spirit, the tiger being emblematic of *yin* and the Western land of the setting sun. As queen of the West, she presides over the realm of the dead, for all souls must make their journey from earth to heaven by passing along the universal axis of Kunlun. Hence the characters for the number four (四) as associated with the metal element, and death (死) are homophones, both pronounced *si*.

Xi Wang Mu rules not only the dead, as portrayed in early myth.[49] Later myths tell us that she resides on Kunlun Mountain, feeding the immortals peaches that bestow immortality.[50] The immortality conferred by the queen mother is the eternal promise of a new beginning bestowed on our primal brother and sister after the flood. For no matter how far estranged from original nature we become, there is always the possibility of returning to the truth that is the primordial *dao*.

The Golden Gate and the Mysterious Pass

> *The gates of the mysterious female,*
> *These we call the roots of heaven and earth.*
> – DAO DE JING[51]

In Daoist mythology, the entrance to the kingdom of the mysterious Xi Wang Mu, queen mother of the West, is pictured as a golden gate *(jinmen:*金門*)* and a place of "ultimate safety."[52] At this gate, she receives both the souls of the dead and the survivors after the deluge. And through this gate, life is eventually resurrected, symbolized by the reunification of the primordial sister *(yin)* and brother *(yang)*. The domain of Xi Wang Mu has been described as a womb or tomb, serving as both birthplace and burial ground of all creation.[53] From the womb of the queen mother the life-giving waters flow, and to her tomb, all return in the flood's wake.

In Daoist literature, the concept of a door, gate, or pass represents the interface between being and nonbeing, early and later heaven, and the one and the ten thousand things. Through this gate, all of creation passes as it emerges from and ultimately returns to the womb/tomb of the *dao*. In alchemical and philosophical texts, the gate is called variously the "golden portal" or "metal gate" *(jinmen)*, and the "mysterious pass" *(yuanguan:*元關*).*[54] The *Dao De Jing*, in Chapter 1, calls it "the door to all hidden mysteries," and in Chapter 6, the "gate of the mysterious female."[55] *The Book of Balance and Harmony*, a thirteenth-century text by Daoist philosopher Li Daoqun, calls this pass "the heart of heaven."[56]

The light given off as things are created and destroyed in passing through the queen mother's gate is represented by the character *ming* (明:illumination), which depicts the sun and the moon symbolizing the interaction of *yin* and *yang*.[57] Li Daoqun, referring to the pass, states, "The heart of heaven and earth—where is it stored? *Yin* and *Yang* stimulate it to manifest a sphere of light."[58] As a mental and spiritual construct, the character *ming* signifies the turning point between the delusion of the material world (indicated by the sun) and the inner illumination of the sage (indicated by the moon). It is interesting to consider that, from a position on earth, as beings leave the void, they are illuminated from the front and appear bright. The sun shines on them, and we are able to see their faces clearly. The face symbolizes the outer, named self and our distance from the original nature of the void. From a point standing in the void, as beings return, they appear backlit by the sun and only their silhouettes are seen, their features undistinguished in the dark shadows.

The functional location of the mysterious pass is between the metal and water element along the *sheng* cycle. The significance of this transition is elaborated in Chapter 7 in terms of *Yijing (I Ching)* hexagrams 23 and 24 and the husband/wife imbalance as it describes the terminal separation of *yin* and *yang*.

Unity: The Harmonization of Opposites

A common theme which has emerged in our review of Chinese myth is that the essential tendency of *dao* is to restore harmony, once original nature is lost, by unifying apparent opposites. In the Daoist enumeration of being this appears as the *chongqi* empowering the interpenetration of heaven and earth. In myth, Kunlun Mountain serves this purpose and is the meeting point of the primordial brother and sister who rekindle the human race after the floods through symbolic reunification of the primordial *yin* and *yang*. Emperor Yu, in quelling the floods, restored spiritual unity to his nation through the fulfillment of his own destiny. Finally, the mysterious pass serves as the interface between nonbeing and being, fusing *yin* and *yang* and mediating the emergence and return of the ten thousand things.

These themes are present in Chinese physiology and in the principles of healing inherent in the inner tradition. Physiologically, the function of *mingmen*, the "gate of destiny," empowers the interpenetration of *yin* and *yang*, *jing* and *shen*, and early and later heaven. It is the spontaneous interaction of these influences that fuels evolution and promotes health. The path of healing in the inner tradition involves harmonizing excessive and deficient emotional states, such as belligerence and timidity, back into virtues such as benevolence. It is the cultivation of virtue in life that empowers our own reunification with primordial *dao*.

Luan *and* Hun: *Culture and Chaos*

The torch of chaos and doubt—this is what the sage steers by.
— ZHUANGZI [59]

That early Daoists look back to a golden age when people lived in accordance with the principles of the *dao* is reflected in the opening lines of the *Nei Jing Su Wen*. The Yellow Emperor, in his first question to Qibo, says,

> I have heard that in ancient times the people lived [through the years] to be over a hundred years, and yet they remained active and did not become decrepit in their activities. But nowadays people reach only half that age and yet become decrepit and failing. Is it because the world changes from generation to generation? Or is it that mankind is becoming negligent [of the laws of nature]?

Qibo responds,

> In ancient times those people who understood *dao* [the way of self-cultivation] patterned themselves upon the *yin* and the *yang* [the two principles in nature] and they lived in harmony with the arts of divination. [60]

Chapter 80 of the *Dao De Jing* describes a society based on the perfect order of the primal *dao*. In such a society, "the people fear death such that they do not move far away" from their true natures. [61] For Daoists, the character *hun* (混), meaning "chaotic," refers to the period of primordial paradise, considered a time of exemplary social order. *Hun* represents the unity of the three, which comprise heaven and earth as they are mediated by the *chongqi*.

In early Daoism, the term *luan* (亂) denotes the chaos that pervaded the world after the fall of humankind from original nature and the ensuing establishment of society and culture. The *Dao De Jing*, in advising the sage to "govern when there is yet no disorder *(luan)*," is imploring humanity to stay close to the *dao* as a guiding influence in life and to shun contrived social conventions.[62]

The character *zhi* (治) means to "govern" or "set in order," but another meaning is to "treat or heal an illness."[63] An original usage of the character *zhi* refers to the order created by Emperor Yu who controlled the floods and healed his nation. For Daoists, healing is a matter of returning to the perfectly incomprehensible chaos-order of the *dao*. They believe, as the *Nei Jing Su Wen* states, that "to follow [the laws of] *yin* and *yang* means life; to act contrary to [the laws of *yin* and *yang*] means death. To follow these laws results in order *(zhi:治)*; to act contrary to them results in chaos *(luan:亂).*"[64]

Confucian texts, however, use the character *luan* to indicate the order imposed on the untamed world by social convention.[65] For the Confucianists, the character *hun* holds negative connotations as it is associated with a world not governed by humanity. Daoists, in their willingness to steer by the "torch of chaos and doubt," are happy to accept life as a mystery that is fundamentally unknowable. Ordinary people, in their attempt to establish values, tend to view life as chaotic, doubtful, and needing clarification.[66]

The Daoists consider inborn nature as being essentially good, representing the highest that heaven wills for each human being. Our primordial endowment from early heaven, *jing, yuanqi,* and *shen,* is synonomous with the guiding influence of heaven's intent as it exists within each of us. These influences represent all potentialities in each human's life as well as the means to manifest those potentialities through appropriate use of our will. Illness is thought to be the result of socialization and acquired belief systems that smother the influence of our primordial endowment. As the influence of early heaven wanes, spontaneous function is replaced with habituated conditioning as each grows increasingly distanced from original nature.

The Confucian view, in contrast, exemplified in its extreme by the writings of Xunzi (Hsun Tzu, c. 312 B.C.E.), is that human inborn nature is a negative influence and humans can only become good through the process of socialization. He concludes his text by admonishing us, "Environment is the important thing! Environment is the important thing!"[67] The Confucian stance is that human nature is wild and chaotic, and only through education and rigorous social protocol do humans have the capacity to rise above the state of wild animals.

Having its roots in Daoism, the inner tradition of Chinese medicine places emphasis in both diagnosis and treatment on the quality of the patient's inherited constitution. This constitutional approach allows the practitioner to see past the habituating influences acquired during life and to reaffirm the guiding light of the heavenly constitution. In the rest of this text we will see how the themes of individual destiny and the loss and return of original nature are manifest in the inner tradition.

Questions

Humans create meaning about the nature of life that either empowers or diminishes their place in the world. This mythology defines the relative weaknesses and strengths of all culture and science based on it.

1. What are the foundational myths of your culture?

2. What are the meanings you have created in your own life?

3. What ways do your patients create meanings in their lives?

4. Are the meanings that you see being created in any way related thematically to the myths of your culture?

5. To what extent do these myths empower, or diminish, health?

6. All human attributes result from a combination of inherited and acquired influences. What is the relative emphasis placed by your tradition of practice upon the role of inherited and acquired characteristics in contributing to a patient's degree of health or illness?

NOTES

1. Chapter 20; in Chen, 1989, p. 103.
2. Girardot, 1983, p. 47.
3. See the appendix for a discussion of the qualitative difference between the paradigms of Western and Chinese medicine.
4. Chapter 42; in Girardot, 1983, p. 56.
5. Lagerwey, 1987, p. 8. The use of the term *lingbao* (靈寶) is based on the Daoist trinity *yuanshi* (元始), *lingbao* (靈寶), and *daode* (道德). *Yuanshi* equates to zero, the primordial cause of being. *Lingbao* equates to pure potential, and *daode* signifies

the manifestation of potential. Personal communication from Jeffrey Yuen.

6. Girardot, 1983, p. 49.
7. Wieger, 1965, p. 326. Chinese characters are composed of several components, including radicals, which may impart a sense of meaning, and phonetics, which impart information regarding pronunciation. A character may itself contain two or more elements that are themselves characters. The character *ming* (明), for example, meaning "illumination" is composed of the character *ri* (日) meaning sun and *yue* (月) meaning moon.
8. Personal communication from Jeffrey Yuen.
9. Chapter 25; in Girardot, 1983, p. 49.
10. De Harlez (1891); cited in Girardot, 1983, p. 50.
11. Watson, 1964, p. 101.
12. Chapter 14; in Chen, 1989, p. 88.
13. Chen, 1989, p. 62.
14. Mathews, 1931, p. 218.
15. Girardot, 1983, p. 57.
16. Girardot, 1983, pp. 47–76.
17. Chapter 14; in Chen, 1989, p. 88.
18. A quote by Wang Bi (226–249 C.E.), author of a highly regarded commentary on the *Dao De Jing* (cited in Girardot, 1983, p. 50).
19. Chapter 25; in Girardot, 1983, p. 49.
20. Chen, 1989, p. 117.
21. Chen, 1989, p. 94.
22. Chen, 1989, p. 60.
23. Watson, 1964a, p. 38.
24. Chapter 1; in Chen, 1989, p. 51.
25. Chen suggests that the *Dao De Jing* offers not a human-centered view, but a nature- or *de-* ("virtue") oriented view of existence. These two notions can be reconciled by the fact that humans, indeed, are a part of nature. When human beings preserve their *de* and fulfill their destiny, the *de* of all existence is preserved (Chen, 1973, pp. 457–470).
26. Chapter 19; in Chen, 1989, p. 101.
27. Huiyuan (334–416 C.E.), a Buddhist; in Liebenthal, 1952 (January), pp. 327–397.
28. Einstein and Infeld, 1938, p. 31.
29. Zhuangzi; in Watson, 1964a, p. 95.
30. Characters *hun* and *chong* both contain the water radical (氵), linking them with the primordial sea and the primal whirlpool of the *dao*.
31. See Christie, 1975, p. 47; Girardot, 1983, p. 92.
32. Quote from the *Shu Yi Ji*; in Girardot, 1983, p. 193.
33. Veith, 1949, p. 187.
34. Quotation from the sixth-century *Shu Yi Ji*; in Girardot, 1983, p. 194. This cosmology is further developed in the answer to the eighty-first question of the *Bai Wen Bian*: "In what ways is man similar to heaven and earth?" The entire text is an exposition on the macro- and microcosmic relationship of the universe and humankind in the language of spiritual alchemy and Chinese physiology (Homann, 1976, pp. 32–33).
35. Chapter 31; in Chen, 1989, p. 137.
36. Chapters 4 and 25; in Chen, 1989, pp. 60, 117.
37. Watson, 1964a, p. 38.
38. Lagerwey, 1987, p. 11.
39. Watson, 1964a, p. 27.

40. Girardot, 1983, p. 24 ff.
41. Christie, 1975, p. 87.
42. Lagerwey, 1987, p. 41. Lagerwey supposes that Feather Mountain is the mountain of birdmen, as Daoists are often called.
43. T'ang, 1962 (January), p. 208.
44. Annals of *Wu and Yueh,* 2.3b; in Lagerwey, 1987, p. 160.
45. Lagerwey, 1987, p. 151.
46. Girardot, 1983, pp. 173–174.
47. Acupuncture point Bladder-60 is named "Kunlun Mountain" and Bladder-10 is named "heavenly pillar," referring again to Kunlun. Both points are located on the bladder meridian, which is consistent with the bladder's role in regulating water flow within the body and the cosmological function of Kunlun in regulating the balance of the primordial *yin* and *yang.*
48. Kohn, 1992, p. 110.
49. The Scripture of the Mountains and Seas *(Shan Hai Jing)* is the sole text that presents her as a demon and mother of the plague. Since the second century B.C.E., she has been portrayed as an immortal who possesses recipes for long life (Bonnefoy, 1991, p. 243).
50. From the early Daoist text *Huai Nan Zi,* written in the former Han dynasty (122 B.C.E.) by guests of the court of Liu An, the prince of Huai Nan.
51. Chapter 6; in Henricks, 1989, p. 198.
52. Lagerwey, 1987, pp. 39–41.
53. Ibid., p. 41.
54. Anderson, 1989, p. 50.
55. Henricks, 1989, p. 58.
56. Cleary, 1989, p. 38.
57. Chen, 1989, p. 155. Chen states, "*Ming* is the mystical light of the round, illuminating both the coming out and the return of all beings" (Chen, *Tao Te Ching,* p. 155). Note that the Chinese characters meaning "to invent" are *faming* (發明), which is literally "to produce a thing by illuminating it." Also note that another character pronounced *ming* (冥) may be translated as "darkness" and "obscurity," and in religious Daoism and Buddhism refers to the underworld.
58. Cleary, 1989, p. 109.
59. Watson, 1964a, p. 37.
60. Veith, 1949, p. 97. Veith translates the couplet *shushu* as "arts of divination." Another interpretation is "arts [or methods] of destiny."
61. Chen, 1989, p. 228.
62. Chapter 64; in Chen, 1989, pp. 202–203.
63. Mathews, 1931, p. 141.
64. *Nei Jing Su Wen,* Chapter 2; in Unschuld, 1988, p. 11.
65. For a detailed comparison of Daoist and Confucian uses of the term *luan,* see Girardot, 1983, p. 114.
66. See Watson, 1964a, p. 38, n. 11.
67. Watson, 1963, p. 171.

2

MING:
OUR CONTRACT
WITH HEAVEN

*Heaven and earth were born at the same time I was,
and the ten thousand things are One with me.*
– Zhuangzi[1]

As the *dao* moves away from and returns to itself, the four seasons cycle endlessly around the earth, and humans move through life from birth to death. Our movement through life is powered by a wave of destiny *(ming:命)* that we are given the choice to either fulfill or repudiate with every heartbeat. Heaven, by conferring a destiny on humans, establishes us as one of three primal powers—heaven, human, and earth. Humans, in assuming their role as mediators between the two cosmic poles, must, like the *chongqi*, blend perfectly the qualities of heaven and earth. The process of maintaining the unity of heaven and earth, and our unity with heaven and earth, culminates in the fulfillment of the personal destiny established for each of us.

We turn our attention next to the nature of destiny as it occurs in the inner tradition of Chinese medicine.

The Language of Destiny

When examining the meaning of concepts such as destiny, virtue, and human will within the context of Chinese medicine, it is important to acknowledge a fundamental difference between the English and Chinese language. Chinese calligraphic characters are not words in the sense of having a specific and narrow definition as words usually do in the English language. Rather, they represent broad concepts and aspects of being, broadly interpreted. A Chinese character may stand for a concept that has been interpreted and translated differently by different authors. No one English word can serve as an equivalent for the concept inherent in any given character. Etymological analysis, however, may yield a sense of the "quality of being" represented by a character.

To best understand the concept inherent in a given character, we must examine as many contexts as possible in which it has been used. The meaning of a character is never precise; it is always open ended and evolving, just as human understanding about the nature of existence is evolving.

A character such as *ming*, for example, may be translated into English as "destiny," "orders," "commands," or as "life." The concept of destiny is not fixed in meaning but evolves as the human conversation about destiny unfolds. The notion of what constitutes an individual's destiny may reflect, at different points in history, the social, political, and philosophical milieu of the period in consideration.

We may add our own observations of *ming* to the discussion as it appears relevant to us in our time. For example, the character *ming* has been translated as equivalent to the English word "life" in all modern Chinese medical texts and in English texts on traditional Chinese medicine. The choice to ignore this character's deeper meaning of "destiny" reflects, I believe, the materialistic and perhaps atheistic bent of the modern world.

Ming: *Our Contract with Heaven*

The magical treasures of Chinese antiquity were understood to have a bipartite existence, one half being placed on earth and the other existing in heaven. Possession of the terrestrial half enables one to summon the celestial half and thus through the union of heaven and earth to cause renewal. Hence ancient Chinese shamans were often represented as partially paralyzed, becoming whole only when possessed by celestial spirit.[2]

Scholar Tang Zhunyi (T'ang Chun-I) defines *ming* as existing "in the mutuality of heaven and man, that is, in their mutual influence and response, their mutual giving and receiving. "[3] The *dao* as our treasure is a pact made with heaven, and the *Dao De Jing* tells us that "the sage holds the left tally" in the arrangement.[4] The left tally signifies the inferior position in an agreement, the position of the debtor.[5] Hence the sage must recognize the fulfillment of his destiny as a debt owed to heaven.

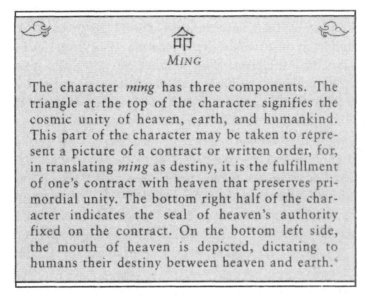

MING

The character *ming* has three components. The triangle at the top of the character signifies the cosmic unity of heaven, earth, and humankind. This part of the character may be taken to represent a picture of a contract or written order, for, in translating *ming* as destiny, it is the fulfillment of one's contract with heaven that preserves primordial unity. The bottom right half of the character indicates the seal of heaven's authority fixed on the contract. On the bottom left side, the mouth of heaven is depicted, dictating to humans their destiny between heaven and earth.[6]

Fulfillment of Destiny as Our Contract with Heaven

The Daoist treasures *jing, qi,* and *shen* constitute the internal world of the individual. By joining one's internal spiritual endowment inherent in these treasures with their corresponding aspects as they exist externally in heaven, the sage fulfills personal destiny. In religious Daoism, the idea of these treasures is expressed in the term *lingbao* (靈寶). *Bao*, meaning "treasure," signifies the terrestrial half of the treasures and is identified with *jing*, the essential *qi* of the human being.[7] The character *ling* denotes the magical potency of the primal *dao*. The notion of the *dao* as a bipartite treasure existing both in the individual and in heaven is signified in the etymology of the character *fu* (付), meaning "to give." This character depicts in its right half a hand giving an object to a man, the sage, who is represented by the left half of the character. The sage on the left is indebted to the hand of heaven on the right that "gives" the sage inborn nature and, therefore, a unique destiny. Hence it is said that "the sage holds the left tally."

The character *fu,* meaning "to give," is a homophone of, and etymologically related to, another character *fu* (符), meaning "a deed in
two pieces," suggesting again a contract held by two parties.[8] This
character signifies the Daoist talismans and charms, whose possession
summons heaven's protection. Lagerwey believes this sense of *fu* as
protective talisman is similar to the original definition of the word
"symbol" in Greek. There, the word "symbol" suggests a piece of bone
or another object broken in two, each half held by any two contract-
ing parties in order to have proof of the identity of the presenter of the
other.[9] A talisman, then, is a bipartite symbol existing both on earth
as an inscription on paper or made in some other form, and in heav-
en as spiritual influence. The symbol protects the wearer by
summoning that aspect of heaven to which it corresponds. It is interesting to note that Sun Si Miao (C.E. 581?–682), perhaps the most
famous historical figure in Chinese medicine, wrote extensively on the
healing power of talismans.[10]

The characters *fu* ("to give" and "talisman") are each etymologically related to, and are homophones of, another character *fu* (腑),
which appears in the couple *zangfu,* indicating the paired *yin (zang:*臟*)*
and *yang (fu:*腑*)* organ systems, respectively. This character may be
translated as "treasury" or "storehouse" and signifies a place where
records are kept.[11] It holds special significance in the realm of
Chinese medicine.

In Chinese medicine, twelve primary organs are identified for treatment. The twelve organs are the heart, small intestine, bladder, kidney,
heart protector, three heater, gallbladder, liver, lung, large intestine,
stomach, and spleen. The term "official" stems from Chapter 8 of the
Nei Jing in which each organ is personified as an official in charge of
specific functions.[12] I use the term to refer to the sum total of a given
organ's sphere of influence in all realms of a person's being. The specific "functions" of each official are mapped onto the body as specific
acupuncture points. Points related in function to that of a given official can be connected by an imaginary line, called a *meridian.* For
example, the fourteen points that most closely relate to the function of
the liver official correspond to the liver meridian.

Each official may be thought of as a storehouse for the terrestrial or
human half of the heavenly contract. The internal organs correspond
in number to twelve spirits *(shen),* who reside in the Big Dipper constellation in the northern sky and impart destiny to humankind. When
these twelve internal "officials" find union with their heavenly counterparts, health is maintained and destiny fulfilled. Hence Emperor Yu,

the embodiment of commitment, patterns himself on the polestar and, in so doing, aligns his own heart with the heart of heaven. In uniting the kingdom, Yu binds the hundred spirits by splitting a rock in two with thunder, the halves representing his contract with heaven and his mandate to rule.[13]

The Nature of Destiny

> *The more fully men cultivate their virtue, the more*
> *fully heaven will confer its mandate on them.*
> – TANG ZHUNYI [14]

It is the nature of the fulfillment of the human contract with heaven that concerns us here. Let us see how the ancient Chinese philosophers discussed the notion of destiny. The earliest use of the character *ming* as "destiny" is the concept of *tianming*, or "heavenly mandate," as used in the *Shu Jing* (Book of Documents). *Ming* is conferred here when heaven approves of our cultivation of virtue. Further and continued cultivation of virtue is needed in order to retain our *ming*. In this sense, *ming* is synonymous with an emperor's authority to rule as bestowed by heaven.

Tang Zhunyi emphasizes that the acceptance of our destiny is the starting point of something to be done, rather than a terminal point of something already accomplished.[15] Heaven mandates a unique mission for each of us to fulfill in this life. Recognizing and accepting this mandate is only the first step in fulfilling the contract. Only through continually bringing our original nature into the world may we cultivate virtue and preserve our *ming*. *Ming* is the source of each individual's power and authority in life.

The *ming* of heaven is continuous and never ending. If an individual has received heaven's mandate but failed to maintain virtue, then heaven, in order to maintain the continuous outworking of its decree, must confer it on someone else.[16] Heaven does all it can to nurture the unique seed planted within each of us. But its only vested interest is that this unique aspect of the *dao* be expressed in the world. It does not care who expresses its will, so long as its will is expressed.

Ultimately, heaven will sacrifice the individual before it sacrifices its own expression of spontaneous self-becoming. This is exemplified by the death of Gun, who failed to quell the floods. Heaven passed on its mandate to his son Yu, who completed the task and ascended the throne. Hence Zhuangzi states, "though the grease burns out of the torch, the fire passes on."[17] The notion that heaven confers its mandate on those who cultivate virtue is the source of the belief that humankind is one of the three primal powers of transformation, along with heaven and earth.

Confucius advocated standing in awe of the heavenly *ming* and its relationship to the fulfillment of duty:

> There are three things of which the superior man stands in awe. He stands in awe of the ordinances *(ming)* of heaven. He stands in awe of great men. He stands in awe of the words of sages.[18]

> Where duty is, there also lies a man's mandate to himself; and this is where the heavenly *ming* is.[19]

For Confucius, the way to fulfill our contract with heaven lies in willing for ourselves what heaven has willed for us. Scholar Tang Zhunyi sums up Confucius's view of *ming*:

> Therefore, the determined and human-hearted man does not feel that his purpose and human-heartedness are possessions of his own; they are rooted, rather, in Heaven. In his sublime state of mind at the moment, he is in union with Heaven: his task of self-examination and realization of his purpose, for which he commands and looks to himself, is absolutely identical with the entire situation sent to him by Heaven. His unceasing exalted spirit, encouraged and nourished by duty, is one with his unceasing duty commanded by Heaven, a duty that increases daily, continuously shining forth and flourishing in his heart. In such a state of mind, where his duty is, there, too, is his *ming;* there is no way to avoid his duty, and, similarly, no way to avoid *ming*. The two become one in their absolute goodness.[20]

Confucian scholar Mencius (c. 371–289 B.C.E.) emphasized "establishing *ming*" and humankind as conduits for heaven's will. His concept of destiny might be stated in this way: "What I command to myself is what Heaven intended to command to me; thus, the heavenly *ming* is established through me."[21] The sage serves as a channel for establishing the will of heaven in this world so as to fulfill his contract. It is through joining heaven within (the commands stored in *jing*) with heaven without (the situations sent to one by heaven) that humans are able to blend in the *qi* of heaven and earth and take their place as one of the three primal powers of the universe.

When humans' will *(zhi)* is perfectly aligned with the will of heaven *(ming),* then people become a conduit for the authentic *(zhen)* divine *qi* of heaven and earth. *Zhenqi* is the *qi* that is present when individuals each manifest destiny by being true to their authentic self.[22] According to Porkert, the *zhenqi* sustains the integrity of an individual and protects and defends him against exogenous and endogenous attacks and disturbances.[23] Hence the term *zhenqi* contains the notion that one's very source of health and integrity spring from the fulfillment of destiny.

For Mencius, the way to understand heaven is through understanding our own original nature *(xing)*, which, in turn, is known through the utmost devotion of our heart. The way to serve heaven, however, is to preserve our heart within and nourish our own original nature.[24] Through acting as a vessel for the *dao* and bringing the heart of heaven fully expressed into the world, we fulfill our destiny.

Zhuangzi emphasizes this point in the following statement:

> In all things, the Way does not want to be obstructed, for if there is obstruction, there is choking; if the choking does not cease, there is disorder; and disorder harms the life of all creatures. All things that have consciousness depend on breath. But if they do not get their fill of breath, it is not the fault of Heaven. Heaven opens up the passages and supplies them day and night without stop. But man on the contrary blocks up the holes.[25]

Heaven plants the seed of original nature within and from the moment of the first breath attempts to nourish that seed at every opportunity. Humans by rejecting their life circumstances and ignoring their internal mandate separate themselves from all that is truly nourishing in life. False interpretations of both the nature of self and life smother the fires of heaven's intent and obstruct the flow of reality through the sensory orifices into one's depths. When illness and death come prematurely it is not the fault of heaven and may only be attributed to human ignorance.

The *Dao De Jing* equates returning to our destiny with tranquility and returning to the root of life:

> *The ten thousand things—side-by-side they arise;*
> *And by this I see their return.*
> *Things [come forth] in great numbers;*
> *Each one returns to its root.*
> *This is called tranquility.*
> *"Tranquility"—This means to return to your destiny.*
> *To return to your destiny is to be constant;*
> *To know the constant is to be wise.*

Not to know the constant is to be reckless and wild;
If you're reckless and wild, your actions lead to misfortune.
To know the constant is to be all-embracing;
To be all-embracing is to be impartial;
To be impartial is to be kingly;
To be kingly is to be [like] Heaven;
To be [like] Heaven is to be [one with] the Dao;
If you're [one with] the Dao,
to the end of your days you'll suffer no harm.

                – DAO DE JING[26]

Here we are given a seven-stage prescription for the maintenance of health through fulfilling destiny. In the Daoist enumeration of being, seven is the number signifying the loss and return of original nature. The ultimate fate of all things is to return to the *dao*. We are given the chance to do this at each moment in life by fulfilling destiny and cultivating virtue. To be a perfect channel for the will of heaven is to return *ming* to the world.

For Laozi, *ming* refers to the potential motivating force of the very life of each sentient being, the energy of life itself, rooted and originating in itself.[27] As the *chongqi* is "the original dynamism of the world," *ming* is the wave of destiny that propels us through life. Just as the *chongqi* blends perfectly all qualities of heaven and earth to preserve the integrity of the primal *dao*, so too does the individual who fulfills destiny.

Destiny and Healing in the Inner Tradition

Simply put, the notion of the fulfillment of individual destiny, as it exists in the inner tradition of Chinese medicine, may be stated as follows:

At the moment of conception, heaven plants a seed of potential deep within each individual. Throughout life, heaven continually nourishes this seed so that it manifests fully in the world. The fulfillment of our destiny entails being able to acknowledge the nature of the seed heaven has planted, a seed synonymous with our deep nature and inborn constitution.

Upon acknowledging the seed, we must then take actions in the world to cultivate and manifest this inborn potential. In manifesting destiny, we must accept all the events of our life as heaven's attempt to nourish the seed of potential it has sowed. Already mindful of this, the sage aligns his own will *(zhi)* with the will of heaven as it is expressed within as inborn potential and without as life's events. He makes the most of life by viewing external events, painful or pleasurable, as lessons to be learned in the path to mastering his destiny. In fulfilling his destiny, the sage becomes a channel for the creative flow of the *dao*.

Our contract with heaven is broken the moment we start closing doors to self-expression and "obstructing" the flow of *qi* between heaven and earth. Like a great flood, the *dao* will overwhelm any obstacle (inappropriate attitude or belief) placed in its path as it strives to assert its true nature. If an individual continues to resist the flow of the *dao*, then symptomatology may develop in the inner kingdom. These symptoms appear as obstructions in the "rivers" of the inner kingdom—the functions, officials, and meridians of the physical body.

The practitioner of the inner tradition helps to "unblock the passageways" by choosing medicines of the highest class that correspond to heaven, thereby promoting the patient's full self-expression, a necessary step if *ming* is to be established and vitality maintained.

The sage is able to establish *ming* and make the best of life not because life fails to challenge the sage, but because of a willingness to see all challenges as the will of heaven. Instead of adding to life's pain and generating illness over life's difficulties, the sage remains unmoved and "goes with the flow." Like Yu, he channels the flow of life so that it rises through him, placing no obstacles in its path. "The man of the great way wins no fame, the highest virtue wins no gain, the great man has no self. To the most perfect degree, he goes along with what has been allotted to him."[28] For the sage to act any other way is to "hide from heaven, turn your back on the true state of affairs, and forget what you were born with."[29]

Although heaven may will a unique nature for each of us, it is not certain that individuals can be true to this nature and manifest their destiny. This is a matter of human will and, ultimately, it is the choice of each person. Destiny itself is placed within at the moment of conception and is therefore unchangeable by human will. Humans, through their own will, must align themselves with the will of heaven in order to fulfill their destiny. This alignment must occur both internally and externally as we cultivate and preserve our inborn nature and accept the situations sent to us by heaven.[30]

Hence the role of our will is merely to acknowledge the nature of our destiny and to initiate actions in the world consistent with the manifestation of destiny. Zhuangzi affirms this by saying, "To know what you can't do anything about, and to be content with it as you would with destiny—only a man of virtue can do that."[31] For Zhuangzi, people of virtue cultivate their inner nature and do not resent heaven for their internal endowment of their basic nature or their external endowment of their life circumstances. "Resign yourself to what cannot be avoided and nourish what is within you—this is best. What more do you have to do to fulfill your mission? Nothing is as good as following orders [fulfilling destiny]—that's how difficult it is!"[32]

Against Destiny

Chinese Medicine is a great treasure-house! We must make all efforts to uncover it and raise its standards.
– MAO ZE-DONG[33]

In 1958 Chairman Mao issued a decree that the Chinese government would supervise the development of a state-run medical system in which traditional Chinese medicine (TCM) would be practiced side by side with Western medicine. In 1972 a governmental health committee stated, "We must therefore strive to comprehend the original significance of the doctrines of *yinyang* and the Five Phases and develop it critically from the perspective of dialectical and historical materialism, in order to uncover the medical treasure-house of our homeland even better."[34]

The development of TCM through the 1970s was constrained by the requirement that it adhere to the ideological views of Marxism. Dialectical materialism, which denotes Marxism, literally means a discussion of those aspects of life that are materially real. The movement to scientize Chinese medicine meant subjecting it to the scrutiny of the analytic method. Analytic science, although ideal for studying the quantitative aspects of structure, is incapable of meaningfully assessing human physiological functions that encompass physical as well as emotional and spiritual realms of being. Eventually, TCM was formulated into a medicine which sought to parallel that of Western medical practice. The central focus during the 1970s became the application of acupuncture to produce surgical anesthesia and for pain relief.

Through gross manipulation of source material, the Marxists rewrote the history and theory of Chinese medicine to reflect the interests of the state in perpetuating communism. This is exemplified in an essay entitled "The Struggle for and Against a Belief in Destiny in the Medicine of Our Land,"[35] published in 1974 in the Shanghai journal, *Dialectic of Nature*. Unschuld calls this piece a "particularly striking example of questionable historical writing."[36] The following is a small abstract of the essay which Unschuld has translated in its entirety:

But why would Confucians seek to link illness and divine destiny so forcefully? Because the slave holders have been destined by fate to be god's deputies among men. Thus when the Confucians determined that the source of illness in the human body was "divine destiny," and when they required that man passively submit to such divine intervention, their intention in reality was to illustrate that whether someone was born rich or poor, of a high or low station, and so forth, was always determined by destiny, and that consequently man must obey divine dictates, seek to accept his destiny, and tolerate the repressive rule of the slave holders. All this, however, was intended to facilitate survival of the seriously threatened existence of slavery itself.[37]

In standardizing their state-run medical system, the ruling party sought to eliminate all aspects of Chinese medical theory that empowered the fulfillment of individual destiny. This was accomplished in part by linking the notion of destiny with the impoverishment that had been experienced by the masses since the dawn of Chinese civilization itself. The Marxists did make some strides helping to overcome superstition and modernize their nation. However, in crafting their state-run medical system they failed to value the deeper spiritual aspects of healing that lie at the heart of traditional Chinese medicine.

The Difference Between Destiny and Fate

He who comprehends the greater destiny becomes
himself a part of it. He who comprehends the lesser
destiny resigns himself to the inevitable.
– ZHUANGZI[38]

Despite the assertions of the communist author just cited, the sense of destiny we have used here in no way implies a course of events fixed or immutable in the face of human will. What is fixed is the unique, innate nature of each being. This nature must be continually aligned, through the action of human will, with the events of the moment. It is this alignment that allows the *dao* to express its spontaneous nature through us in a creative rather than a determinate fashion.

That heaven wills only the highest for each individual is made clear by Mencius. It is the responsibility of each person to discern the nature of his or her own destiny, he says, for heaven does not send misery to our life of its own accord. Pain in life is only brought on by turning our back on heaven's will and our own nature. "Therefore," Mencius warns us, "one who knows destiny will not stand beneath a poorly built wall. . . . It is no man's true destiny to die in fetters."[39]

Daoist philosopher Liu Yiming (Liu I-ming) offers an alchemical meaning of destiny and restoring our original nature. He stresses being a master of one's destiny rather than just going along through life a slave to fate, unaware of both our inner nature and our motivations for acting:

> People of great wisdom reverse the operation of the natural process; they are not bound by the natural process, not molded by *yin* and *yang*, not compelled by myriad things, not changed by myriad conditions. Planting lotuses in a fire, hauling a boat through mud and water, they make temporary use of things of the world to practice the principles of [*dao*], by the human [*dao*], completing the celestial [*dao*]. They uproot the mundane senses conditioned by history and sweep away all acquired influences. They rule their own destinies and are not ruled by fate. Restoring the whole, original being, they avoid compulsive routine, transcend all worlds, and become incorruptible.[40]

Another notion of destiny in the sense of the preordained events in life is expressed in the Chinese character *shu* (數), meaning, literally, "numbers." This character is related to the "lesser destiny" referred to by Zhuangzi, denoting common fortune-telling rather than the deeper philosophical concept of destiny *(ming)* we are discussing here.

In this text, the term "destiny" refers only to the highest destiny manifested willfully by the sage. I use the term "fate" to denote the lesser destiny to which the masses resign themselves.

Destiny and Immortality

Alchemy, like any of life's disciplines, has both an internal and an external aspect.[41] External alchemy in China, as in the West, was concerned with the quest to turn lead into gold. This endeavor laid the groundwork for modern understanding of metallurgy and the basic physical properties of many substances.

Inner alchemy, however, is the quest for immortality. Inner alchemy itself has its inner and outer aspects. On a superficial level, inner alchemy may be said to deal with our search for eternal life. But the deepest aspect of internal alchemy is concerned with the fulfillment of destiny and the spiritual evolution of the practitioner. Immortality may be seen here as the cultivation of virtue that results from bringing an individual aspect of the *dao* into the world fully expressed. The person who fulfills destiny in this way makes a unique, undying contribution to the world and, in so doing, gains immortality.

Summary

Emphasis on the importance of fulfilling destiny is a meeting ground between Chinese cosmology, philosophy, alchemy, and medicine. As the *chongqi* blends heaven and earth, so too does the individual who fulfills destiny. By aligning between these two cosmic poles the sage, in essence, becomes a pillar of the universe and in so doing cultivates undying virtue.

Turning our back on innate purpose compromises the integrity of our primordial influences as our guiding light in life. Rejecting the circumstances encountered in life we are effectively separated from the influence of heaven both within and without. In this way, the influence of the heavenly *yang* diminishes, the mundane influences of acquired *yin* accumulate, and the path to illness and death is trod slowly one step at a time.

The fulfillment of destiny in Chinese medicine is influenced by, and impacts, the interrelated functioning of several dynamic aspects of being. Next, we examine the language of Chinese physiology as it applies to the fulfillment of destiny.

Questions

The Chinese concept of destiny implies that each person has an innate purpose to manifest in life.

1. Who are you?

2. When you answer question 1, how much emphasis do you place on acquired traits (who you have become) relative to innate traits (who you are)?

3. Why are you here?

4. What are you doing about it?

NOTES

1. Watson, 1964a, p. 38.
2. Anderson, 1989, pp. 56–57.
3. T'ang, 1962 (January), p. 195.
4. Chen, 1989, p. 226.
5. Lin, 1942, p. 308; as cited in Chen, 1989, p. 227.
6. Wieger, 1965, p. 47.

7. Anderson, 1989, p. 57.
8. Wieger, 1965, p. 594.
9. Lagerwey, 1987, p. 155. Paraphrased from Lagerwey's quote of Liddell and Scott, a Greek/English lexicon, s.v. H.G. Liddell, *A Lexicon: Abridged from Liddell and Scott's Greek-English Lexicon* (Oxford; New York: Clarendon Press, 1977).
10. Class with Ted Kaptchuk, 1990.
11. Wieger, 1965, p. 125.
12. Larre and Rochat de la Vallee, 1987.
13. Lagerwey, 1987, p. 159.
14. T'ang, 1962 (January), p. 202.
15. Ibid., p. 201.
16. Ibid., p. 203.
17. Watson, 1964a, p. 49.
18. T'ang, 1962 (January), p. 209.
19. Ibid., p. 213.
20. Ibid., p. 215.
21. T'ang, 1962 (April), p. 34.
22. Larre and Rochat de la Vallee, 1985, p. 63.
23. Porkert, 1982, p. 171.
24. T'ang, 1962 (April), p. 33.
25. Watson, 1964a, p. 138.
26. Chapter 16; in Henricks, 1989, p. 218. I changed Henrick's translation of the character *ming* from "fate" to "destiny."
27. T'ang, 1962 (April), p. 44.
28. Watson, 1964a, p. 101.
29. Ibid., p. 48.
30. This according to Mencius (see T'ang, 1962 [January and April]).
31. Watson, 1964a, p. 66. I changed Watson's translation of the character *ming* from "fate" to "destiny."
32. Ibid., p. 58.
33. Unschuld, 1985, p. 251.
34. Ibid., 1985, p. 253.
35. In Unschuld, 1985, pp. 340–352. I have changed Unschuld's use of the word "fate" to "destiny."
36. Ibid., 1985, p. 254.
37. Ibid., 1985, pp. 340–352. I have substituted the word "destiny" for Unschuld's use of the word "fate."
38. Morgan, p. 28.
39. Mencius, Book VII, Part I, Chapter II; in Legge, 1970, pp. 448–449.
40. Cleary, 1986a, pp. 54–55.
41. For a detailed account of "external" alchemy, see J. Needham and L. Gwei-Djen, *Science and Civilisation in China: Chemistry and Chemical Technology,* Vol. 5 (Cambridge: Cambridge University Press, 1983).

3

THE
LANGUAGE
OF DESTINY

*Words exist because of meaning; once you've gotten the meaning,
you can forget the words. Where can I find a man who has forgotten
words so I can have a word with him?*
– ZHUANGZI [1]

ACCORDING TO LAOZI AND ZHUANGZI, LANGUAGE
creates reality. The language of Chinese medicine in many modern texts reflects a materialistic ideology. Discussion of Chinese physiology is often presented in a linear, mechanistic fashion that is derivative of Western biomedicine. Many concepts, along with fine shades of meaning of characters essential to understanding the foundation of the inner tradition of Chinese medicine, have eroded over time.

In this chapter I define the terms and concepts central to understanding the deep nature of Chinese medicine as a science that advances the evolution of the human spirit. We begin by examining the fundamental nature of *yin* and *yang* and the concepts of early and later heaven as they relate to inborn and acquired constitution. My emphasis is on the idea of heaven's will, as it exists both internally (as the *jing* and *yuanqi*) and externally (as personal life circumstance and environment), and human will *(zhi)* relative to the fulfillment of destiny. Further, I elaborate on the concepts of original nature *(de)* and spirit *(shen* and *ling).*

Yin *and* Yang

Yin   陰

The Chinese character *yin* depicts the shady side of a hill. Cosmologically, *yin* is synonymous in its characteristics with *dao*, in that it is the soft, receptive, and quiescent aspect of life. In humans, our storehouse of primordial *yin* is the ocean out of which all of our manifestations in life are drawn. *Yin* is the basis of the bones and the nervous system, which may be thought of as deriving their strength and integrity from our primordial source. *Yin* is also the basis of all fluids, such as blood, saliva, and the fluid that keeps all mucous membranes moist and healthy. *Yin* comprises the physical substrate of the body. Hence Porkert terms *yin* the "structive" aspect of being.[2]

Our inherited endowment of *yin*, referred to in this text as *yuanyin*, must last a lifetime. Signs that one's store of *yin* is becoming depleted are varied and include hot flashes, heat in the palms and soles of the feet, night sweats, excessive thought, restless spirit, heart palpitations, a peeled tongue (shiny with no coat), and a tight to wiry pulse.

Acquired *yin* represents the habituating influences of later heaven, which extinguish one's original nature. This includes primarily the false interpretation of reality and acquired belief systems that do not empower the manifestation of true self. Physiologically, this may correspond to the production of unhealthy fluids in the body, such as damp and phlegm, which become burdens and thus hinder the ascension of the spirit.

Yang   陽

The Chinese character *yang* depicts the sun shining above the horizon. Cosmologically, *yang* is synonymous in its characteristics with the nature of heaven as it activates and actualizes the hidden potentials inherent in *dao*. *Yang* is the sun shining down on the ocean of *yin* and drawing life ever out of it. *Yang* is that fire toward which all beings strive in their evolutionary path. It is the impulse that sparks all physiological activity and movement. In humans, *yang* represents the activating influences of the mind as it works through the nervous system. Thus our *shen*, the heart fire that activates and initiates all action, is an emanation of *yang*. Porkert terms *yang* the "configurative" aspect of physiological function.[3] Our inherited endowment of *yang*, here referred to as *yuanyang*, is the creative evolutionary seed placed within the kidneys at conception.

Our natural endowment of *yang* must also last through the course of our life. In fact, in Chinese medicine, the moment of death may be defined as that instant when our last bit of *yang* dissipates. Corpses have *yin*; they are cold and have form. But they have no *yang*—movement or warmth. *Yang* deficiency includes symptoms of coldness and of physiological processes slowing down due to the deficient *yang's* inability to initiate and sustain activity.

Early and Heaven   先天 後天

As each human life unfolds along the thread of the *dao*, it exists in each moment as the sum total of all its inherited and acquired characteristics. The potential for manifestation in life that we acquire prior to the moment of drawing our first breath falls under the influence of early heaven. Early heaven may be thought of as our genetic and karmic endowment. *Karma* (from the Sanskrit *kri*, "to do"—literally, "deed") means all that we bring to this life from past lives and ancestors including the spiritual lessons which move with us from one life to the next. The *qi* we acquire from food, air, and life experience after the first breath falls under the influence of later heaven. Hence early heaven consists of all that we bring to this life, whereas later heaven is all that we receive during life.

Think of early heaven as the seed of potential that heaven plants deep within us at the moment of conception. It provides primordial influences at conception that become the foundation of all of life's manifestations. These influences are the *jing* (essence), *yuanqi* (our inherited endowment of *yin* and *yang*), and *shen* (spirit). In the sense of being potential, early heaven corresponds to *yin*. Think of later heaven as all that heaven sends during our life in its ceaseless attempt to nourish the seed it has planted. In this sense, the contribution of later heaven is to activate our inborn potential and it may be considered as corresponding to *yang*.

Early heaven is not always associated with *yin* and later heaven with *yang*. In the spiritual alchemy of Liu Yiming,[4] early heaven is thought to correspond to *yang* because the *jing, yuanqi,* and *shen* are the celestial influences that govern humans' ascension in life, providing the motivating force that guides evolution and the fulfillment of destiny. These positive *yang* influences support the fires of *mingmen*, ensuring the integrity of the physiological process governed by this "furnace of evolution."[5] In Liu Yiming's view, the habituating influences acquired in later heaven result in negative interpretations of our life experience and thus correspond to *yin*. These are the "mundane" influences that dampen the fires of *mingmen* and extinguish heaven's spark. Zhuangzi warns, "Do not through human doing extinguish the heavenly constitution."

The study and practice of Chinese medicine involves being able to hold simultaneously in our consideration seemingly contradictory principles such as these without feeling the need to consider one view correct and others incorrect. It can thus be said that inasmuch as early heaven represents absolute potential, it is *yin*, and inasmuch as it consists of the true primordial influences that govern human evolution, it is *yang*. In the same way, later heaven, inasmuch as it represents the positive, active role of heaven to nourish our inborn potential, is *yang*. Inasmuch as the habituating influences acquired during later heaven tend to obscure the influences of early heaven, it is *yin*.

Early Heaven

The influences associated with early heaven—*jing, yuanqi,* and *shen*—are granted to the individual at the moment of conception. The essential nature of this endowment can never be damaged by the effects of our environment or acquired experiences. Although life may obscure their true nature, they remain pure and always reflect the underlying unity of the *dao* as it exists as truth in each person's depths. *Yin* and *yang* may separate in the course of our life, but as long as one bit of primordial *qi* remains intact, consciousness of our original nature as a guiding force in life can be restored.

De: *Original Nature*

To serve your own heart so that sadness or joy do not sway
or move it; to understand what you can do nothing about
and to be content with it as with destiny—
this is the perfection of virtue.
– Zhuangzi[6]

The name Laozi means literally "old infant." The title of his text, the *Dao De Jing,* may be translated as "The Path *(dao)* of Virtue *(de)*

Classic *(jing)."* As a text, the *Dao De Jing* instructs us on the preservation of and return to original nature *(de)* in the world. The concept of *de* has two fine shades of meaning depending on whether it is applied to an infant or adult. As applied to the infant, *de* may be translated as "original nature" in reference to the complement of primordial influences that guide its life. In the adult, *de* may be translated as "virtue," referring to the sage's manifestation of his or her innate capacities in the world.

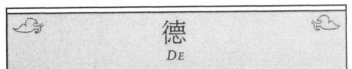

德

DE

The character *de*, often translated as "virtue," is composed of three key components. The first is a picture of a man walking (彳) and implies movement or action. The second means "perfectly right" (惪) and suggests that a thing scrutinized by the eye (罒) from all directions (十) has shown no deviation (一). The last component denotes the heart *(xin: 心).*[7] The character *de* may be interpreted to mean that the virtuous person's behavior perfectly reflects his or her heart, which, under scrutiny, shows no deviation. The power of *de* may be said to grant the ability to be straight, keeping true to one's essence and maintaining an invariable direction such as the downward flowing tendency of water.[8] The imagery of the character *de* also has an overtone suggesting the empowerment of intuition. According to the etymology of the character, intuition may be defined as the ability to directly bypass one's mind and know spontaneously with one's heart the heart of all things.

Chen says, "*De* stands for the original endowment of nature prior to moral distinctions and conscious effort."[9] "*De* is the pristine state of nature unburdened by the distinctions between good and evil."[10] *De* is original nature as seen in the infant, unsullied by life's experience and the accretions of mundane consciousness. The *Dao De Jing* tells us, "One who contains *de* in fullness, is to be compared to an infant. . . . Such is the perfection of its life-force *(jing)."*[11] Indeed, the infant is thought to emulate the state of the one. Because "the infant is all *qi* but no mind *(xin)*,"[12] it may "cry all day without getting hoarse."[13] The infant has boundless energy to move through life's transitions because it has no mind to react to or judge its response to life. It is the perfect channel for the creative flow of the *dao*.

Heaven supplies us with our natural endowment along with an environment in which to cultivate it. It is each person's duty to preserve the original nature of heaven both within and without. By mandating for ourselves what heaven has mandated for us, each of us joins heaven internally and externally, uniting them as one. To preserve original nature in both self and the world is to cultivate true virtue.

> Dao *gives birth*,
> De *rears*, . . .
> De *is treasured*,
> *Not by decree* (ming),
> *But by spontaneity.*
>
> . . . .
>
> *Therefore*, dao *gives birth*,
> De *keeps, grows, nurtures, matures, ripens, covers, and buries.*
>
> – *DAO DE JING*[14]

The last line here outlines seven stages in the evolution of *de* from conception to death, seven signifying the return to original nature at its source. Heaven may will us a unique nature, but it cannot force us to manifest that destiny. Thus it is not certain that each person follows and manifests his or her inner nature. Only by preserving our infant-like spontaneity may we fully cultivate the virtue planted within. Just as an emperor cannot command people to be upright, so heaven cannot mandate each of us to treasure the gift of *de*.

Our *de*, then, constitutes that aspect of heaven, as it exists within each of us, that the vicissitudes of life may never harm. *De*, as the primordial influence of heaven, remains pure and untouched in each person's depths. *De* as a concept contains the philosophical underpinnings of such physiological concepts as *jing* and *yuanqi*. As we see later, the quality of each individual's destiny is characterized by the transformation of an unbalanced emotion back into its corresponding virtue.

The Three Treasures: Jing, Qi, *and* Shen

Our endowment of *jing, qi,* and *shen* are the three Daoist treasures. Together, they constitute the *hun* spirit associated with the liver, governor of human evolution and our ascent toward heaven during life. These gifts from early heaven form the constitutional foundation of our path during life.

Jing: *The Terrestrial Storehouse*

The *dao*, our treasure, is "bipartite," existing partly in ourselves and partly in heaven. This split treasure is a pact made between heaven, the celestial half, and the terrestrial half on earth, known as *jing*, our inherited endowment.[15] By possessing the terrestrial half, *jing*, we may summon the celestial half, creating healing and fueling evolution by this union of heaven and earth. This view is supported in the *Dao De Jing*, which suggests the *dao* contains the seed *(jing)* of the authentic *(zhen)* self:

> *Dark and dim,*
> *In it [the* dao*] there is life seed* (jing).
> *Its life seed being very genuine* (zhen),
> *In it there is growth power* (xin).
>   – DAO DE JING[16]

Zhuangzi tells us that heaven blows "on the ten thousand things in a different way, so that each can be itself."[17] Heaven mandates for us in every cell, in every aspect of who we are, a unique quality of being that we are destined to bring into the world. Noting this full self-expression *(ziran)* in the infant, in whom is contained *de* (original nature) in its fullness, the *Dao De Jing* states, "such is the perfection of its life force *(jing).*"[18] This mandate is imprinted on the *jing*, the fluid that governs the smooth unfolding of our individual destiny as we move from the beginning of life to the end. In order to assure communication with heaven, our *jing* must be carefully preserved.[19] *Jing* is the microcosmic emanation of the *dao* as unity, the seed of all being, and the wellspring of life's manifestations. The potential inherent in *jing* may manifest only to the degree that it meets with *shen*, the functional expression of complementary quality. *Jing* holds the potential for the manifestation of heaven's will as it exists uniquely within each human being.

精

JING

The character *jing* has three components. On the
left (米) is the character for grains of rice, which
symbolize essence. On the right is the character
qing (青), itself composed on top of the character
for plants growing (生), with an alchemist's pot
(月) containing cinnabar (一) located underneath. The image of the alchemist's furnace
recalls the image of *mingmen*, the "gate of destiny," where *jing* and *shen* interpenetrate to fuel
the fulfillment of destiny. As a totality, the character *jing* calls forth an image of the essential
generative and transformative power of the *dao*
seen in the new growth of spring.

Yuanqi

> But the emergence of one thing *[yuanqi]* in the ocean of nothing *[jing]*
> provoked the conversion of nothing into something, and that some-
> thing *(yuanqi)*, which is also nothing, is at once positive, insofar as it
> makes everything possible, and negative, insofar as it is no-thing, as
> opposed to one thing. It is, in short, two. . . .[20]

The *yuanqi* is the representation of heaven and earth as imprinted
on the *jing* at the moment of conception. As an individual's *shen* rises
out of *jing* to recreate this polarity internally, the *yuanqi* emerges as an
individual's innate complement of primal *yin* and *yang* within the left
and right kidneys, respectively. *Yuanqi* is associated with the one in
Daoism, and the character *yi* [一], denoting "one," corresponds to
heaven. *Yi* is the first stroke in the character *yuan* [元], as well as in the
characters *shen* [神] and *ling* [靈], which denote spirit. Therefore,
yuanqi may be understood to represent the unified influence of heaven
as it exists in humans. However, considered relative to *jing* as pure
potential, *yuanqi* is "two," the original *yin* and *yang* of the kidneys.

The relationship of *jing* to *yuanqi* is similar to that of the unnamed
dao to the named *dao*, in that the unnamed *dao* precedes the named
dao. The unnamed *dao* is one and represents unified potentiality
beyond human conception. The named *dao* is also one, but it is one as
conceived by humans. Considering the named *dao* relative to the
unnamed *dao*, it is now two, and thus begins the evolutionary ladder

of material existence. Hence Lagerwey equates the unnamed *dao* with pure potential *(ling)* and tells us that the *yuanqi* is "One . . . a single pearl in the midst of a boundless ocean."[21]

Jing is the microcosmic representation of *ling,* the undifferentiated potential in the macrocosm.[22] This undifferentiated potential is the vast ocean from which all of life's manifestations emerge. The *yuanqi* is the primordial *qi* that rises out of this ocean. In one sense, the *yuanqi* may be considered synonymous with *jing* inasmuch as it too represents undifferentiated potential.[23] However, if we consider *yuanqi* relative to *jing,* then the *yuanqi* becomes two as suggested by its presence as the *yuanyin* and *yuanyang* in the left and right kidney, respectively.[24] Recapitulating the *dao's* ontogeny, these three—the *jing, yuanyin,* and *yuanyang*— remain, in health, forever interpenetrated in a state of primal unity.

Note that terms like *yuanqi* and *jing* are used differently by different authors in different texts throughout history. In my interpretation of *jing* as representing primordial unity and the *yuanqi* as representing duality, I am attempting to define these terms in a way that is both theoretically and clinically relevant. Clinically, the degradation of *yuanqi* may be discussed in terms of the separation of original *yin* and *yang,* which implies duality. However, *jing* as unity does not "separate." It is merely depleted as our inherited complement of *yin* and *yang* unravels.

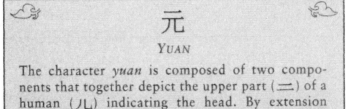

元

YUAN

The character *yuan* is composed of two components that together depict the upper part (二) of a human (儿) indicating the head. By extension *yuan* denotes a principle or origin. The *dao* is the principle that is the origin and motivation force of all things. *Yuanqi* denotes our inherited endowment of *qi* that flows from this primordial source.

Shen: *The Celestial Storehouse*

The radiant spirit of heaven shines down on the primordial sea from whence it came. This heavenly brightness *(shenming:*神明*)* is the spirit *(shen),* the "ultimate rationally conceivable cause of living organization *(sheng:*生*)*."[25] One visual analogue of this interaction is an electrical storm in which heaven extends itself toward earth in a pulse of lightning. In fact, *shen* is related etymologically to a character denoting lightning and thunder.[26] Interestingly, this description of creation is strikingly close to that of modern evolutionary theory. The current wisdom hypothesizes that life began on earth as a result of lightning striking the primordial "hot thin soup." With this catalysis, amino acids joined to form complex proteins, which, in turn, created single-cell organisms, thus beginning the evolutionary tree of life.

Just as Emperor Huang Di (黃帝) was the center of the nation in the legendary period, so *di* (帝), the polestar, is the center around which the heavens spin. The whirling of the heavens is powered by the Big Dipper, the giant spoon-shaped constellation in the northern sky that stirs life along. The celestial half of the contract between heaven and earth lies in the Big Dipper, which is considered the central administration of human destinies and life-giving center of the universe.[27] Here, the "primordial spirits of fundamental destiny" *(ben ming yuan shen)* (本命元神) allocate life to us based on astrological calculations and individual merit.[28]

Each of us is born under the protection of one of the spirits who reside in the Big Dipper's seven stars. "They [the seven stars] move in the center of the heavens and look down to control the four quarters in order to establish the four seasons and [to distribute] evenly the five elements."[29] Interestingly, a homophone of *xing* (星) meaning "star" is the character *xing* (性) meaning "constitution." This connection suggests that our constitution is granted by the stars.

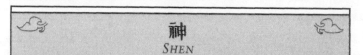

SHEN

The character *shen* is composed of two elements. On the left, heaven is pictured [一] above the portents of the moon, stars, and sun [朿]. Through these portents, the will of heaven is made known to humankind.[30] On the right are two hands [丨], "giving or taking downwards."[31] The hands are extending a rope, giving the idea of expansion or extension.[32] Taken as a whole, this character gives the sense of heaven extending its will toward earth and the consciousness of humankind. Humans, in turn, extend their own *shen* toward their *jing* in the act of self-discovery. As the *yang* aspect of heart spirit, *shen* empowers the creative and expansive nature of heaven within each individual.

Shen *in the Microcosm*

The will of heaven is exercised through its *shen*, which imprints on the *jing* the unique spiritual disposition presiding over each of us at the moment of conception. It is at this moment that our constitution and destiny are imparted. This imprint, stored in the *jing*, constitutes our unique endowment from heaven, which, in turn, gives rise to our personal *shen* (heart spirit). Our individual *shen* must then illuminate the *jing* over "the entire route of one's destiny," binding our core to the core of heaven.[33] Porkert tells us that "*shen* is primarily the actively organizing configurative force and transformative influence that determines and upholds the specific character of an individual."[34] Larre expands this to say, "The *shen* are that by which a given being is unlike any other; that which makes an individual an individual and more than merely a person. . . . The relation of the individual to heaven is a way of binding oneself to the core of one's existence."[35]

In human physiology, the upper burner (the area between the xiphoid process and throat including the heart and lungs) corresponds to heaven.[36] The *shen*, as an emanation of heaven in humans, is present as the heart spirit. This spirit resides in each of the *zang (yin)* officials (heart, spleen, lung, kidney, liver) as an emissary and emanation of the heart official. The five *shen* and their corresponding organs are listed in Figure 3.1a and depicted in Figure 3.1b. The five *shen* help empower us to manifest our destiny between heaven and earth. They allow us as individuals to change our lives through the conscious intention to do so.[37] The *shen*, as an emanation of the heart, is the active impulse from the pole of heaven, as it exists within each person, to ignite our inborn potential *(jing)*. The quality of this interaction is determined by the *zhi*, or will of humans.

Ling

Let us go back to the Beginning:
Before the Beginning was the Dao. *Let us call the* Dao
zero, neither negative nor positive: pure potential (ling).[38]

As pure potentiality, the *dao* ultimately must be identified with the attributes of *yin*. In Daoist spiritual writings, the character *ling* refers to the *dao* as "pure potentiality." Porkert tells us that "*jing* in medical contexts exactly takes over the role played by *ling*, 'structure force,' 'structure capacity,' in philosophical and Daoist technical writing. . . ."[39]

Although the term *ling* is almost unknown in medical literature, its character figures prominently in the names of five acupuncture points. These are Heart-2, "blue-green spirit"; Heart-4, "spirit path"; Kidney-24, "spirit burial ground"; Gallbladder-18, "receiving spirit"; and Governor Vessel-10, "spirit tower."

Jing and *ling* differ in quality. *Jing* is stored in the kidneys and is treated chiefly through points related to the lower burner; *ling* is treated through points related to the upper burner.

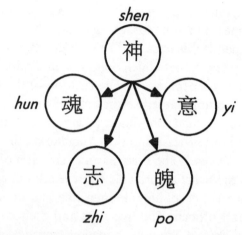

The Five *Shen*	
Organ	Spirit
Heart	shen
Spleen	yi
Lung	po
Kidney	zhi
Liver	hun

Figure 3.1
THE FIVE *SHEN*

Each of the yin *organs is associated with a spirit that represents the heart* shen *as it manifests through the function of each organ. The* shen *of the spleen is the* yi, *which grants the capacity of thought and ideation. The* shen *of the lung is the* po, *which consists of the seven emotions (fear, fright, anger, joy, worry, sadness, and grief). The* po *represents animal instincts and urges and empowers us to receive and assimilate life into self. The* shen *of the kidneys is the* zhi, *or human will, which empowers self-knowledge and the ability to align our will with the will of heaven. The* shen *of the liver is the* hun, *which consists of the* jing, qi, *and* shen. *It is the evolutionary spirit that governs our ascension in life.*

The character *ling* has been changed in modern Chinese to one that hides the meaning of its etymology (灵). There is no discussion of *ling* as an aspect of spirit present in the modern texts from China. These texts, which reflect the materialistic ideology of Marxism, discuss only *shen*. This reflects the predilection of the modern Chinese to shun a concept of spirit that has a shamanistic derivation and implies that the individual has the power to evoke changes in heaven (the governing

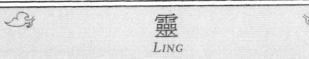

LING

The etymology of the character *ling* reveals its inner meaning. At the top, four drops of rain fall from clouds under heaven [☲]. In the middle, three mouths [☷] appear, and, at the bottom, two female shamans[40] [☵] offer jade and dances to heaven. The image is a ritual dance for rain. The notion expressed in the character is that through the appropriate performance of ritual, heaven is summoned, effecting change in the world. Hence *ling* has the associated meanings "spiritual," "mysterious," "supernatural power or effect," "transcendent," and "marvelous."[41] Mathews defines *ling* as "The spirit of a being, which acts upon others."[42] In religious Daoism, *ling* is the aspect of spirit that manifests itself after death to protect its descendants.[43]

regime). The concept of spirit inherent in *shen*, that heaven sends down the portents of what will be, is probably a more comfortable notion to the leaders of a totalitarian state.

The concepts of spiritual power present in *ling* have been decried not only in the modern era. Xunzi (born 312 B.C.E.) directly attacked the notion of *ling*: "When performance of the great rain dance is followed by rain, what does this mean? [I] say it means nothing. It is as though the rain dance had not been performed and it had rained. . . . understanding them [rituals] as ornamental leads to good fortune; understanding them as spiritual leads to ill fortune."[44] Perhaps Xunzi is railing against the superstitious masses who both fear omens from heaven (such as falling stars) and employ "witch doctors" to protect them from evil. The concept of *ling* is still a potent symbol for the spiritual power of one who has fulfilled destiny and, in this highest sense, should not be discarded.

Ling *as Spirit*

Spirits [shen] *attain the One thus are efficacious* [ling]

. . . .

Spirits (shen), *without that which makes them efficacious* (ling), *would, I'm afraid, be powerless.*

– *DAO DE JING,* Chapter 39

We have already learned that *shen* may manifest only to the degree that it meets with *jing* or *ling.*[45] *Ling* is the *yin* aspect of heart spirit as it complements *shen.* The *Lingshu*[46] states, "The *jingqi* of *yang* is called *shen*; the *jingqi* of *yin* is called *ling.*"[47] *Ling,* as the complement of *shen,* is the capacity of a substratum to make concrete the active influences to which it is exposed.[48] *Ling* may be thought of as the microcosmic representation of the *dao* as unlimited evolutionary potential as it exists in each human being. As the *yin* aspect of heart spirit, *ling* empowers potency, or the ability to manifest our inner potential effectively in the world.

In medical and philosophical texts with strong Confucian influences, the characters used to express the concepts of heart (*xin*) and mind (*xin, zhi*) are associated with the active *yang* aspect of spirit, *shen.* In such Daoist texts as the *Zhuangzi,* the heart and mind are often associated with *ling,* the *yin* aspect of heart spirit. Hence, when Zhuangzi advises us that our hearts and minds must remain tranquil in the face of life's challenges, he states, "Life, death, preservation, loss, failure, success . . . [T]hese are the alterations of the world, the workings of destiny [*ming*]. . . . They should not be allowed to enter the spirit storehouse [*lingfu* (靈府)]."[49] The term *lingfu,* "spirit storehouse" or "storehouse of potency," refers to the heart.[50] Zhuangzi also uses the characters *lingtai* (靈台), or "spirit tower," to refer to the heart.[51] *Lingtai* is also the name of acupuncture point Governor-10, located on the back in the upper burner at the level of the heart and between the heart *shu* points on the bladder meridian.

The use of the term *ling* associated with the heart in some Daoist texts is, I believe, consistent with the passive nature of Daoism and on the *Dao De Jing*'s emphasis on following the *yin* principle in nature. The use of *shen* associated with the heart in Confucian texts may be considered consistent with the relative Confucian emphasis on the *yang* principle in nature as exemplified in the *Yijing.*

Ling *as Potency*

Ling may be best understood as a spiritual emanation of the potency contained in *jing.* *Jing,* transformed through the internal alchemy that leads to the fulfillment of destiny, becomes *ling* and mixes with the heart spirit *(shen)* in the upper burner. Once we have fulfilled our individual destiny, we may be empowered with the potency *(ling)* to invoke changes in the world by influencing the will of heaven.

When *shen* interacts with *jing,* the will of heaven becomes a spiritually potent force in human beings. That is to say, our *shen* may illuminate the nature of heaven's will as it is stored in our depths. In this way, we are granted an opportunity to live in a way consistent with heaven's intent. When *shen* interacts with *ling,* then we humans become a spiritually potent force in the universe. This power allows "transformation to follow; wherever he (the sage) abides."[52]

Just as heaven cannot "force" us to fulfill destiny, as individuals we cannot "make" heaven respond to our commands. We are only in the position, through the appropriate performance of ritual, to say, "I have fulfilled my contract and now I request from you rain." *Ling* does not give us the ability to make things happen but empowers us to create the appropriate context in which the desired result may occur. Ultimately, the performance of ritual in this way becomes an act based on the open receptivity that comes from the inaction *(wuwei)* of aligning our will with the will of heaven. Creating this state of openness is the most *yin* action that we may take. *Ling* is the power of the substrate (human) to evoke the presence of activating impulse (heaven). It is our individual power to evoke heaven to manifest in a way that is aligned with our own intention and will.

Later Heaven

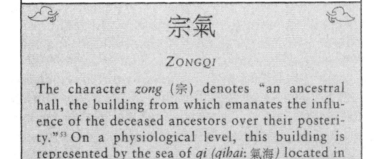

宗氣

ZONGQI

The character *zong* (宗) denotes "an ancestral hall, the building from which emanates the influence of the deceased ancestors over their posterity."[53] On a physiological level, this building is represented by the sea of *qi* (*qihai:* 氣海) located in the chest where the primordial breaths *(yuanqi)* and ancestral breaths *(zongqi)* are gathered together under one central authority.[54]

Chapter 4 of the *Dao De Jing* describes the movement of the *dao* as a "whirling emptiness" and calls it the "ancestor *(zong)* of the ten thousand things." *Zongqi* powers the rhythmic motion of the body, which is most evident in respiration.[55] This process occurs in utero, as evidenced by the beating of the fetus's heart, and the moment of the infant's first breath fully establishes this interaction in later heaven. For it is at this moment that the infant separates from the mother and, with the umbilical cord cut, begins along its own path of destiny, taking a unique place in the lineage of its ancestry. Interestingly, it is from the moment of first breath, and not the moment of conception (which would be difficult to calculate), that astrological calculations are made.

The motion of the breath suggests the reciprocity between humans and heaven. It is this relationship that enables us to nourish what heaven has placed within us *(yuanqi* and *jing)* and receive what comes to us from heaven from without (air, food, and life experience). Hence the spontaneous mixing of early heaven with later heaven may be considered the physiological and spiritual foundation of fulfilling destiny.

Shen *in the Macrocosm*

Throughout life, heaven continues to extend its influence by sending situations to each of us that are conducive to the nourishment of our unique inborn potential. The metaphor of being stirred through life by the dipper, caught in the whirling vortex of fate, is what the *Dao De Jing* and the Chinese alchemical texts refer to as "going along," that is, going through life with mundane consciousness, having lost our original nature.

The alchemical texts use the image of "reversing" the direction of the Big Dipper's movement as a metaphor for the return to original nature. According to Zhang Boduan, "After birth, it [original nature] is polluted by external influences and seduced by external things; the dipper handle points outward, not inward; the enlivening energy is outside, the killing energy is inside. Following the course of nature, the young mature, the mature age, the aged die; this goes on and on in repetitious cycles, with no hope of escape. If one knows the mechanisms of life and death and turns around the dipper handle, one can change one's orientation, one arrives at one's homeland and can thereby take over the evolutionary cycle and thus join the four forms and the five elemental energies. . . ."[56]

Through the willful act of centering, by aligning ourselves with the polestar, the Big Dipper spins around us, making us masters of our own destiny rather than pawns of fate. For it is only by maintaining a constant center (the polestar) that movement can occur in an organized fashion. Seven is the number of return, and the seven stars of the Big Dipper signify that it is the destiny of all things to return to the *dao*.

Zhi: *Human Will*

Our *shen* is imparted at the moment of conception and, inasmuch as *zhi* is one of the five *shen*, it too is imparted at this time. However, the emergence of human will as a guiding force in life occurs later as the infant becomes a child and, therefore, falls under the influence of later heaven.

The will of heaven is stored within our essence *(jing)* as innate nature and manifests externally as the situations we encounter in our lives. Although heaven determines a unique nature for each of us, it is not determined that each individual will be true to this nature and manifest personal destiny, for that is a matter of human will *(zhi)* and, ultimately, the choice of each person. Using our own will *(zhi)*, we must align ourselves with the will of heaven in order to fulfill our destiny *(ming)*. This alignment must occur both internally and externally as we cultivate and preserve our inborn nature and accept the situations sent by heaven. The infant's spontaneity springs in part from the continual alignment and identity of its will with the will of heaven. The separation of human will from heaven's will occurs as we lose our original nature and attempt to impose our own will on the world. The role played by human will in contributing to health and illness is elaborated in Chapter 4.

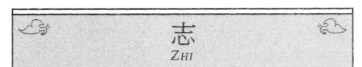

ZHI

The character *zhi* has been variously translated as knowledge,[57] mind,[58] will, purpose,[59] ambition,[60] memory,[61] intention,[62] resolve, and determination.[63] The character *zhi* has two components. The upper component (士) pictures a plant growing, giving the idea of development, progress, and continuity. The lower component indicates the heart *(xin)*. Wieger translates *zhi* as "the will; a purpose that is fixed, that develops itself" and notes that the heart is "the seat of the intellect and will."[64]

Acquired Jing

At conception, heaven imparts a complement of inherited influences to each individual that represents our foundation for all growth and possibility in life. Like a trust fund, we must manage our innate store of *jing* wisely, living largely off interest and conserving the principal until old age. For once spent, our innate endowment can never be replenished. Surely herbal *jing* tonics, which emulate the qualities of *jing*, may be taken supplementally. But these tonics cannot impart *jing* of the unique quality received at conception.

Heaven, in its unceasing attempt to nourish the seed it has planted within, radiates sunlight toward humankind. This nourishing *yang* is contained in air, food, and water and represents the highest good that comes to support us throughout life. The function of respiration and digestion is to abstract this acquired *yang* from all that we receive, in order to supplement the body's store of *jing*. It is this acquired *jing* that we must draw on until old age when our reserves of inherited *jing* may be tapped.

Just as we must contact the highest in all physical sources of nourishment in life, so too must we find heaven's intention in each life experience. Every situation holds some kernel of potential to help us nourish the manifestation of destiny received at conception. Therefore I list positive interpretation of our life experiences as another source of postnatal *jing*.

Summary

"[T]he sage concentrates his jingshen, *swallows the heavenly* qi, *and is in touch with the brilliant radiance of* shen."
– NEI JING SU WEN[65]

Jing, qi, and *shen* are the three Daoist treasures, the inborn constitutional influences that make up the internal world of the individual. They are the microcosmic counterparts of the primordial, creative breaths of the universe: heaven, earth, and *qi*.[66] The *dao* divides from the one into the two to give each of us an inborn nature corresponding to heaven (*yang*) and to earth (*yin*). The duality of heaven and earth is simultaneously present in the polarities of *shen* and *jing*, *yuanyin* and *yuanyang*, and early and later heaven.

The heavenly aspect of inborn nature is *shen*; the earthly aspect is *jing*.

Humans must establish their *zhi* (human will) as a conduit for *shen* (heaven) to interact with *jing* (earth). If destiny is to be fulfilled, this interaction must occur in a way that illuminates *(ming:*明*)* the commands *(ming:*命*)* that heaven has stored in the depths of self *(jing)* at conception. Hence the sage focuses and concentrates *shen* on *jing* in the spontaneously creative act of discovering self anew in each moment.

All that comes to us in life holds a kernel of truth sent by heaven to nourish that seed placed within at conception. It is up to each of us to contact, and make use of, the highest that life has to offer. For it is in joining heaven within and heaven without that health is promoted, virtue is cultivated, and destiny is fulfilled.

We next turn our attention to the importance of human will in the inner tradition.

Questions

1. How does the language defined in this chapter correspond to the meaning attributed to such terms in your own tradition of practice?

2. How may terms unique to your own tradition of practice be expanded to encompass the values inherent in the discussion of language in this chapter?

NOTES

1. Watson, 1964a, p. 140.
2. Porkert, 1982, p. 23.
3. Ibid.
4. The works that serve as the basis for this discussion are Liu's commentary on a Sung dynasty alchemical text, *Jin Dan Si Bai Zi Jie* (Four Hundred Characters Explaining the Golden Elixir) by Zhang Boduan, and Liu's text, *Symbolic Language: Breaking Open Doubt*. The latter text comprises the translated work in this book. In these texts Liu explains the hidden symbolism of Chinese alchemical writing. He enumerates seven stages each of losing original nature, returning to it, and becoming a sage. Written in the early 1800s, Liu's work is of deep significance in understanding the spiritual and psychological aspects of Chinese physiology and the inner tradition of healing in Chinese medicine. These two works have been translated into English (see Cleary, 1986a).
5. As Liu Yiming refers to *mingmen*. Cleary, 1986b, p. 260.
6. Watson, 1964a, p. 56. Watson translates *xin* as "mind" and *ming* as "fate." I have translated them as "heart" and "destiny," respectively.
7. Weiger, 1965, pp. 36–37.

8. Ibid.

9. Chapter 63; in Chen, 1989, p. 184.

10. Chapter 63; in Chen, 1989, p. 201.

11. Chapter 55; in Chen, 1989, p. 185.

12. Chen, 1989, p. 187.

13. Chapter 55; in Chen, 1989, p. 187.

14. Chapter 51; in Chen, 1989, p. 175.

15. Anderson, 1989, pp. 57–61.

16. Chapter 21; in Chen, 1989, pp. 106–107. Chen translates *xin* as "growth power." *Xin,* the virtue associated with the earth element, is more frequently translated as "faith" or "trust." But Chen tells us that trust is based on heaven's eternal promise of a new beginning, such as occurs with new growth each spring.

17. Watson, 1964a, p. 32.

18. Chapter 55; in Chen, 1989, p. 185.

19. Anderson, 1989, p. 57.

20. Lagerwey, 1987, p. 8.

21. See Lagerwey, 1987, p. 8.

22. Porkert, 1982, p. 177.

23. Ibid., p. 173.

24. Larre and Rochat de la Vallee, 1985, p. 63.

25. Porkert, 1982, p. 181.

26. Wieger, 1965, p. 138.

27. Anderson, 1989, p. 25.

28. Ibid., p. 61.

29. Ho Peng Yoke, cited in ibid.

30. Wieger, 1965, p. 29.

31. Ibid., p. 137.

32. Ibid., p. 138.

33. Larre et al., 1986, p. 115.

34. Porkert, 1982, p. 181.

35. Larre et al., 1986, p. 169, n. 1.

36. One paradigm of Chinese physiology divides the torso into three regions of associated physiological function, known as the upper, middle, and lower "burners," or *jiao*. The upper *jiao* extends from the base of the sternum to the collarbone. It contains the heart and lungs and is responsible for receptivity. The middle *jiao* extends from the umbilicus to the base of the sternum and contains the organs of the digestive system: the liver, gallbladder, stomach, and spleen. It is responsible for assimilation. The lower *jiao* extends from the pelvic bone to the umbilicus and contains the bladder, kidneys, and large intestine. It is responsible for elimination.

37. Personal discussion with Ted Kaptchuk, 1990.

38. Lagerwey, 1987, p. 8.

39. Porkert, 1982, p. 177.

40. The character *wu* [巫] refers to female shamans; male shamans were referred to as *xi* [覡]. Fung, 1983, p. 23.

41. Wieger, 1965, p. 182.

42. Mathews, 1931, p. 586.

43. Dore, 1987, p. 160.

44. Eno, 1990, p. 202

45. Porkert, 1982, p. 181.

46. In Ki and Yunkyo, 1985, and Wu, 1993. The *Lingshu* (Spiritual Axis or Spiritual Pivot) is the second half of the *Nei Jing Su Wen* written in the "Warring States" period (480–222 B.C.E.).

47. Chamberlain, 1980, p. 16.
48. Porkert, 1982, p. 193.
49. Watson, 1968, pp. 73–74. I have paraphrased Watson here and changed the word "fate" to "destiny."
50. In the *Bai Wen Bian* (Homann, pp. 10, 77), the term *lingfu* is used in reference to containing the "penetrating fire" that fuels alchemical transformation. In this usage, it would appear related to the functioning of *mingmen*. Note that in the upper *jiao, shen* and *ling* are consumed. In the lower *jiao, shen* interacts with *jing.*
51. Watson, 1968, p. 255.
52. Mencius; in Eno, 1990, p. 455.
53. Wieger, 1965, p. 101.
54. See Larre et al., 1986, p. 114; and Larre, 1985, pp. 61–63.
55. Porkert, 1982, p. 171.
56. Cleary, 1986a, p. 19.
57. Porkert, 1982, p. 128.
58. Unschuld, 1986, p. 367.
59. Wieger, 1965, p. 203.
60. Worsley, 1979.
61. Fung, 1983, p. 291.
62. Kuang-ming, 1989, p. 241.
63. Bloom, 1985, p. 312.
64. Wieger, 1965, p. 203.
65. My translation of *Nei Jing Su Wen* from the Chinese text in Lu (1978, p. 15). Porkert (1982, p. 194) translates the term *jingshen* in this section as "configurative forces capable of manifestation." The term *shenming* here suggests the sage is in touch with the radiance of personal heart spirit and the radiance of the macrocosmic *shen.*
66. Anderson, 1989, p. 22. The *hun* spirit is comprised of the *shen, jing,* and *qi* (see Williams, 1974, p. 462).

4

ZHI:
HUMAN WILL

⸻

EAVEN MANIFESTS TO US BOTH AS INBORN NATURE
(de) and as the events and conditions we contend with every
day. Although heaven may plant the seed of original nature in each person, it cannot ensure that each individual will be true to this nature and
thus fulfill destiny. Fulfilling our destiny is ultimately our personal
choice. Each of us, using our will *(zhi)*, must choose to be aligned both
inwardly, in terms of awareness, and outwardly, in terms of action,
with the will of heaven. By accepting the circumstances sent by heaven
as those we would choose for ourselves, inborn nature is preserved as
well as cultivated, and destiny is fulfilled. This chapter examines the
role played by human will in the cultivation of virtue and the fulfillment of destiny.

I define the highest aspect of *zhi*, human will, as "our purpose growing into the world directed by the heart's focused intention." Wieger
notes that the heart is "the seat of the intellect and will."[1] The close
relationship between the will and heart is indicated by the presence of
the heart radical (心) in the character *zhi* (志). But where is the *zhi* of

the heart to be found? It is found in the kidneys stored with the essence. The *Nanjing* tells us that the kidneys store the *jing* and the will and that the will is the spirit *(shen)* of the kidneys.[2] Each of the *yin* officials contains one of the five *shen (shen, yi, po, zhi,* and *hun),* which comes to the official through the heart as the emperor is present in his ministers.[3] Therefore, *zhi* may be thought of as an emanation of the heart spirit present in the kidney official.

According to Confucian philosopher Zhuxi (1130–1200 C.E.), "the will lies in the deepest recesses of the [heart] mind and, therefore, the doctors say the will belongs to the kidneys."[4] The heart's function is to guide the development of insight and intuition. It accomplishes this by facilitating knowledge of our destiny as stored in our "heart of hearts," which I consider to be synonymous with *jing,* the kidney essence. Hence the function of *zhi* is to facilitate the interaction of *shen* with *jing* in a way that illuminates destiny as stored in our depths.

The character *zhi* appears in the name of acupuncture point Bladder-52 (47),[5] *zhishi* (志室), which translates as "ambition room"[6] or "room of will."[7] Bladder-52 also has another name: *jinggong* (精宮), or "palace of essence."[8] The traditional practice of using the same acupuncture point to treat the *jing* and the *zhi* confirms the intimate relationship between these dynamic aspects of being.

Of Heart, Mind, and Will

The character *xin* denoting the heart is often translated into English as "mind." Many authors also translate the character *zhi* as meaning "mind." I define the heart as that official which empowers us to know spontaneously the nature of reality as it occurs in each moment. Reality is defined as that interpretation of events, and response to them, that empowers the fulfillment of individual destiny. I define the mind to be our capacity to interpret data flowing both from the world inward to the heart and from the heart outward to the world. The will is the heart's capacity to focus our mind either internally or externally and to initiate action by commanding the *qi* to move the body.

In health, these three—the heart, mind, and will—are one. The functions of the mind and will are transparent in communicating the nature of the world to the heart and the nature of the heart to the world. In illness, however, these three functions can be seen to act independently as the will initiates action, ignoring the heart in a vain attempt to satisfy the mind's desires.

Throughout this text I translate the character zhi as meaning "will." I translate the character *xin* as heart when it denotes the balanced functioning of that official. I translate *xin* as mind when it denotes separation of our capacity to know (heart) and to think (mind). The concept of unity and separation between heart and mind is discussed in Chapter 10.

Internal and External Will

As with many concepts in Chinese medicine, *zhi* has both an internal and an external aspect. When the will is turned inward, the mind is channeled into an act of introspection to know and then to manifest through the governing of *qi* (which leads to actions) heaven's will as stored in the *jing*. With the manifestation of heaven's will, the individual establishes *ming* (命) in the world and emanates the light of inner illumination *(ming:* 明*)*. This light can be seen in the brilliance of the heart spirit sparkling in the eyes. When the will is turned outward, the *jing* is consumed as the individual expends *qi,* striving to satisfy the mind's worldly desires. Actions performed solely in the service of ambition undermine the integrity of the individual, ultimately leading to ruin and never to the fulfillment of destiny.

Human Will and Self-Discovery

The fate of all humans is to be separated from our original nature as we move away from infancy and gain self-consciousness. The path back to original nature and the subsequent fulfillment of destiny requires focusing the will inward in an act of self-discovery. The firm will of the sage leads to choosing the path of self-discovery from among the other "thousand forks and ten thousand roads" in the world.[9]

Confucian scholar Mencius emphasizes the establishment of will in "making a total commitment to self-realization" and purifying the will so that it can be focused exclusively on personal cultivation. For Mencius, the purpose of the will is to search for the lost heart.[10] He tells us,

> How lamentable is it to neglect the path and not pursue it, to lose this heart and not know to seek it again! . . . The great end of learning is nothing else but to seek for the lost heart.[11]

For Confucius, the will meant directedness of mind. He believed that focusing the will on learning was the first step in cultivating *ming* and following the heart.[12] Zhuxi echoes these sentiments. He believes the heart is composed of only the most refined and spirited *qi*,[13] and the will must be directed toward manifesting by learning "the good nature with which one is born."[14]

> ### CONFUCIUS AND HIS STAGES OF SPIRITUAL DEVELOPMENT
>
> *At fifteen I had my will* [zhi] *bent on learning.*
> *At thirty I stood firm.*
> *At forty I had no doubts.*
> *At fifty I knew the decrees of heaven* [ming].
> *At sixty my ear was an obedient organ*
> *for the reception of truth.*
> *At seventy I could follow what my heart desired,*
> *without transgressing what was right.*[15]
>
> Confucius's first step in spiritual development was to fix his will upon self-discovery. By fifty, he understood his destiny as appointed by heaven; and by sixty, he was able to listen to his heart and the hearts of others.[16] By seventy, he felt no more conflict because he had resolved that what heaven had willed for him and what he willed for himself were the same. Confucius's *de* was reestablished by his seventieth year, a year with numerical significance because seven is the number denoting the loss of, or return to, original nature.

Once the true self has been rediscovered, then taking actions consistent with one's intention (with the heart's purpose, or the will) is necessary if the goodness within is to manifest. All actions are predicated on the movement of *qi*, and it is through an individual's actions, guided by the will, that the quality of our heart and mind are revealed.

When Mencius was queried by his student Gong Sun Zhua about how he maintained an unperturbed mind, he responded,

> The will *(zhi)* is the leader of the *qi*. The *qi* pervades and animates the body. The will is first and chief, and the *qi* is subordinate to it. Therefore, I say, maintain firm the will, and do no violence to the *qi*.[17]

For Mencius, the will is the mechanism that helps the mind to manifest its direction and intentionality through appropriate action. The *qi* must be guided gently by the will, so that it does not become overly constrained or damaged, both conditions that would unsettle the heart and mind. Hence "the conscious mind must lead and direct [the *qi*, by means of the will] without forcing or distorting the normal and natural development of the complete individual."[18] By warning that "what produces dissatisfaction in the mind is not to be helped by *qi*,"[19] Mencius asserts that our resources should not be spent in actions that strive to satisfy the mind's desires. With actions properly directed, the will may be turned inwardly for self-discovery and recovery of our lost heart. Our will may also be directed outwardly as we strive to establish our name *(ming)* in the world. When the will is turned inward, then *ming* (命:destiny) is established; when will is turned outward, then *ming* (名:personal name) is established. Zhuangzi warns against constraining the will by striving for fame.[20] The Chinese characters that translate as fame *(youming:*有名*)* mean, literally, "to have name."

The External Will

To go forward with strength is to have ambition (zhi).
– DAO DE JING [21]

If directed toward external concerns, the will may be used to accomplish things on the worldly level. Ultimately, however, there may be negative consequences if the will becomes too strong and depletes the vital resources of *jing* and *qi*. Mencius admonishes, "Let not the mind *(xin)* forget its work, but let there be no assisting the growth of that nature (the *qi*)."[22] Mencius compares the habits of people who deplete their *qi* by overexercising their will to the farmer who killed his entire corn crop by pulling on the stalks in order to help them grow.[23] When his son heard his father complain that he was tired from having worked the entire day helping the corn to grow, he ran to the fields to find the entire crop withered and dying. Mencius tells us that there are few in the world who do not deal with their *qi* as if they were helping the corn to grow.[24]

In this spirit, both the *Dao De Jing* and the *Zhuangzi* give firm warnings to seekers of longevity that vigorous breathing exercises may overly constrain the will and the *qi*, leading to an early death. The *Dao De Jing* warns, "for the mind to control the breath *(qi)*, that's . . . forcing things."[25] This idea is also supported by Daoist scholar Liu Yiming and spiritual alchemist Li Daoqun, who warned adepts of spiritual alchemy not to be led astray by these techniques, which are false teachings that may shorten life.[26] In my clinical experience, psychotherapeutic exercises that utilize forced and rapid breathing, such as "rebirthing" and "primal scream" therapy, are overly draining and, if practiced regularly, contribute to serious functional imbalances, such as "*qi*-wild" conditions which denote separation of the *yuanqi*.[27] Zhuangzi reminds us that the true sage is able "to attain loftiness without constraining the will" through such practices.[28]

Negative consequences can also occur if the will is weakened. The *Nei Jing Su Wen* attributes the shortened life span of humans to a will weakened by overworking: "[Human's] passions exhaust their vital force *(jing)*; they do not know how to find contentment within themselves; they are not skilled in the control of their spirits *(shen)*. They devote all their attention to the amusement of their minds *(xin)*."[29]

Hence a weakened will may allow the *jing* to be depleted by the mind's ever expansive "passions" and "desires." Contrast this to the sage's will, as described in the *Nei Jing Su Wen*:

> They were tranquilly content in nothingness and the true vital force *(zhenqi)* accompanied them always; their vital original spirit *(jingshen)* was preserved within; thus, how could illness come to them? They exercised restraint of their wills and reduced their desires; their hearts were at peace and without any fear; their bodies toiled and yet did not become weary.[30]

The sage lives long by preserving and nourishing the authentic self *(zhenqi)* and focusing *shen* on *jing* in a way that enhances endowment rather than depletes it. If the sage represents the heart—the emperor charged with control of one's entire being[31]—the following passage may be interpreted as describing the functional relationship between the heart, mind, will (ambition), and kidneys (bones):

> *Therefore, when the sage rules*
> *He empties the minds of his people,*
> *Fills their bellies,*
> *Weakens their ambitions* (zhi) *and strengthens*
> *their bones."*
>
> – DAO DE JING [32]

As advice to the heart as emperor, the verse just cited could be interpreted as saying, when the heart rules well, the mind is empty of the desires that tend to lead us away from our original nature. When we are content nurturing the self, our willpower (ambition) will not be overly strong and deplete the *jing*. If willpower is under control, then our bones will be strong, evidence of our fullness of *jing* and the strength of our kidneys.

Strong bones result from well-functioning kidneys whose essence is intact. An overly active will and overriding ambition may deplete this essence as we work beyond the body's natural capacity. Wilhelm warns, in his discussion of The Creative, the first hexagram of the *Yijing,* that "many a great man has been ruined . . . ambition *(zhi)* has destroyed his integrity."[33]

The *Nanjing* also discusses the relationship between physical and emotional health as governed by will: "When the *yin* and *yang* (tie vessels) cannot maintain their respective ties, one feels uncomfortable and loses one's mind [*zhi:* will]. One is weak and cannot support one's stature."[34] Lu Guang explains, in his commentary on the *Nanjing,* that "[uncomfortable] means that a person is afraid. When one is afraid, the tie vessels relax. Hence, a person will no longer be able to support his bodily [stature]. When one is afraid, one loses one's mind (will: *zhi*); one has a tendency to forget, and one will be confused."[35] Thus fear (the emotion associated with the kidneys) weakens the will with a corresponding loss in bodily stature. This weakening of the body corresponds to a weakening of the kidney and heart spirits *(zhi* and *shen),* which can leave us forgetful and confused. With a weakened will, it is easy to forget our way "home" to original nature.[36] A compromised will cannot channel the confused *shen* into the depleted *jing*. The result is "aimlessness" and "recklessness," words Zhuxi used to describe the behavioral consequences of a weakened will.[37]

Xunzi tells us, "Man from birth has the capacity to know things; this capacity has its memory *(zhi)*. This memory is what is meant by stored away impressions."[38] Xunzi's use of the character *zhi* to denote memory suggests the following physiological relationships. The *zhi* serves as a conduit for the *shen* to extend into the *jing,* our stored potential. When the *jing* of early heaven is accessed, we may find therein a memory of original nature and our "commands" from heaven. When the *jing* of later heaven (acquired potential) is accessed, then we may remember our life's experience. If the functional relationship between *shen* and *jing* as mediated by will is compromised, loss of memory is the predictable result.

The Balance Between Will and Potential

Short well ropes won't dip up deep water. In the
same way I believe that destiny has certain forms
and the body has certain appropriate uses.
You can't add to or take away from these.
– ZHUANGZI [39]

Each human is endowed with innate capacities that cannot be added to or subtracted from. Our deepest potential is manifested by extending, by means of the *shen,* a "rope" of appropriate length to draw from our inner well, or *jing.* Sometimes the rope is too long or too short, drawing more or less *jing* than is appropriate or needed. Zhuxi recognized this. Ailing and close to the end of his life, he nevertheless found that his mind and will were in full command and unable to relax. His will continued to deplete his *jing* without regard for his weakened physical state:

> Although there are certainly times when people's physical powers (*xueqi:*血氣, "blood and qi") are strong or weak, the willpower (*zhiqi:*志氣) never fails. If one constantly maintains this will, then even if one's physical powers fail utterly, the will is not implicated.[40]

Even in his weakened state, and with the knowledge that he ought to rest, Zhuxi observed that his mind "is that of a person who has already gotten up and is unwilling to remain in bed." Although death was near, he was well aware that his mind and will continued to drain his body's resources. Even Zhuxi was unable to rein in his will in service of his overall good. As with any function, the will may be severely hypo- or hyperfunctional in circumstances of extreme imbalance. Thus, when the life force has been spent, the will may either crumble or continue to function like a runaway train. I have seen this frequently in my clinical practice: Rather than learn from their illness and change their ways, patients with serious imbalances display, in force, the very behaviors of excess that contributed to their illness.

The concept of recognizing personal limits and staying within our capabilities has profound implications for both patient and practitioner in the inner tradition of Chinese medicine. The pattern of working beyond our capacity is seen in many people with chronic fatigue syndrome and similar imbalances. Treating strong-willed people symptomatically using acupuncture and herbs for purposes of tonification can be dangerous. Like a compulsive gambler, these individuals spend any resource given them, and treatment may only result in helping them expend their last reserves of *qi* and *jing*. The practitioner must educate patients to redirect their will internally toward self-development and conservation, investing their newfound strength in internal healing rather than accomplishments in the external world.

This pattern of expending stores of inherited *jing* may be seen at its extreme in people who overexercise. Addicted to the heady feeling of challenging the will to achieve increasingly greater physical feats, they push themselves to deeper and deeper levels of deficiency. As their "endurance" increases, *qi* becomes depleted and their heart rate may dip to dangerously low levels. The result may be damage to the heart and circulatory system as well as the kidneys, with symptoms such as cardiac conditions and low back pain (weakened stature) with its corresponding kidney pathology. Mencius describes an exercise such as running as an example of the *qi* moving the mind (*xin*), rather than the desired state of the heart, using the will, gently moving the *qi*.[41] Zhuxi echoes Mencius's concern, adding, "those who are moved by their physical powers (blood and *qi*) . . . 'do violence to themselves' and 'throw themselves away.'"[42]

The phenomenon of expending blood and *qi* in heavy exercise, known popularly as "runner's high," corresponds to increased production of endorphins, endogenous opiates that dull our ability to feel pain. Their secretion may allow people to ignore the pain that signals the body it is working beyond capacity. I have found that convincing people to exercise less is one of my most difficult tasks in clinical practice. Habits in life tend to arise from attempts to escape an emotion or feeling that we are unable to confront directly. People engaged in a path of healing often transfer their negative habits, such as drinking or smoking, into more socially acceptable habits, such as heavy exercising. Most often, they have merely transformed a "bad" into a "good" habit, and the habitual behavior remains. Any behavior done to extremes is unhealthy, and heavy exercising especially will pay poor long-term dividends as an investment in health.

Comparing External and Internal Forms of Exercise

External exercises are those that require the use of will to override our inner sense of knowing when enough work has been done. These generally involve any regimen that involves a sustained cardiovascular workout and high pulse. The net effect of this type of exercise is always to deplete the body of one or more vital substances such as *qi*, blood, *yin, yang,* and ultimately *jing*. In time the *qi* supporting the function of the heart is drained as the heart rate diminishes and the circulatory system goes into a state of shock.

The hallmark of internal exercises is that vital substances are not consumed but are transformed so a person has more, not less, reserves when they are done exercising. Hence, when practiced appropriately, exercises such as yoga, meditation, *taiji,* and *qigong* all cultivate reserves so that our internal capacity is strengthened for having performed them.

These same principles apply to the physiological function of the organ systems in Chinese medicine. In illness, an organ merely consumes our sources of vitality as it strives in vain to support its own function. In health, an organ transmutes the *qi,* blood, *yin,* and *yang* it consumes. The net effect of its metabolic function is to enhance the overall qualities of these reserves, which it then contributes to support the function of the organism as a whole.

Summary

By focusing the will internally on the spiritual path of self-inquiry, the sage is led to the fulfillment of destiny. Individuals may choose, like the sage, to concentrate the will within themselves, or they may choose to focus on external goals such as winning fame and fortune. But an overly active will occupied externally constrains the *qi* and diminishes resources until the *jing,* life's reserve of inherited essence, is depleted. Eventually, the will weakens as the *jing* dries up, accompanied by a corresponding loss of presence of mind and bodily stature. The mechanisms underlying the function of human will may be summed up as follows:

1. *Jing* is inherited from early heaven as the internal resource and potential of one's life. An individual's specific endowment of inherited influences, received at conception, is the storehouse of heaven's will and virtue *(de)* and may be either expended or conserved by the choices made throughout life. This inherited constitution is the unique legacy of the *dao.*

2. *Jing* is also acquired from food, air, and the positive interpretation of experience. This accumulated essence, the contribution of later heaven, is the only source to supplement the inherited constitution. Inherited *jing* should be conserved whenever

possible. Any endeavor in life should expend only a small percentage of inherited *jing* relative to acquired *jing*. This means
that people should stop their daily work after accomplishing a
sufficient amount and before depleting their resource of
acquired *qi*.

3. Human will *(zhi)* is most appropriately used to gently channel
the active impulses *(shen)* from the heart *(xin)* into the depths
of self *(jing)* so that original nature *(de)* may be returned and
destiny *(ming)* fulfilled. In any of life's endeavors, the heart's
function is to intuitively acknowledge truth. Truth is defined as
that which empowers the fulfillment of one's own destiny.
Internally, truth is the essential nature imparted to us at conception and externally it is the knowing that every situation, no
matter how painful, offers the opportunity for self-cultivation.
Our will is the bridge between internal and external truth. It is
what allows us to act in a way which allows heaven to cultivate that seed it has planted within. The heart must acknowledge those aspects of every situation that offer us the opportunity to cultivate increased awareness of self. The will must then
be aligned between the reality that heaven sends and our innate
capacity to respond to that situation in a way which cultivates
virtue. It is our will that may guide the *qi* and thus empower us
to act in a way which is in line with the intention held jointly
by heaven and our heart of hearts.

4. People with an overly strong will tend to work past the capacity of their acquired resource and burn a disproportionate
amount of inherited *jing* as they utilize their *qi* trying to satisfy their mind's desires. However, actions that are habitually
driven rarely, if ever, lead to fulfillment. Resources are diminished through both excessive physical work, which depletes *qi*
and *yang*, and overwork of the nervous system, which creates
psychic reactions—the "internal devils" of fear, fright, anger,
joy, worry, sadness, and grief—in turn, depleting the internal
store of *yin*.[43]

5. *Jing* is depleted in direct proportion to individual expenditure
of will utilized to work beyond our capacity. The *zhi* in this
case does not guard the essence but depletes it (see Figure 4.1).

6. Continued overwork or overexercise ultimately leads to failure
as both *jing* and *qi* become depleted, with a corresponding

weakness in the bones and physical stature. The will eventually weakens as it grows unable to focus the confused, forgetful, and fearful mind on the depleted *jing*. This process is circular: The more the will weakens, the more it is unable to focus the already confused mind. The mind, becoming increasingly confused, may then dictate actions that further weaken the will and deplete the *jing*. The will may also hyperfunction and drain resources at an increased pace.

7. According to the Daoist enumeration of being, the seventh stage is a return. For the sage, this means self-realization and a return of the *dao*—the source of the authentic self—to the world as personal destiny becomes manifest. For the individual who has squandered his or her treasure, the seventh stage

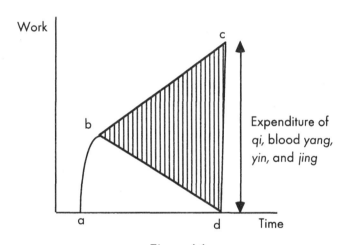

Figure 4.1

RELATIONSHIP OF WORK, WILL, AND *JING*

This figure depicts the relative expenditure of inherited to acquired resources over time. A person working from time a to time b expends qi *acquired from food, air, and other life resources. At time b, acquired resources have been spent, so work from time b to time c is accomplished using willpower to tap inherited reserves as acquired resources decrease over time to point d. The shaded triangle indicates that our life resources of* qi, blood, yin, yang, *and, ultimately,* jing, *are expended in direct proportion to use of the will to work past our natural capacity. Overwork of the physical body leads to* jing *depletion through a path of* qi *and* yang *deficiency. Overwork of the nervous system leads to* jing *depletion through a path of* yin *deficiency.*

It is essential that the practitioner guide each patient to learn when the point is reached of working beyond natural capacity. Learning to expend and conserve our resources wisely is a foundation of all true healing.

means death and the return of the lost self to the mysterious workings of the *dao*.

The authentic heart is lost in the individual's inevitable fall from original nature. The memory of this true nature is stored in *jing* as a mandate from heaven that blows "on the ten thousand things in a different way, so that each can be itself."[44] By fixing the *zhi* and turning inward, directing the mind "down into" the *jing,* the depths of self, the lost individual may rediscover heaven's commands and return his or her heart back into the world, fully expressed. With our destiny thus fulfilled, we may become a channel for the creative flow of the *dao,* the very source of life and vitality.

Next, we turn our attention to the function of *mingmen,* the "gate of destiny" in mediating the physiological relationships on which the fulfillment of destiny is based.

Questions

1. What are the ways you tend to use willpower to push past your limits?

2. What is the motivation that drives you to use your will in this way?

3. What price do you pay for overusing your will?

4. In what situations have you used willpower in a way that empowered you?

5. If you were to turn your will inwardly in an act of introspection, where would you look and what would you look for?

6. What concepts and beliefs do you hold that would obscure the goal of this inquiry?

NOTES

1. Weiger, 1965, p. 203.
2. Chinese text in Unschuld, 1986, p. 367.
3. Larre, Schatz, and Rochat de la Vallee, 1986, pp. 115, 169.
4. Bloom, 1985, p. 312.
5. Several systems are used in Chinese medicine for numbering the order of points on the meridians. On the bladder meridian, for example, some traditions notate Bladder-52 as Bladder-47. I follow the more common numbering system found

in modern Chinese texts. For the sake of clarity, the alternate number appears in parentheses after the point's first mention in the text.

6. Worsley, 1982, p. 79.
7. Ou-Ming, 1982, p. 295.
8. Porkert, 1982, p. 249.
9. Zhuxi; in Bloom, 1985, p. 312.
10. Tu, 1985, p. 223.
11. Legge, 1970, p. 414. Note: I have substituted the word "heart," rather than use Legge's translation of mind, for the character *xin*.
12. *Analects* 2:4; in Legge, 1971, p. 146.
13. Gardner, 1990, p. 51.
14. Ibid., p. 166.
15. Legge, 1971, p. 146.
16. For a discussion of the relationship of listening, the fulfillment of destiny, and the function of Small Intestine-19, see Chapter 13.
17. Gardner, 1990, p. 166. In my translation, I have paraphrased and not quoted. I kept the pinyin for *qi* and deleted the term "passion-nature" that Gardner had used to translate the character *qi*.
18. Bloom, 1985, p. 303.
19. Legge, 1970, p. 188.
20. Watson, 1968, p. 168.
21. Chapter 33; in Henricks, 1989, p. 252. I am following the interpretation of Chen (1989, pp. 136–137) that to act with "strength" and "ambition" goes against the Daoist ideal of inaction *(wuwei)*. Compare with Henricks, 1989, p. 252.
22. Legge, 1970, p. 190.
23. Ibid., 1970, pp. 190–191.
24. Ibid., p. 191.
25. Chapter 55, *Dao De Jing;* in Henricks, 1989.
26. Cleary, 1986, p. 55; 1989, pp. 33–36.
27. Jarrett, 1995a, 1995b, 1995c.
28. Watson, 1968, pp. 167–168.
29. Veith, 1949, p. 98; Chinese text from Lu, 1978, p. 2. The character *yu,* translated as "passions," also means "desires." Here the character *xin* is translated as "mind" and not "heart." As discussed later, all habitual behavior is predicated on the separation of the heart from the mind.
30. Veith, 1949, p. 98.
31. The *Ling Shu* states, "That which controls all things is called the heart" (see Unschuld, 1986, p. 372).
32. Chapter 3; in Henricks, 1989, p. 192.
33. Wilhelm, 1968, p. 8.
34. Unschuld, 1986, p. 333. Unschuld translates *zhi* as "mind." I have translated it as "will."
35. Ibid. Although the characters are not provided in his commentary, my assumption that Unschuld used the word "mind" as a translation of *zhi* is well founded on its frequency of occurrence throughout his work. I have changed this to "will" and inserted it in parentheses.
36. Poor memory is traditionally associated with deficient *jing* or scattered *shen*. The *zhi* helps focus the *shen* and protect the *jing*.
37. Gardner, 1990, p. 105.
38. Quoted in Fung, 1983, p. 183.
39. Watson, 1964, p. 115. I have changed Watson's translation of *ming* from "fate" to "destiny."

40. Bloom, 1985, p. 313.
41. Legge, 1970, p. 18.
42. Bloom, 1985, p. 313.
43. The term "internal devils" suggests that the presence of a given emotion has become so deeply habituated, no room is left for any other form of personal expression.
44. Watson, 1964, p. 32.

5

THE
SPIRITUAL ALCHEMY
OF *MINGMEN*

If one does not depart from everlasting virtue,
One again returns to the state of the infant.
– DAO DE JING[1]

The Sage and the Return

Early Daoist texts hold the sage and the infant as examples of individuals who preserve their unity with *dao*. The infant is living in harmony with *dao* at the moment of first breath, but moves increasingly away from it as self-consciousness develops. The sage cultivates virtue in order to reestablish as a guiding force in life the original nature that was experienced as an infant. This involves a process of reestablishing connection to the true self empowered by the *jing, yuanqi,* and *shen* and sweeping away acquired influences that suppress the expression of the primordial endowment. In this way the sage reclaims the very source of health and vitality.

The physiological processes that support the health of the infant and the sage occur within *mingmen,* or the gate of destiny. Here I discuss these processes and their relationship to the function of *mingmen* in mediating the fulfillment of individual destiny.

The Physiology of Mingmen

> When superior people who practice the *dao* refine themselves and
> master their minds, illumination arises in inner openness, and the liv-
> ing potential is activated. They should quickly gather it into the fur-
> nace of evolution, conscientiously forestall danger, carefully seal it
> and store it securely, fostering its growth from vagueness to clarity,
> until there is eventually a return of the celestial energy to pure com-
> pleteness. This is the same idea as the ancient kings shutting the gates
> on the winter solstice.[2]

In Chinese myth, Kunlun Mountain is conceived as the root of heav-
en and earth and the interface between the primordial *yin* and *yang*. A
strong similarity exists between this function of Kunlun Mountain, the
mysterious pass, as it is conceived cosmologically in the *Dao De Jing*,
and *mingmen* as it is conceived in Chinese physiology.

The mysterious pass is strictly a functional concept, and Liu Yiming
emphasizes that it has no fixed position in the body.[3] Liu's intent is to
admonish adepts of "false teachings" for fixing their attention during
meditation on certain parts of the body where they consider the pass
to be located. But the mysterious pass is not material; it has no location; rather, it is a functional process that permeates every aspect of
being internally and in the cosmos. As we see later, the functional location of the mysterious pass is found in the transition from the metal to
the water element along the *sheng* cycle.

The description of the mysterious pass as an immaterial function is
remarkably similar to descriptions of *mingmen* in Chinese medical literature. The light of *ming* given off in the operation of the pass may be
likened physiologically to the fires of *mingmen*. Situated between the
kidneys, *mingmen* provides the mechanism for the infusion of all physiological dualities in a way that creates life and fuels evolution. All
such dualities including water and fire, *jing* and *shen,* heaven and
earth, *yin* and *yang,* and early and later heaven reflect the loss of the
dao's original nature as unity. Within the context of the human being
these dualities may be reunited into one in the fires of *mingmen*.

Humans, as the vessel for the interacting influences of heaven and
earth, play a crucial role in maintaining the integrity and unity of the
primordial *qi*. The foundation of human life has its source in the interpenetration of heaven and earth, and water and fire. For only in organic
life can water and fire mingle without extinguishing one another. This
is the inner alchemy that fuels the "furnace of evolution" and, ultimately, the ascension of the human spirit to heaven and immortality.

Zhi, *Destiny, and the Alchemy of* Mingmen

> The three energies together are unified in the One. There is essence [*jing*], there is spirit [*shen*], and there is energy [*yuanqi*]. These three are originally one. They are founded in heaven and earth and form the root of all human energy. Human beings receive spirit from heaven, essence from earth, and energy from the middle harmony of heaven and earth. Joined together they are the one. . . . The three support each other and form an integrated whole. –*Taiping Jing Shengjun Bizhi* [4]

Physiologically, the unfolding of human destiny depends on several processes that involve the interpenetration of *yin* and *yang*, early and later heaven, and *jing* and *shen* (see Figure 5.1). The name of acupuncture point Governor Vessel-4, known as *mingmen* (命門), or the "gate of destiny," refers to the alchemical melting pot of these processes located between the kidneys. *Mingmen* contains and focuses the infusion of our inheritance of primordial *yin* and *yang* (the *yuanqi*), which, at our core, joins each of us to the primordial *dao*.[5] The interaction of this authentic water and fire conforms to the deep, inner nature of each individual—the "authentic self."[6] Concurrently, the inherited constitution is intermingling with the acquired constitution, and the *shen* is interacting with the *jing*. These three processes occur simultaneously and are functionally related.

It is important to note that acupuncture points Governor Vessel-4 (*mingmen*, "gate of destiny"), Bladder-23 (the kidney *shu* point), and Bladder-52 (*zhishi*, "room of will") are all at the same anatomical level in a straight line at the space between the second and third lumbar vertebrae.[7] This supports the idea of the functional relationship between the *jing*, will, kidney, and the function of *mingmen*.

The Interpenetration of Yin and Yang

The *yuanqi* is our endowment of primordial *yin* and *yang* located in the left and right kidney, respectively. Having risen out of the *jing*, it represents the primordial *dao* differentiated into the dual poles of *yin* and *yang*. The function of the *yuanyang* is similar to the *shen* inasmuch as they both activate potential. The function of the *yuanyin* is similar to the *jing* inasmuch as they both represent pure potentiality.

Humans are endowed with potential to manifest as well as the capacity to will that to happen. However, the fetus does not will its evolution; that is governed and presided over by early heaven. While

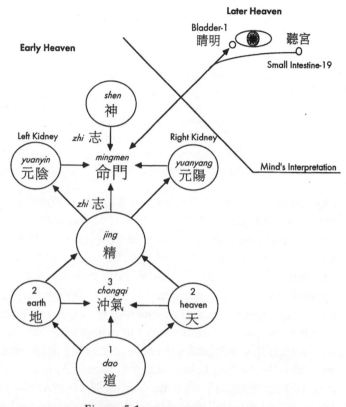

Figure 5.1

PHYSIOLOGICAL RELATIONSHIPS AND CORRESPONDENCES
BETWEEN THE MACROCOSM AND MICROCOSM

*Whatever exists in the macrocosm has corresponding manifestations in the
microcosm. The figure depicts the basic correspondences between cosmological (macrocosmic) and physiological (microcosmic) processes. The lower half
illustrates the primal unity of heaven, earth, and qi in the macrocosm. The
upper half shows the unity characterizing the relationship between the* jing
and the yuanqi *(differentiated into* yuanyin *and* yuanyang).

In the macrocosm the *dao is one, its separation into dual poles of heaven
and earth are two, and heaven, earth, and* chongqi *are three. In the microcosm* jing *is one, its separation into dual poles of* yuanyin *and* yuanyang *are
two, and yin, yang, and* mingmen *are three.*

Just as the chongqi *blends heaven and earth, so too does* mingmen *blend
together our complement of* jing *and* shen, yuanyin *and* yuanyang, *and early
and later heaven. The contribution of the sensory orifices (mouth, ears, nose,
and eyes) in transmitting later heaven (acquired* jing) *into our depths is represented by the exit and entry points Small Intestine-19 ("listening palace") and
Bladder-1 ("eyes bright").[8] It is the mind's interpretation of events that sullies
the fires of* mingmen *and compromises the influence of early heaven in our
life. As we see in Chapter 9, it is the notion of constitutional type that allows
us to assess the elemental nature of the "tint" on the window that each of us
sees life through and colors our perception of experience.*

in the womb, the *yuanqi* guides the entire differentiation of the embryo and fetus. During life, the *yuanqi* serves as the inner fire that fuels all developmental processes such as making blood, the growth of bones, emotional and psychic development, and the ascent of the spirit.

If the function of an official is severely compromised for a prolonged period of time, its complement of *qi*, blood, *yin*, and *yang* will be depleted. Eventually, the primordial *yin* and *yang* that supports the function of the official will begin to separate as they are consumed in a desperate attempt to sustain functioning. At this point the severe dysfunction of the official represents a break in functional integrity that depletes the entire organism of its physiological resources.

The single term *yuanqi* denotes a unity that contains implicitly the duality of *yin* and *yang*. The image of the primordial *yin* and *yang* separating is a physiological metaphor for the consequences of having lost touch with our original nature that is synonymous with the unity of primordial *dao*. With the separation of *yin* and *yang*, *jing* is increasingly depleted and the human being becomes highly vulnerable to illness.

Early and Later Heaven

Who an individual is at any moment is the sum total of all inherited and acquired characteristics. These interpenetrate each other in a way that the two influences present as a single entity. Every attribute a human may possess has as its basis a relative degree of genetic potential, yet the degree to which potential manifests is influenced by a multitude of environmental factors. As discussed previously, the Daoists place emphasis on the role of innate human nature in promoting individual health. In contrast, the Confucians emphasize the importance of acquired conditioning and living according to social convention.

Modern analytic science tries in vain to sort out the relative contributions of genetics and environment to specific behaviors and illnesses. For example, it is possible to demonstrate that the severed optic nerve of a goldfish is able to regenerate and connect with the correct cells in its brain so that normal vision is restored. Much research has been performed to determine if the regenerating cell is able to find its way back to the optic tectum because of genetic cues internal to the nerve or external environmental cues such as chemical and electrical gradients. The relative contributions of genetics and environment to illnesses such as schizophrenia are also still topics of considerable research. Despite years of investigation, it is clear that the contributions of genetics and environment to any specific human attribute are inexorably bound to each other in a way that they cannot be quantitatively separated with any degree of precision.

In the beginning verse of the *Nei Jing Su Wen,* the Yellow Emperor addresses Qibo and queries him as to why in ancient times people were vital into their old age yet at the present time people lived to only middle age with failing health. Qibo responds, "There was temperance in eating and drinking. Their hours of rising and retiring were regular and not disorderly and wild. By these means the ancients kept their bodies united with their souls, so as to fulfill their allotted span *(ming)* completely, measuring unto a hundred years before they passed away."[9] This answer demonstrates an awareness that health is a result of both living properly through the appropriate use of one's will, as well as the specific nature of one's innate capacities (destiny).

If one believes in the notion of karma, then every life circumstance that touches an individual must have some basis within the person from the moment of conception. Any functional imbalance or illness has as its foundation a patient's inborn constitutional predisposition. Yet it is the way each of us lives life, as well as the events we are subjected to, that influence the degree to which our potential for manifesting illness or virtue is realized.

The attempts of analytic science to quantify the relative contribution of genetics and environment to any specific human attribute have proven futile. However, the Chinese sciences predicated on the study of function do allow a qualitative assessment of our inborn nature and the degree to which it is manifesting in life. The different systems of Chinese medicine afford us a qualitative appraisal of the relative contributions of early and later heaven to individual health.

Several paradigms of practice focus on the degree to which acquired influences are contributing to illness. These systems include the four divisions of heat-induced illness, the six stages of cold-induced illness, and the six-pathogen model. The eight-principle system allows for the discernment of physiological relationships according to a thermodynamic model. With this model we may assess the relative quantity of physiological resources such as *qi,* blood, *yin,* and *yang.* We may also determine the location of pathology in terms of organ involvement and position in the body from its depth to its surface. In regard to the inherited constitution, the eight principles allow for the determination of the relative quantity of constitutional influences instilled at conception or depleted during life. Hence we may speak in general terms of deficient *yin, yang,* or *jing* either as a result of being born with a poor endowment of these capacities or having expended them through excessive work.

The five-element system is unique in allowing for a qualitative assessment of the elemental nature of constitutional endowment. An individual's five-element constitutional type is commensurate with his or her life lesson and purpose for being on the planet. Knowledge of constitutional type informs us of how individuals are prone, from the moment of conception, to attributing meaning to life and embodying their belief system as pathology. For it is the false interpretation of our life experience that ultimately smothers the expression of our constitutional potential and extinguishes the fires of *mingmen*.

Although it is certainly important to resolve acquired disharmonies, the patient's constitutional endowment is always the foundation of health and well-being. Only through the balanced consideration afforded by all the systems mentioned here may the practitioner arrive at an integrated diagnosis. Such a diagnosis may assess the relative degree to which innate capacities and acquired characteristics are contributing to the momentary picture of a patient's health.

A foundational assumption in the inner tradition is that the quality of our inherited constitution represents the guiding influence that treatment seeks to restore in the patient's life. If we find the highest good in all that life has to offer, then acquired influences may supplement our inherited endowment. However, we may fail to accept life as an opportunity for cultivating virtue and instead attribute disempowering meanings to challenging and painful experiences. In this case, the fires of *mingmen* will be extinguished and life will be governed, not by the reality of heaven's intention, but by self-generated belief systems and coping mechanisms. With the function of *mingmen* smothered under such mundane influences, the *yuanqi*, and *jing* and *shen*, may separate, leading to both illness and the ignorance on which it is predicated.

Shen *and* Jing: *The Heart/Kidney Axis*

Think of the *yuanqi* as the core of fire burning at the center of the earth as opposed to the *shen*, which may be likened in function to the sun. *Yuanqi* guides physiological processes that occur beneath the level of conscious awareness. *Shen* allows us to inquire willfully into our own natures and therefore direct the development of our purpose in life. Initially in life it is the *yuanqi* that guides human development. The fall from original nature happens as this seed is covered by erroneous interpretations of life experience. The *shen* provides us with the capacity to return to original nature by focusing our intention inwardly toward the *jing*.

Inherited *jing* represents an internal standard corresponding to true self against which all that comes to us in life may be judged. Hence the *shen* provides insight into the quality of our innate nature so that we may recognize throughout all of life that which is congruent with our well-being. The *shen* constitutes our capacity for conscious awareness and the *jing* constitutes the depth of our innate endowment. The act of willing the interpenetration of *jing* and *shen* is a physiological metaphor for introspection and self-discovery.

Our *shen* illuminates our depths and thus draws out potential so that it may become manifest in the world. The term *jingshen*, as an adjective, suggests the power evidenced by an individual who is manifesting destiny. Such power is in evidence in the conductor of an orchestra or in leaders such as Mohandas Gandhi and Martin Luther King, Jr. If we fail to make the essential connection between *shen* and *jing*, the result is ignorance of self and failure to contact the potential that life holds for nourishing destiny. As we see later, the integrity of the heart/kidney axis is fundamental to the notion of health and balance in the inner tradition.

The Role of Will in Mediating the Function of Mingmen

The quality of how *mingmen* functions is determined in large part by the human will *(zhi)*. Daoist scholar Liu Yiming believes the very foundation of inner alchemy is the stability of the human will. He affirms that the stability of will sets up the foundation of our ability to seek the authentic self and fulfill destiny.[10] Indeed, the nature of our will may determine whether we fully express the authentic self or whether our habitual behavior extinguishes the flames of *mingmen*.

The relationship between *mingmen* and the *zhi, jing,* and *shen* is addressed in Li Jiong's commentary on the *Nanjing*. He tells us that a spirit resides in the "room of will" (Bladder-52) on either side of *mingmen* which guards the gate of destiny and does not allow any evil to enter.[11] He further emphasizes that "room of will" is where the *shen* and *jing* reside.[12] The *Lingshu* adds that it is the function of the will to guard the essence.[13] Hence the *zhi* is the spirit of the kidneys that manages our reserve of *jing* and, in so doing, protects the integrity of the gate of destiny.

Think of the *zhi* as an active conduit between the heart and the kidneys that directs the interaction of the *shen* and *jing*. The quality of an individual's will defines the directionality of this interaction, that is, whether the *shen* interacts with the *jing* inwardly, in a way that leads to the fulfillment of destiny, or outwardly, in a way that leads to material gain and depletion of inner resources.

The *zhi* may be turned internally, to guard the gate of destiny and essence. For the heart's purpose to become manifest and transform life, it must combine with the potential of heaven's purpose as stored in the *jing*. The spiritual alchemy of the sage is the process of the heart spirit *(shen)* extending into the *jing*, directed there by will *(zhi)*. It allows the heart to know and manifest the true nature, as vested by heaven, in the depths of self *(jing)*. With the manifestation of heaven's will, the individual establishes *ming* (destiny) in the world, which gives off the light of inner illumination *(ming)*. This light is evidenced by the brilliance of one's heart spirit sparkling in the eyes. The quality of *shen* coming through the eyes is addressed by acupuncture point Bladder-1 *(jingming)* named "eyes bright."

When the *zhi* is turned externally, the *jing* is consumed as we expend *qi,* striving to satisfy the mind's worldly desires. Here, the spirit *(zhi)* does not guard our treasure *(jing)*. When we act habitually, the spontaneous function of *mingmen* is compromised and the fabric of our life begins to disintegrate.

Summary

The interactions between our original endowment of *yin* and *yang,* early and later heaven, the *shen* and *jing,* and the intermingling of water and fire combusting within the alchemical furnace of *mingmen* are the physiological foundation of human health and evolution. The continued integrity of these interactions ensure that life unfolds smoothly, health is maintained, and destiny fulfilled. As long as these interactions occur without deviation, our *qi* may be said to be "true" *(zhen),* and it is the *zhenqi* that supports the integrity of the authentic self.[14]

Acquired influences in life that do not conform to true self dampen the fires of *mingmen* and obscure our constitutional endowment as a guiding influence in our lives. Such mundane influences may include poor sources of nourishment, impure air, and disempowering interpretations of our experiences in life. It is of paramount importance for the practitioner of the inner tradition to recognize and educate the patient regarding the nature of these belief systems. For it is our erroneous attribution of meaning in life that smothers the fires of *mingmen* and perpetuates separation of the three primordial treasures. By resolving the functional basis of this separation, the fundamental integrity of the relationships on which health is predicated may be restored.

Next, we review our journey through life as humans inevitably lose, and are afforded the opportunity of returning to, original nature.

Questions

1. In your own tradition of practice, what are the fundamental processes that are thought to maintain the integrity of each individual's health?

2. To what degree do people's belief systems affect these processes, and what is the mechanism for such interaction?

3. What are the ways that your tradition of practice offers you the opportunity to intervene in your patients' health at the level of their belief system?

NOTES

1. Chapter 28; my translation.
2. Cleary, 1986b, p. 260. "Shutting the gates on the winter solstice" is a reference to hexagram 24 (*fu*, "return") in the *Yijing*. For a discussion of this hexagram as it pertains to the loss and return of original nature, see Chapter 7.
3. Cleary, 1986a, p. 81.
4. The Secret Instruction of the Sage on the Scripture of Great Peace, Tang dynasty. In Kohn, 1993, p. 194.
5. Larre, Schatz, and Rochat de la Vallee, 1986, p. 112.
6. Larre and Rochat de la Vallee, 1985, p. 46.
7. A strong reserve of *yuanqi* may be accessed for each of the *yin* and *yang* officials through a corresponding point on the bladder meridian known as that official's *shu* point.
8. In circulating through the meridians, *qi* leaves a meridian at its exit point and enters the subsequent meridian at its entry point. *Qi* leaves the small intestine meridian at Small Intestine-19 and enters the bladder meridian at Bladder-1. The exit/entry points on the head are all located directly next to the sensory orifices. The inner functions of these points may empower the accurate perception of reality. For a discussion of entry and exit points, see Jarrett, 1994b.
9. Veith, 1949, p. 97.
10. Cleary, 1986a, p. 113.
11. Unschuld, 1986, p. 384. In paraphrasing Unschuld I have translated the character *ming* as "destiny" rather than "life" and the character *zhi* as "will" rather than "mind."
12. Ibid.
13. Ting Deyong, quoting the *Lingshu* in his commentary on the *Nan Jing*; in Unschuld, 1986, p. 371.
14. Larre, 1985, p. 63; Jarrett, 1992b, p. 357.

6

THE
ONTOGENY
OF LIFE

Heaven and earth were born at the same time I was,
and the ten thousand things are one with me.
– ZHUANGZI[1]

The Life of Humans

It is the destiny of each named being to recapitulate the ontogeny of
the *dao's* loss of, and return to, original nature. Humans move through
life from conception, to incubation, birth, and each subsequent stage
of development, to finally return to the *dao* upon death of either the
real or created self, just as the *dao*, as one, separates and differentiates
into the two, the three, and then the ten thousand things, only to return
to its original state of unity.

Unnamed infants perfectly manifest the virtue of eternal *dao*. The
very act of naming draws the infant out of the void to begin the journey away from the *dao* and into self-consciousness, returning to the
dao later in life only if the willful choice is made to recapture original
nature. As self-awareness dawns with naming, the senses open, and the
dao as the primordial influence that governs our life begins to fade.
Corresponding to the number of holes (sensory orifices) drilled in the
head of Emperor Huntun, Daoist philosopher Liu Yiming describes a

seven-stage progression through life as humans become distanced from their original nature. This chapter discusses the ontogeny of human life using Liu's model of seven developmental stages.

STAGE I: EARLY HEAVEN: THE EMBRYO AND THE FETUS

> Before one's father and mother give birth to one's body, when the male and female *qi* of *yin* and *yang* interact, a point arises which comes forth from emptiness. This is called the true, unified, ancestral (*zu*) *qi* of early heaven. This *qi* enters the *jing* and the blood (*xue*) and fuses (*daoyong*) them back into a chaotic (*hun*) unity. Having no form (*xing*), yet it gives birth to form. Having no substance (*zhi*), yet it gives birth to substance. Internally, the five *zang*, six *fu*, five palaces (*gong*), and hundred bones change and transform, becoming complete [according to the principle of] natural spontaneity (*ziran*).[2]

In this passage, Liu Yiming describes the process by which the embryo recapitulates the numerical ontogeny of the *dao*. In the ancient Chinese view of conception, the *jing* of the father met and fused with the blood of the mother. This is a functional description of the modern concept of a sperm fertilizing an ovum. The development of the fetus follows perfectly the *dao*'s own spontaneous self-becoming. The characters *daoyong* (匋烙) are used to describe the process whereby *jing* and blood are fused. These characters give a sense of the type of fusing that occurs when molten metals are joined in a kiln. *Dao* indicates a kiln, and *yong* means to smelt or fuse metals. Together they mean to "melt" or "transform." In his works, Liu uses the words "obscure" and "void" to describe the state of the womb, comparing embryogenesis to the incubation of the *dao* itself. Hence he designates this period to be early heaven.

In the womb, there is a point of life that is ancestral *qi*, corresponding to the *dao* in its perfection. In reference to this *qi*, the term *zhen* indicates it is the *qi* of fulfilled destiny that perfectly blends the qualities of heaven and earth. These three, *jing*, blood, and *qi*, are blended back into a chaotic unity that perfectly mirrors the chaotic nature of the *dao*. Liu emphasizes that it is only this *qi* of early heaven which causes the fetus to develop with no contribution from later heaven. Note that the character *zu* (祖), used here for "ancestor," denotes the first ancestor in a lineage, whereas the character *zong*, as in *zongqi*, denotes the subsequent lineage.

In describing the process of embryogenesis, Liu tells us,

Although there is human form, there is no human way. Heaven, earth, the ten thousand things, water, fire, and weapons, all these together cannot harm one here. The seven emotions, six desires, five rebels, and four directions are not able to enter. Ultimately, in reality, there is only the unity of the void. When the ancient immortals taught people how to cultivate their *dao* and return to what they were like before their mother and father gave birth to them, they meant returning to the emptiness of the void, beyond sense. Where there is no sense, there is the ultimate limitlessness of *dao*.

During this time of early heaven the fetus incubates within the womb of *dao*. It is to this state of "emptiness" inherent in the womb that the sage, through spiritual development, strives to return.

Later Heaven: The Journey from Birth to Death

STAGE II: THE INFANT

In having "no sense," the fetus perfectly mimics the primordial chaos of Emperor Huntun. After ten months, the fetus, "like a ripe melon," falls off the stem and is born.[3] Breaking out of the amniotic sac of the primordial *dao*, the newborn emerges through the "gate of the mysterious female." Liu Yiming goes on to describe birth:

> With a cry [the infant] receives the *qi* of later heaven which enters through its mouth and nose and descends into the sea of *qi* [*qihai*] [in the chest], mixing there with the *yuanqi* of early heaven. Early heaven is the body, later heaven is the [basis of] its function. Later heaven depends on early heaven to inhale and exhale, while early heaven depends on later heaven to nourish the vascular system [*xuemai*]. Furthermore, at the moment of this single cry, the conscious spirit (*shen*) transmigrates in through these openings and merges with the *yuanqi* of early heaven to form a chaotic (*hun*) unity.

At the moment of the infant's first breath, the primordial influence of early heaven begins to mix with the acquired influence of later heaven. The nourishing essence from food and respiration meets in the chest to form the *zongqi*, which then activates and begins to actualize the "genetic" potential stored within the *yuanqi*. In this balanced condition, as the primal *yinqi, yangqi,* and *zongqi* fuse, the two (early and later heaven) "merge into non-differentiation"—and then there exists "one reality alone."[4] As with the *dao* and the fetus, the three merge and return together to the one. This explains why the *Dao De Jing* tells us, "one who contains *de* in fullness is to be compared to an infant,"[5] for *de* is original nature as seen in the infant, unsullied by life's experience and the accretions of mundane consciousness. In Liu's view, all influences in life gained prior to the first breath correspond to early heaven and all influences gained after the first breath correspond to later heaven. In his discussion of spontaneous versus conditioned awareness, *yang* is positive and corresponds to the influence of early heaven; *yin* is undesirable and corresponds to the habituating influence of earthly experience.

It is interesting to consider why early heaven is not thought of as being constituted of the endowment received at the moment of conception, with later heaven being all that comes afterward. If we consider early heaven to be the time prior to the infant's first breath, this suggests that the time spent in the mother's womb does not involve a contribution from later heaven. In modern times, we are well aware that the mother's lifestyle and habits during her pregnancy, such as diet and alcohol consumption, may indeed strongly impact the healthy development of the fetus. After all, the womb provides a physical environment in which the inborn potential of the fertilized egg and subsequent fetus are nourished.

I believe the relative designations of early and later heaven being differentiated by the infant's first breath have to do with theoretical considerations in Chinese cosmology. Cosmologically, early heaven corresponds to the "paradise time" of the undifferentiated *dao* as it incubates creation. Later heaven corresponds to the birth of being as the ten thousand things and the resultant fall of creation from original nature.

STAGE III: THE CHILD

Dao *is hidden and without name.*
– DAO DE JING[6]

The emergence of all creation occurs at the moment the *dao* gains self-consciousness. In the ontogeny of the human being, this is the moment of birth—not the child's physical birth, but the birth of self-awareness. The seeds of self-awareness are sown when the infant receives a name *(ming)* in the third month of life (one year after conception). The act of giving a personal name differentiates the infant from all the other people and things—much as the two are differentiated from the one, to become the ten thousand things. Named, the infant grows into a child, creating an identity based on individuation and separation from the unity of primordial being. As feelings of separation grow, original nature *(de)* and awareness of the *dao's* primordial influence in one's life are lost.

It is the role of the father to bestow a personal name, an act that draws the child out of "seclusion"—out of the arms of the mother and the comfort of the womb—into the world. Granet posits that "the child is not really in a position to possess a superior soul until it is capable of laughter. . . . the father teaches it to laugh and . . . gives it that personal name which the Chinese rites show to be identical to the superior soul, with destiny, and with life itself. At the third month the child, which up until then has been kept in seclusion, is at last presented to the father who greets it with a smile."[7] Interestingly, the soft apertures (fontanelles) in the infant's skull close during the third month of life. The fusing of the two halves of the skull to form a unified whole suggests metaphorically that the infant has differentiated from the *dao* and both accepted and internalized destiny as bestowed by heaven.

The child's first laugh corresponds to the awakening of its *shen,* which represents the child's initial spark of self-awareness. The child does not laugh until it is presented to the father, who then names it. This is when the *hun* (evolutionary soul) is activated and the child begins the process of gaining self-awareness.[8] In this scenario, the mother corresponds to earth and *yin,* providing nourishing sustenance to the child, as representative of the womb of *dao.* As representative of the manifest world and intellect, the father activates the infant's *shen* *(yang)* through the presentation of personal name, stimulating progress toward self-awareness and movement away from the mother, the *dao.*

The sage seeks to retain the infant-like state and treasures "feeding from the mother." The sage is happy to stay connected through the umbilical center in order to receive limitless nourishment from the womb of *dao.* By so doing, the sage consciously rejects the state of self-awareness offered by the earthly father and chooses rather to be nourished by the primordial *qi* bestowed by heaven.

Both infant and sage emulate that faceless idiot Emperor Huntun, who had no name, no logic, and no ability to distinguish things until he received the "gift" of sensory awareness. But, Liu Yiming tells us, unlike Emperor Huntun, the child has discriminations and cognition "as if floating clouds are dotting the sky."[9] By this, he means that although the child still largely retains the spontaneous character of the *dao,* original nature is beginning to be sullied by the conditioning influence of later heaven. The child, in possession of an intellect, has begun to process and interpret life experiences.

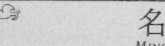
MING

The Chinese character *ming*, translated here as "name," is composed of a mouth (口) on the right and the character for "evening" (夕) on the left, "because, at dusk, it is necessary to give one's name to be known."[10] The Chinese characters for logic *(mingxue:名學)* mean, literally, the study of names. To distinguish *(mingming:命名)* means to give a thing a destiny by naming it.

Zhuangzi advises us not to seek a name for ourselves in his story of a man who refuses an offer to rule an empire in order to avoid acquiring a name:

> You [the host] govern the world and the world is already well governed. Now if I take your place, will I be doing it for a name? But name is only the guest of reality—will I be doing it so I can play the part of the guest?[11]

Here the host remains centered at home and thus preserves his innate qualities intact. The guest stays just a short while, then disappears into the dark night like any "thing" that gains momentary fame. The *Dao De Jing* tells us that "the most famous has no fame."[12] The *dao*, which is all pervasive, is yet elusive and remains obscure. It cannot be said to have fame or *youming*, which translates from the Chinese, literally, as "to have a name." The *dao* as "the valley spirit" is "free from danger" because it does not elevate itself to a lofty position from which it may "fall." Hence *Zhuangzi* advises us that to do good, "stay away from fame [having a name]. . . . and live out your years."[13]

STAGE IV: THE YOUNG ADULT: *YIN* AND *YANG* DIVIDE

Those who discriminate, fail to see.
– ZHUANGZI[14]

The fetus, infant, and child—the first three stages in the seven-stage ontogeny of the human—all retain, to some degree, the spontaneous self-expression of the *dao* as unity. The child, however, by gaining a name and an intellect, has set the stage for the loss of original nature. At the following stage, the young adult begins to attribute meaning to life in a way that inhibits the inborn spontaneity inherent in the infant or child. Liu states,

> Man gradually grows from childhood . . . *yin* and *yang* divide each dwelling on one side, in the center of truth there is artificiality; here knowledge and experience gradually develop, and good and bad are discriminated.[15]

Knowledge and experience in the world develop as the adult spends life pursuing worldly accomplishments. Having lost primal unity with *dao,* the adult becomes another one of the ten thousand things.

It is knowledge of the self as being separate from the unity of the *dao* that the *Dao De Jing* considers to be the source of illness:

> *From knowing to not knowing*
> *This is superior.*
> *From not knowing to knowing,*
> *This is sickness.*
> – DAO DE JING[16]

So the dynamic process of separation from one's true nature, as one grows from young adulthood into adulthood, begins with the separation of *yin* and *yang* that occurs with the gain of self-consciousness. This is the initial crack in the functional balance of our constitutional endowment which serves as the foundation for all healthy growth and development in life. Losing touch with the true nature imparted by heaven, we react to life by creating a false self built out of belief and colored by our interpretations of life. The spontaneity imparted by a properly functioning *mingmen* slowly dwindles as its fires are extinguished by the accretions of experience in later heaven. With the fire of *mingmen* dampened, our primal endowment of *yin* and *yang* continues to separate. Early and later heaven cease to interact spontaneously as inner nature is forgotten.

Eventually, we reject the opportunities and circumstances sent by heaven in its attempt to cultivate the seed it has sown deep within. Simultaneously, the *jing* and *shen* separate; the will *(zhi)* depletes the *jing* as our mind struggles to reject heaven's will, both internally and externally, and to assert its own will on the world through force. As the mind depletes the *jing*, the kidney's function grows correspondingly weaker. The very source of life is now expended in our striving for worldly accomplishment. Here the "gate of birth" closes and the "door of death" opens, with a corresponding separation between metal and water on the *sheng* cycle. The failure to make this most vital transition corresponds to failure in all spheres of human function. This condition known as the "husband/wife" imbalance is presented in Chapter 7 in relationship to the separation of *yin* and *yang* as discerned through Chinese pulse diagnosis.

STAGE V: THE SEPARATION OF THE FIVE ELEMENTS[17]

As *yin* and *yang* separate, the functional dynamics of one's constitution become apparent. Liu explains,

> When *yin* and *yang* divide, the five elements become disordered (*luan*). The five elements, metal, wood, water, fire, and earth, represent the five *qi*.[18] The five elements of early heaven create each other following the *sheng* cycle. These five elements fuse to form a unified *qi*. From them issue forth the five virtues (*de*) of benevolence, righteousness, propriety, wisdom, and integrity. [The five elements] of later heaven overcome [*ke*] one another following the [*ke*] cycle. This manifests as the five rebels of joy, anger, grief, happiness, and desire.
>
> When the five elements are united, the five virtues are present and *yin* and *yang* form a chaotic unity. Once the five elements divide, the distinguishing spirit (*shishen*) gradually arises, and the encrustation of the senses gradually takes place; truth flees and the false becomes established. Now, even the state of the child is lost.

Liu goes on to say that the five organs (*zang*) serve as inns for the conditioned elements of later heaven, but are not the gardens of virtue in which the five elements of early heaven reside.[19] This can be interpreted to mean that the negative effects of acquired experience accrue in the different internal organs, conditioning the five elements and eventually harming their function. In contrast, the primordial five elements empower all aspects of the "being" to flourish.

Eventually, a major event occurs in each young life that knocks the child's elemental balance off in such a way that harmonious functioning is not easily returned to. At that instant, the primordial *yin* and *yang* divide and the five elements, formerly infused one with the other, become aberrant. The child or young adult becomes "stuck" in one of the five movements of the *dao* as a predominant form of self-expression. As one's elemental balance becomes skewed toward a fixed expression, the integrity of the *sheng* cycle is lost and the elements "overcontrol" one another in a dysfunctional relationship, following the *ke* cycle.[20]

As this major event occurs, the qualitative experience of the element associated with constitutional type surges through the child and becomes strongly apparent in every aspect of being. This is the moment that one's constitutional type becomes explicit. The qualitative feeling of this element's expression in all domains of being, including its correlated emotion, is instantly paired in the child's mind with the interpretation of the event that is simultaneously occurring. No longer able to react spontaneously to all situations "sent by heaven," this event is interpreted as suggesting a fundamental truth about the child's own nature and the nature of life itself. The child learns that it is painful and not safe to express, or be in the presence of, a given quality of feeling and its related emotional state.

For example, qualities of feeling associated with the wood element could include tight shoulders, burning in the epigastrium, resentment, anger, and thwarted creativity. These physical, emotional, and spiritual states all merge and become paired with the pain felt at the moment of trauma. In the future, the child will react habitually whenever the expression of the wood element is experienced in self, other, or nature. Now the child begins closing doors to full self-expression as natural spontaneity dwindles.

Liu specifies a distinct relationship between the presence of the five Confucian virtues (benevolence, righteousness, propriety, wisdom, and integrity) when the five elements are balanced, and the inappropriate presence of emotion after the five elements have divided. To restore original nature in each constitutional type, a life transformation must occur that moves the individual from the inappropriate expression of a given emotion to the embodiment of its associated virtue. The relationship between the elements, emotions, and virtues are given in Figure 9.3.

STAGE VI: ACQUIRED CONDITIONING RUNS AFFAIRS

As the individual's definition of self becomes increasingly colored by a particular interpretation of the events that have occurred in life, contact with true nature is lost. This corresponds to the dampening of the fire of *mingmen*, which gradually becomes "encrusted" with our erroneous beliefs about our own nature and the nature of life. Day by day, spontaneity dwindles as we become creatures of habit, enslaved by mistaken beliefs and assumptions.

As stated earlier, the infant's journey away from true self begins with laughter. Laughter is also a sign of the continuing separation from the *dao* later in life. The *Dao De Jing* tells us,

> *When the inferior person hears of* dao, *he roars.*
> *If* dao *were not laughed at,*
> *It would not be* dao.
>
> – *DAO DE JING*[21]

Once we become unable to recognize true nature within or without, laughter and mockery may be our only response when confronted with the *dao*. Individuals become stuck largely in one form of emotional expression characteristic of the directionality of their constitutional imbalance. At this point, people become prisoners of their own beliefs and habitual behaviors. Every new situation encountered in life is now interpreted in relation to past experience, and the capacity to respond spontaneously has died.

Liu explains this dynamic that develops as we move through the stages of adulthood: "The influence of mundanity *(yin)* enters . . . and the influence of heaven *(yang)* gradually wanes. Indulgently pursuing desires, one eventually becomes subservient to them." This acquired temperament *(qizhi:*氣質*)*[22] can be attributed to the conditioned five elements belonging to later heaven. According to Liu, true nature *(zhenxing:*真性*)* is found in the destiny appointed by heaven *(tianming)*. It belongs to early heaven and is beneficial to people. Temperament emerges from acquired conditioning and is created by humans; therefore it is harmful to people. Zhuangzi advises that we must not live in a way that damages the constitution which has been decreed by heaven.[23] He is emphatic that we should not develop what is natural to humans (temperament), for this only injures life. Only by developing what is natural to heaven *(ming,* destiny) does life benefit.[24] For to do any less than fulfill our destiny is "the crime of hiding from heaven."[25]

STAGE VII: PURE MUNDANITY, NOTHING CELESTIAL

Men, in time, return again to the mysterious workings.
So all creatures come out of the mysterious
workings and go back into them again.
– *ZHUANGZI*[26]

The seventh stage of development corresponds to what may be the irreversible loss of our original nature. According to Liu,

> As [the conditioning] of later heaven runs affairs, *yin* [mundanity] enters and *yang* [celestial influence] retreats, day by day, year by year. Internally, ten thousand thoughts bring calamity; outside, the ten thousand things entice. With the inside and outside under attack, the *yangqi* diminishes to the point of exhaustion and the entire body becomes pure *yin,* the three treasures [*jing, qi,* and *shen*] are depleted, and the *hun* and *po* spirits become troubled. How is one able not to die?
>
> Ignorant people think that when their days are numbered and their destiny is cut short, this [mandate] resides with heaven, but this is not so. Man's life depends on celestial influence *(yangqi);* if there is one bit of *yang* remaining, one will not die. If there is one bit of mundanity *(yinqi),* which is not pure [i.e., still retaining a part of heaven or *yang*], then one will not die. If one goes along and lets mundanity extinguish the influence of heaven *(yangqi),* this is personally searching for death. How could this involve [the destiny appointed] by heaven?

This developmental stage represents a turning point in our path through life. Ultimately, the fate of all things is to return to the *dao.* At the seventh stage, we may "wake up" and begin on the path of returning to full self-expression. This represents a "death" of the mundane, imagined self as we rediscover our destiny, thereby returning the *dao* back into the world and our self back to the *dao.* If, instead, we continue on the path of alienation from original nature, then *yin* and *yang* and the five elements will reach a terminal point of separation with early death being the unavoidable result. The alchemist Ge Hong considers people alienated from original nature to be traveling through life like "walking corpses."[27] The death of the physical body may also be thought of as a return to original nature as the individual's spirit travels home to the eternal *dao.*

It is not inevitable that as individuals we will each irrevocably become lost in our own habitual delusions. The return to fulfilling our heaven-appointed destiny may occur at any moment. Physical illness may proceed beyond the reach of therapy so that death is inevitable. However, even in the process of dying, destiny may be fulfilled through aligning our will with the will of heaven. Remember Confucius's statement: "If a man in the morning hears the *dao,* he may die in the evening without regret."[28] Only by ignoring our destiny and turning away from the heart of heaven may we lose the way home. For destiny is the lamp, burning brightly in heaven's heart, which may guide us ever onward toward our true selves. Destiny is the thread that, if followed, will always guide us home to the eternal *dao*.

Summary

The loss of original nature is implicit in human life, which ultimately follows the movements and ontogeny of the *dao*. Each individual has a unique nature willed by heaven, and each human life follows the basic steps elaborated here. In conclusion, I summarize the process of the loss of and return to original nature.

At conception, our primal *yinqi* and *yangqi* fuse together and heaven imprints on our *jing* a destiny commensurate with presiding cosmological circumstances and the merit of the individual. At that instant, a theme is born around which our life is organized until the moment of death. This theme is synonymous with our constitutional type, reflecting both the potential virtues and challenges inherent in our path through life.

The fetus, gestating in the womb of the *dao*, thrives in its time of cosmic incubation. Having no "sense," the fetus lives in a paradise beyond human comprehension. After birth, this state is retained by the infant, whose primordial endowment gives rise to the perfect expression of the virtues that govern its life. The infant is able to move through all changes in life spontaneously because its reactions to life are unblemished by the interpretations of its mind. Thus the infant exhibits the spontaneous self-becoming *(ziran:*自然*)* inherent in the movement of the *dao*. Both Laozi and Zhuangzi consider this spontaneity to be the precise definition of health.

As the infant gains a personal name, the seeds of self-awareness are sown. Like a bolt of lightning, the infant's first laugh illuminates the world as self is experienced for the first time as separate from the other "ten thousand things." Eventually, the infant transforms into a child who gains knowledge about the nature of life and constructs an image of reality, which is colored by the mind's own interpretations. Inevitably, some trauma occurs, and the five elements that had been working in synchrony become unbalanced. The constitutional theme of the child's life emerges as one of the five elemental expressions. Stuck predominantly in one of the five elemental expressions, the individual begins to behave in habitual patterns consistent with the emerging constitutional type.

No longer able to move and function spontaneously, the child begins to react to life in a way consistent with its own interpretation. Slowly becoming a creature of conditioned habit over time, the child grows into an adult who has lost touch with original nature. Increasingly distanced from true self, the adult's *yin* and *yang* continue to separate, with death of the real or imagined self as the inevitable result. The inner tradition of Chinese medicine may provide a vehicle through which we may glimpse a memory of the forgotten self.

As with every concept in Chinese physiology, Liu's seven stages are functional and do not correspond to precise physical stages in life. Only the first stage, the fetus, conforms to a precisely defined physical manifestation. At the instant the fetus emerges from the womb and takes its first breath, it becomes an infant. These first two stages are well defined, but the delineation in time between the other stages is not so clear. To try to determine the exact moments of transition would be like trying to discern the instant a kitten becomes a cat. Like the dynamic transitioning of the five elements, the subsequent stages blend into and overlap one another. They do not necessarily occur over long periods of time; they may occur at any time in a life, even instantly and simultaneously. One may die in a state of ignorance at the age of 90 or at 23.

The stage at which mundane conditioned influences conquer our store of primordial *qi* and lead to morbidity and death differs with each individual and depends on a wide spectrum of inherited attributes and acquired circumstances. For example, an individual with a poor inherited endowment may be overwhelmed in life by an initial insult of relatively small magnitude. This may lead to serious physical illness (cancer) or spiritual illness (taking one's own life) at a fairly young age. But given a different endowment, the insult might slide away without harm like water off a duck's back, as in the case of an infant who is born fully realized as a reincarnated Tibetan monk (tulkhu) or a bodhisattva. According to Buddhist teachings, this infant became a sage in a previous life and made a conscious decision to reincarnate in order to help humanity. The evolutionary force supporting such a child may be so strong that when a traumatic life event occurs, original nature is lost, but returned to instantly.

Given these general considerations, there are correspondences between Liu's seven stages of life and specific ages that I have discerned in my clinical practice. The stages manifest differently in each life depending on the patient's relative level of awareness.

The life of the fetus (stage I) is governed exclusively by early heaven. During this time, the fetus incubates and develops in a way governed by internal processes initiated at conception. Even though subjected to external input from its environment, the infant's (stage II) development after birth continues to be guided by the influence of early heaven. The infant may be said to have become a child (stage III) at that point in life when its personality begins to emerge. In my experience this happens between the ages of 2 and 3. At this stage, a tendency toward a given type of emotional expression is seen, but the child is not yet stuck in that form of expression.

At some point, generally between the ages of 4 and 12, a life event occurs of such magnitude that he or she cannot fully recover spontaneous function. At this moment, the child makes its initial interpretations regarding its own nature (who "I" am) and the nature of life itself ("Life is not safe," in the case of the fire constitutional type). The constitutional type generally becomes evident at this point. Later in life, the individual may have no memory of the event that triggered this reaction because it occurred at such a young age. The initial interpretation made by the child does not conform to reality and thus causes a separation between *yin* and *yang,* which is described by Liu's fourth stage. Liu's fifth stage generally follows soon afterward and may be concurrent with the fourth. It is during these two stages, ages 12 to 18, that habits take hold as young adults continue to build an imagined self, defining themselves and the world by what they believe to be true rather than by being true to their original nature.

Between the ages of 16 and 21 (stage VI), a second traumatic event often occurs that reinforces the effects of the initial trauma. Generally, this event involves the death of a parent or grandparent, or some difficulty associated with emerging sexuality or an intimate relationship. Later in life, the individual may think of this event (rather than the first, which happened too early to remember) as a defining moment that shaped who he or she is. Pushed deeper into habitual reaction, the adult has now reached Liu's sixth stage, where acquired conditioning now governs life and the primordial influence of early heaven has been extinguished.

At about 30 to 40, another life trauma often occurs (stage VII). This has two possible results. It may reinforce the first two traumas, thus driving the individual more deeply into habitual dysfunction. In this case, one proceeds on the path to ruin, interpreting the event as further proof of one's thesis of who one is and how life is. Or, the pain caused by the event may offer a glimpse of the lost self. One may realize the falsehood of one's interpretations and question who one really is and, in the seventh step, return to one's original nature. But if the individual retreats from the opportunity afforded at this last juncture, the seventh stage leads instead to morbidity and death.

What if an infant is born with physical symptomatology? These symptoms are "constitutional" in the sense of representing an inborn weakness present from conception. Genetic defects such as a cleft palate fall into this category. But symptoms resulting from losing touch with our innate nature generally begin to manifest in Liu's fourth and fifth stages. Acne, asthma, or headaches, for example, may begin at this time. Generally, they are easily treatable using Chinese medicine because the patient's primordial endowment as a guiding influence is still easily contacted during this period.

But by the sixth stage, symptoms have become too materially manifest to be reversed entirely. They may be well managed with treatment but often return if treatment is stopped. By the seventh stage, physical symptomatology becomes irreversible and generally must be handled with life-saving interventions, such as Western medications and surgeries. These types of conditions may include heart disease, atherosclerosis, and degenerative conditions of the spine or nervous system. It is important to note that, even at this late date, our awareness of true self may return in a moment. However, the return of the primordial influences upon which this awareness is based will, in all likelihood, not have the force to effect enough change to materially alter the general course of physical pathology.

Next, we examine the functional dynamics that determine whether an individual awakes to regain original nature or proceeds through life on a path of ignorance only to die estranged from true self.

Questions

Beginning with receiving our personal name, society reinforces the development of our created self-image.

1. What were the major influences in your life that helped define who you are?

2. Which of these influences do you consider to have been positive and which do you consider to have been negative?

3. Did the positive influences give you an attribute you did not already have, or did they cultivate an attribute that lay within you?

4. What has been more difficult for you, the negative situations you have experienced or the meanings you have attached to such circumstances?

NOTES

1. Watson, 1964a, p. 38.

2. The character *hun* refers to the "chaotic" nature of the *dao* and may also mean "to blend." Throughout my translation, I have interpreted the character *hun* as the blending of two seemingly opposite factors back into a unity beyond human comprehension that is patterned on the *dao* of early heaven. For further discussion of this topic, see Girardot, 1983.

3. The human gestation period is calculated as "ten months" according to the Chinese lunar calendar.

4. Cleary, 1986a, p. 62.

5. Chapter 55; in Chen, 1989, p. 185.

6. Chapter 41; in Chen, 1989, p. 154.

7. Ganet, 1930; cited in Chen, 1989, p. 104.

8. *Hun,* denoting the "superior soul," is a homophone of *hun,* which means "to blend" and denotes "chaos." Hence the three treasures, *jing, qi,* and *shen,* blend into one to form the *hun* spirit.

9. Cleary, 1986a, p. 63.

10. Wieger, 1965, p. 164.

11. Watson, 1964a, p. 26.

12. Chapter 39; in Chen, 1989, p. 149.

13. Watson, 1964a, p. 46.

14. Zhuangzi; in Watson, 1964a, p. 39.

15. Translation mine.

16. Chapter 71; in Chen, 1989, p. 215.

17. For a discussion of the five elements, see Chapter 8.

18. Cleary writes that the five *qi* are "sense, essence, vitality, spirit, and energy." Liu Yiming, however, in the edition I have translated, does not define them.

19. Liu Yiming; in Cleary, 1986a, p. 66.

20. The *sheng* and *ke* cycles are discussed in Chapter 8.

21. Chapter 41; in Chen, 1989, p. 153.

22. Another meaning of *zhi,* translated here as "temperament," is "constitution."

23. T'ang, 1962 (April), pp. 29–49.

24. Zhuangzi; in Watson, 1964a, p. 120.

25. Ibid., p. 48.

26. Watson, 1964a, p. 117.

27. Ware, 1966, p. 76.

28. See Book IV, Chapter 8, in Legge, 1971, p. 168.

7

THE
TURNING
POINT

THE INTEGRITY OF LIFE DEPENDS ON THE BALANCED
functioning of the twelve "officials," or organ systems. The constitutional foundation supporting this function is the interpenetration of
our original endowment of *yin* and *yang,* which constitutes the *yuanqi.*
The *yuanqi* is the seed of true nature that heaven plants deep within at
the moment of conception. We must nurture the potential of this seed
to fulfill our destiny. However, our true nature is forgotten as, in the
course of living in mundane consciousness, accumulated habitual
behaviors extinguish the fire of heaven's intent. By receiving our personal name, self-awareness dawns and original nature is lost. Gaining
self-awareness forms the original crack in our balanced functioning and
paves the way for the separation of *yin* and *yang.* When we lose touch
with true nature imparted by heaven, the usual reaction is to create a
false self predicated on erroneous interpretations of life experience. This
leads to the unbalanced functioning of the five elements—water, wood,
fire, earth, metal—bringing us, ultimately, to death.

It is not destiny that a person should die estranged from true nature.

In each life, a turning point arrives when we are given a glimpse of the virtue imparted by heaven. We are then granted the opportunity either to cultivate this deep inner nature or to continue following habitual patterns on the path to worldly gain and spiritual ruin.

The separation of *yin* and *yang* is both predictable and treatable using the diagnostics and therapeutics of Chinese medicine. The condition is evident on the pulses, taken during diagnosis and later in treatment sessions, and is known in the five-element tradition as the "husband/wife" imbalance. Earlier, I described human destiny as it relates to the loss of original nature and to the inner tradition of Chinese medicine. Here I continue this inquiry, this time focusing on the functional dynamics that determine whether a given individual "wakes up" to the memory of his or her lost self or ends life with destiny unfulfilled as *yin* and *yang* move toward a premature terminal point of separation. I examine the separation of *yin* and *yang* as it is relevant to the clinical practice of the inner tradition. But first I consider the separation of *yin* and *yang* as it appears in Chinese creation mythology, the *Yijing*, the spiritual alchemy of *mingmen*, and in Chinese physiology and pulse diagnosis.

The Functional Location of the Mysterious Pass

In Chinese creation mythology, as we learned in Chapter 1, the passageway of the queen mother is known as the golden gate, or the mysterious pass. In the five-element tradition, metal (west, fall) gives birth to water (north, winter), and this transition represents the gate leading to the tomb or womb of the queen mother—the mysterious pass. Both hexagram 23 ("splitting apart") and hexagram 24 ("return," or "the turning point") of the *Yijing* are associated with the mysterious pass. Interestingly, hexagram 23 is paired with the months October and November (fall) and hexagram 24 is paired with December and January (winter). These pairings are consistent with the mysterious pass that exists in the transition from metal (fall) to water (winter).

In the circle of five-element transformation *(wuxing:*五行*)*, wherein the five elements—water, wood, fire, earth, and metal—transform in a cycle, one into the next, the transition from metal to water is the most crucial to perpetuating life. For it is at this juncture that our destiny hangs by a thread. In the brief moment when fall (metal) changes to winter (water), a person's link to life is at its most delicate. I am reminded of a patient with AIDS whom I treated on a daily basis during the last eight weeks of his life until he died. He felt complete in this life and looked forward to death as a new transition and as a way to end his agony. He wanted to know how long he had to live and asked me to predict this based on pulse diagnosis. After determining a severe separation of *yin* and *yang* on his pulse, I predicted that he would die upon the first frost as fall (metal) changed to winter (water). This is precisely what happened.

The transition from metal to water is the turning point when, upon entering the mysterious pass of the queen mother, we are given the opportunity to travel deep within to discover our original nature. If this opportunity is missed and the functional link between metal and water is broken, the dissolution of our life force begins as it returns "back into the mysterious workings of things."

Several Chinese myths recognize the transition from metal (west) to water (north) as crucial to attaining immortality. The epic poem *Da Ren Fu* (Rhapsody of the Great Man) by Sima Xiangru (179–117 B.C.E.) describes Emperor Wu's search for immortality. After many journeys, he reaches Kunlun Mountain in the West for a visit with Xi Wang Mu, the queen mother. From there, he heads to the North and proceeds through the "dark pass" to spiral upward and disappear from the world.[1] Another Daoist myth reiterates this same transition: The gatekeeper at the western pass bids Laozi to write the *Dao De Jing* before he passes through the gate to retire from this world. Laozi has no doubt ascended Kunlun Mountain to dine on the queen mother's fruit of primordial *yin* and *yang*.

The Functional Dynamics of Yin and Yang

The gate of birth and the door of death are both
immaterial, formless passageways. By following mundanity,
one dies; by returning the celestial, one lives—hence the
names gate of birth and door of killing.
In reality, they are just one opening.
– LIU YIMING[2]

The separation of *yin* and *yang* begins when the child or young adult forgets true nature and begins to create an imagined self out of their interpretations of life's events. The dynamics of the separation of *yin* and *yang* are described at length in the *Yijing*. It is the functional transition of hexagram 23 (*bo,* "splitting apart") into hexagram 24 (*fu,* "the return") that holds important implications for the practice of Chinese medicine (Figure 7.1a and 7.1b).[3] Liu Yiming describes this transition as a gate or passageway between life and death, unconscious habitual functioning *(yin)*, and the illumination of spiritual awakening *(yang)*. He names the two hexagrams the "gate of birth" and the "door of killing the self," respectively. Like the Golden Gate leading to the womb/tomb of the queen mother, these two hexagrams form a door to either death or immortality, depending on the intention of the individual who opens it. The choice of which door to open faces each person in each moment as life's challenges are confronted. The decision spells the difference between awakening to the reality planted deep within by heaven or further estrangement from true self.

According to the *Yijing,* the dark forces of *yin* overcome the superior *yang* forces not by direct means but by gradually and imperceptibly undermining them so that they finally collapse.[4] For the path to death is trod slowly one step at a time. With each challenge life hands us, with each heartbeat, we are given the choice of being true to our hearts or turning our backs on destiny. Liu is adamant that even if we are successful in the world, inevitably there can be only ruin if original nature is ignored. If habitual functioning persists, we will eventually exhaust our storehouse of *yang* as the framework of life collapses.

The Door of Death: Splitting Apart

Hexagram 23, translated by Wilhelm as "splitting apart," represents the final stage of separation of the primordial *yin* and *yang*.[5] Here, only one *yang* line is left at the top of the hexagram, which is supported by a weak foundation of five *yin* lines. This portrays a situation where acquired *yin* influences are at the point of extinguishing the heavenly *yang*. The image in hexagram 23 is a mountain that has an insubstantial base, indicated by the five *yin* lines. The dynamics of this hexagram suggest that the foundation of life has been slowly eroded and the internal structure is crumbling. If the last *yang* line of hexagram 23 disintegrates into a *yin* line, the resulting hexagram is hexagram 2, "the receptive," representing earth (Figure 7.1c). Earth represents pure potentiality without any *yang*-activating influences. At this point, life comes to an end as "the house of the inferior man is split apart,"[6] and the essence constituting life returns to the primordial sea whence it came.

The functional dynamics of this condition describe precisely the physiological effects of kidney deficiency that result from squandering

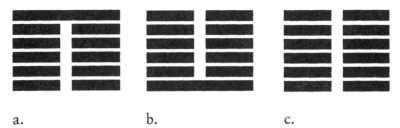

a.   b.   c.

Figure 7.1
HEXAGRAMS 23, 24, AND 2 OF THE *YIJING*

In the structure of the Yijing *hexagrams, a solid line stands for the influence of* yang *and a broken line stands for the influence of* yin. *(a) Hexagram 23. Bo (剝), "splitting apart": The hexagram depicts a house with a faulty foundation that will soon degenerate and crumble. The solitary* yang *line in the top position is the heavenly influence of* yang *slowly eroding by the action of the mundane* yin *influences of later heaven pushing up from below.*

(b) Hexagram 24. Fu (復), "return," or "the turning point": The single yang *line is pushed away by the rising* yin *lines and returns to the bottom, the root of life, to serve as a strong foundation for another round of evolution. The practitioner must recognize and direct the patient's attention to the moment of return if healing is to be complete. The dynamics of the turning point are discussed in Chapter 12 in the context of the healing crisis.*

(c) Hexagram 2. Gun (坤), "earth," or "the receptive": As the last yang *influence in hexagram 23 changes to* yin, *the result is a return to earth. With no* yang-*activating influence remaining, but only potential, life comes to an end. Our essence returns to the origin, the primordial sea of the* dao.

one's inherited constitution. Liu compares the last remaining *yang* influence in hexagram 23 to the pit of a peach. He cautions that life or death is only a matter of gaining or losing this one pit, which is the basis of life's continual renewal and evolution.[7] The peach pit serves as a metaphor for the *yuanqi*, which remains intact as the source and center of one's life and vitality. Liu explains that spiritually developed people have a method of suppressing the mundane influences of *yin* and strengthening themselves by following the *yuanqi*, which is the way of heaven. He explains, "where this one point of *yangqi* is not yet exhausted, they accord with it and stabilize it, getting rid of intellectualism, shutting out conditioning influences, and returning to the fundamental, original foundation."[8]

The single remaining *yang* line in this hexagram may also be likened to our ego at the peak of life, when it is furthest removed from our true foundation in the depths of self (the *jing* and *yuanqi*). Just as someone who is inundated by a flood tries desperately to keep their head above water, so the ego bobs in a swirl of mundane *yin* as we struggle to maintain an image of created self. It is identification with the acquired self that brings us to the brink of ruin. Hence the *Yijing*, in discussing "splitting apart," tells us, "Those above can ensure their position only by giving generously to those below."⁹ By letting go of the false self that separates us from others, we may return to the true self firmly rooted in the depths.

Liu Yiming sums up his discussion of this hexagram by saying, "The secure home for humans is benevolence; taking from those above to give to those below, when the inversion is made, stripping changes into return. Having returned, it is possible to rely on benevolence; the mechanism of enlivening operates, and nature and life are secured."¹⁰ In order to return to original nature and thus secure our foundation in life, we must reestablish the connection between that which lies above (heaven, *shen*) and that which lies below (earth, *jing*). "Taking from those above to give to those below" is an admonishment to humans to follow the way of heaven in life. By taking the *yang* from its position above and returning it to a foundational position below, the "door of death" transforms into the "gate of birth."

The Gate of Birth: The Return

The Yijing hexagram "return" consists of one yang *arising under five* yins: yin *is quietude,* yang *is movement; when quietude reaches its consummation, it gives rise to movement. It is this point of movement that is the mysterious pass.*

– LIU YIMING¹¹

In the *Yijing*, the return of original nature is represented by hexagram 24 and named, appropriately, "return." Comparing it to hexagram 23, one *yang* line has returned to the depths and now serves as a strong foundation for the five *yin* lines above (Figure 7.1b). This suggests that one has avoided splitting apart, and that in choosing the gate of birth one has paved the way for a new beginning. The image given in the *Yijing* for hexagram 24 of "thunder within the earth"¹² stands for the return of the primal *yangqi* to the primal *yin*, which occurs on the winter solstice. Hence the *Yijing* states, "All movements are accomplished in six stages, and the seventh brings return. Thus the winter solstice, with which the decline of the year begins, comes in the seventh month after the summer solstice; so too does sunrise come in the seventh double hour after sunset. Therefore, seven is the number of the young light, and it arises when six, the number of the great darkness, is increased by one. In this way, the state of rest gives place to movement."[13]

The text of hexagram 23 advises to "turn around and return to one's dao."[14] Without a return to this "inner light," life is not renewed and the primal *yin* and *yang* separate, resulting in the dissolution of self described in "splitting apart." The winter solstice signifies the time for retreating deep within one's self and concentrating resources in anticipation of renewed growth in the spring. This is the reason Liu Yiming calls this hexagram the "gate of birth."[15] Wilhelm describes the "return" as the heart of heaven and earth. To the ancient Chinese, "a promise that never fails is the heart of heaven and earth,"[16] for by keeping the promise of an eternity filled with new beginnings, the *dao* fulfills its destiny.

The Law of Husband and Wife

When the "wife" follows the "husband,"
water and fire balance each other.
— Liu Yiming[17]

The separation of *yin* and *yang* signals an alienation from true self on the most fundamental level. Continued separation from self is predicated on the individual's self-concept constructed from erroneous interpretations of life's experiences. Over time, as this crack in the individual's constitutional foundation widens, serious illness manifests in all spheres of function. The functional basis of this illness is a lifetime of false beliefs and interpretations. The presence of the husband/wife imbalance shows that one has been brought to the very brink of destruction. However, habitual delusion is only one possible path to arrive there. A person may have congenitally poor kidney *qi* and therefore be prone to this imbalance from birth. Further, a severe physical trauma may so deplete the kidney that a husband/wife imbalance manifests. These last two scenarios could be described as being beyond the control of the individual and resting with the will of heaven. Even so, the concept of karma still places the responsibility for appropriate action on the patient. By the time an individual reaches a husband/wife imbalance, *yin* and *yang* are fast approaching the terminal point of separation. Precursors of this imbalance in an individual's life are separation from the very sources of life's vitality. Two such sources that have major impact on the overall condition of health are relationship to family and relationship to work.

Patients evidencing a husband/wife imbalance often feel trapped in a situation that is harmful and outside of their control. Often the very basis of personal identity and self-esteem is derived from this harmful work or personal relationship, but in order to leave the situation, they would have to kill their fundamental source of ego identification. Rather than endure the emotional pain associated with such an extreme step, individuals habitually suppress the inner drive for self-expression in the spheres of function consistent with their constitutional type. Eventually, this suppression leads to pathological changes in the structure and function of tissue, forming the organic basis for serious illness. In this scenario, the practitioner expects to see a fundamental "tearing apart" on deep functional levels that corresponds to the separation of the primordial *yin* and *yang*. Self-destructive tendencies can often be seen in other areas of the patient's life as he or she is unconsciously driven toward self-destruction. This may manifest in a tendency to cut or burn oneself, or to "accidentally" harm oneself in more serious ways.[18]

If the individual lives long enough with a husband/wife imbalance and continues to function habitually, then an extreme "*qi*-wild" (*san-mai*:散脈) pattern may appear on the pulse; now *yin* and *yang* are at their terminal point of separation.[19] In addition to the symptoms already described, the patient may evidence both extreme fatigue and an all-pervasive anxiety that emanates from the conscious or unconscious knowing that life is slipping away.[20] Thus the husband/wife imbalance is a clinically useful distinction with both diagnostic and therapeutic implications.

We may go along through life habitually driven, turning our back on destiny and "the door of life," continually entering instead the "door of death" in the face of heaven's challenges. If we proceed in this way, then the separation of *yin* and *yang* will ultimately manifest on our pulse, signaling gross imbalance throughout our being. By this time we are either involved with or soon headed for serious, life-threatening symptomatology. Here we are truly at a crossroads that may spell the difference between life and death.

In the five-element tradition, the separation of *yin* and *yang* as it occurs on the pulse is called the husband/wife imbalance. The "law of husband and wife" may be summarized as follows: When *yin* and *yang* are in relative harmony, then the pulses on the left hand (the husband, *yang*) will be better in both quantity and quality than the pulses on the right hand (the wife, *yin*).

The pulses on the left hand are constituted by the water, wood, and fire (heart and small intestine) elements. The movement of these elements

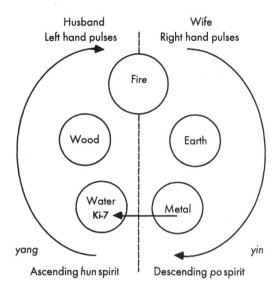

Figure 7.2
THE HUSBAND/WIFE IMBALANCE

The functional movement of the left hand pulses involves drawing the stored genetic potential out of water and manifesting it in the world. This may be likened to a tree (wood, spring) sending down its roots to draw on earthly reserves (water, winter) and channeling them in growth toward the sun (fire, summer). This movement corresponds to the ascension of the hun *spirit to heaven. The right hand pulses correspond to the second half of the year where the expression of life returns back into empowering the potential of the seed. Late summer (earth) and fall (metal) correspond to the time of the harvest and the digestion and integration of life. This movement corresponds to the descent of the* po *spirit as it returns back to the universal pole of earth.*

The dotted line indicates the juncture at which the pulses separate in a husband/wife imbalance. Kidney-7 is the key point for assisting in breaking the husband/wife imbalance and reestablishing the functional link between metal and water. The name of Kidney-7, "returning current," recalls the function of the point in aiding the connection of metal to water and thereby supporting the return of original nature.

is in drawing the potential out of the inherited constitution (water), up through the wood element, toward the pinnacle of life (fire). This movement corresponds to the ascension of the *hun* spirit as it travels to heaven to report on the merit of the individual (see Figure 7.2). The physiological basis of this movement is the kidney fire, which powers the evolutionary thrust of water up to fire.

In the five-element system, the pulses on the right hand correspond to the fire (heart protector and three heater), earth, and metal elements. The direction of movement is from the height of life (fire/summer) back down through the abundance of the harvest, and finally to the return to origin, which is mediated by the metal element. This transition corresponds to the descending movement of the *po* spirit, which is *yin* in nature, as it returns back to the earth.

The pulses of the left hand correspond fundamentally to the quality of function of the organ systems themselves, which finds its basis in the kidney. The right hand pulses correspond to the digestive system. If the pulses on the right hand are significantly better in quality and quantity than the left hand, then we may surmise that the actual functioning of the organ systems has collapsed. This collapse suggests that the resources of *jing, qi,* and *shen* have been severely depleted and are compromised as guiding influences in life. In this case, the digestive system is compensating and overworking in order to extract the maximum amount of essence from food and air so it may support the continued functioning of the organism. The collapse of the organ system corresponds to the compromised function of *mingmen,* which plays a key role in guarding the inherited constitution.

If the functioning of the digestive system, which guards the acquired constitution, collapses, then serious pathology cannot be far off. In this scenario all pulse positions evidence a superficial pounding. However, there is no depth to the entire pulse, indicating that the pounding felt is the patient's final store of *yangqi* dispersing. This "empty" pulse is indicative of an extreme "*qi*-wild" condition in which *yin* and *yang* are at their terminal point of separation. With the true *yin* (the *yuanyin* as imparted by heaven at conception) exhausted, the patient's *yang* floats to the top of the pulse. Now we are truly knocking at the "door of death" as the functional dynamics of the pulse exactly replicates the image of hexagram 23 (Figure 7.1a). This pattern generally is evidenced later in time than the classic husband/wife imbalance just described. It indicates that the functions supporting the digestive system have collapsed so it may no longer compensate for the failure of the organ system.

Treatment

If one knows about white and preserves the black, then
divine clarity comes of itself. The white is the metal
essence, the black is the basis of water.
– ZAN DONG JI[21]

The essential nature of the husband/wife imbalance is that the separation of the *yuanqi* and compromised function of *mingmen* has led to a failure of the *sheng* cycle to make the all-important transition between the metal and water element. Hence the basic principle in treatment of the husband/wife imbalance is to restore the connection between the organ functions represented by right and left pulses. Of particular importance is aiding the transition from the metal to the water element along the *sheng* cycle. This can be done in several ways. The primary strategy is to choose points that tonify the wood and water elements by drawing *qi* from the "right" half of the cycle to the left half. Kidney-7 and Bladder-67 are the primary tonification points that establish the link between metal and water. The secondary tonification point Kidney-3 draws *qi* from earth to tonify water and the secondary tonification point Liver-4 draws *qi* from metal to tonify the wood element. These four points constitute the primary strategy used to break the husband/wife imbalance. Generally, these points are repeated until the patient returns for treatment with a sustained kidney pulse.

In my experience, Kidney-1 and Bladder-1 needled together in the same session have proved valuable in breaking a husband/wife imbalance. Kidney-1 is the source of all power in the kidney meridian and when tonified has the function of helping to restore collapsed *yang*. The function of restoring collapsed *yang* specifically calls to mind the transition between the hexagrams "splitting apart" and "return." Bladder-1, located at the medial canthus and named "eyes bright," aids in stimulating the spontaneous interaction between early and later heaven. For the eyes receive life (later heaven) and channel it down into the fire of *mingmen,* where it meets the *yuanqi* (early heaven). In a given individual any point done at precisely the right moment may help restore the memory of original nature necessary for the restoration of health. Generally, however, when trying to break this particular habitual pattern, only points that tonify the left hand pulses or sedate the right hand pulses are chosen.

Lastly, if the pulses of both hands have collapsed and the patient evidences the "*qi*-wild" pattern described earlier, then a different therapeutic strategy must be chosen. The *yin* of the whole being must be tonified in order to root the *yang*. Conception Vessel-1, named "meeting of *yin,*" represents the source of *yin* in the human being. Governor-20, named "hundred meetings," is the gathering point of the *yangqi*. These two points together represent the central axis of heaven and earth as it occurs in the human being. Treating them together can help restore balance of the primordial *yin* and *yang* and help realign a patient to these dual poles of universal function. Interestingly, an alternate name for Conception Vessel-1 is *jinmen,* or "metal gate," which recalls the entrance to the kingdom of the queen mother. In myth the primordial brother and sister resurrect the human race after riding the crest of the flood through the "golden gate." Similarly, a key function of Conception Vessel-1 is for revival after drowning. The *Neijing* states that the conception vessel originates in the uterus and, as in myth, it is the "metal gate" that provides passageway into and out of the womb of *dao.*

Discussion

Though the grease burns out of the torch, the fire passes on, and no one knows where it ends.
– ZHUANGZI[22]

Heaven does all it can to nurture the unique seed that it has planted within each of us. However, heaven's only vested interest is that this unique aspect of *dao* be expressed in the world. Ultimately heaven will sacrifice the individual before it sacrifices its own expression of spontaneous self-becoming. Heaven does not care who does the expressing of its will just so long as its will is expressed. Hence, there are two ways of returning.

The first involves returning to the root in life represented by the *yuanqi* and manifesting the will of heaven as it is stored there. Here we continually establish the connection between metal and water, which allows for a perpetual return and "coming into being." However, if we turn our back on destiny and the link between metal and water is broken, then we perish, returning instead back into the "mysterious workings" of the eternal *dao.*

In treatment, there are times when the separation of *yin* and *yang* progresses past the point that therapy can restore physical health. However, even then, it is still possible to restore to the patient the consciousness of original nature so that destiny may be fulfilled. Ultimately, healing must be concerned with the evolution of the individual rather than solely with his or her survival—the domain of modern medicine. The practitioner of the inner tradition is always assisting patients in their return to original nature. When heaven wills this as a renewal of life, the practitioner assists in the furthering of that life. When the connection between metal and water separates and the condition has gone beyond what nature can restore, the practitioner still assists patients in their return, back to the greater origin of life which is heaven. *The Book of Liezi (Lieh Tzu)* reminds us, "Dying is the virtue in us going to its destination. The men of old called a dead man 'a man who has gone back.' Saying that the dead have gone back they implied that the living are travelers. The traveler who forgets to go back is a man who mistakes his home."[23]

Summary

The mysterious pass, Kunlun Mountain, the turning point, and the husband/wife imbalance are all concepts describing the mechanism that preserves the fundamental integrity of heaven and earth in the macrocosm and microcosm. The imagery of the separation of the *yuanqi* in Chinese creation mythology is precisely replicated physiologically as the husband/wife imbalance. Further, the dynamics of this pulse pattern are described at length in the *Yijing* commentaries of hexagrams 23 and 24. That the same theme weaves its way through creation mythology, philosophy, alchemy, physiology, and pulse diagnoses underscores the importance for the student of Chinese medicine to have a well-rounded understanding of these domains.

In the microcosm, the integrity of the two universal poles—heaven and earth—is preserved by the interpenetration of the *yuanqi*, early and later heaven, and the *jing* and *shen*. The traditional practitioner must help the patient preserve and restore the quality of these relationships so the fundamental integrity of life's functions may be maintained. This is done by leading the patient toward that forgotten truth of original nature which lies in one's heart of hearts. For true healing lies only in remembering and restoring this original self. How can this spiritual achievement be accomplished within the venue of traditional Chinese medicine? It is knowledge of the patient's constitutional type that equips the practitioner with a view leading ever onward toward the flame of destiny that lies within each patient's heart of hearts as well as the tools to fan it.

Questions

People often hear an internal voice guiding them toward right action but fail to follow the guidance received. Instead, they follow a course of action that gradually undermines the integrity of their health.

1. How often do you hear an inner voice telling you what to do

that you neglect to follow even though you are aware the course of action you have chosen is not the most empowering path you could take?

2. Is there a situation in your life you are resigned to that is compromising your health and well-being?

3. What personal attribute would empower you to listen to your inner voice and find the will to change your situation for the better?

4. Do you have a five-element association for such an attribute?

5. Can you think of a point combination or herbal formula that would empower such an attribute?

6. What officials and elements does it involve?

NOTES

1. Kohn, 1992, p. 100.
2. Cleary, 1986a, p. 95.
3. The names of these hexagrams have been translated variously. Wilhelm terms hexagram 23 as "splitting apart"; Liu Yiming terms it "stripping away." Liu also calls this hexagram "the door of death" and "the door of killing the self" in an attempt to describe it functionally. Wilhelm terms hexagram 24 as both "return" and "the turning point," whereas Liu uses "return" and "gate of birth."
4. Wilhelm, 1968, p. 93.
5. Ibid.
6. Ibid., p. 104.
7. Cleary, 1986b, p. 108.
8. Ibid., p. 106. Note that I have substituted the word "*qi*," which Cleary translates as "energy."
9. Wilhelm, 1968, p. 94.
10. Cleary, 1986b, p. 259.
11. Cleary, 1989, p. 57.
12. Wilhelm, 1968, p. 506.
13. The *Yijing* on hexagram 24; in Wilhelm, 1968, p. 98.
14. Wu, 1991, p. 113.
15. Cleary, 1986a, p. 95. If one does not return to original nature during life, then eventually the flood waters will rise and carry the primal brother and sister (one's *yuanqi* and life essence) back through the golden gate to the tomb of the *dao*.
16. Chen, 1989, p. 152.
17. In Cleary, 1986a, p. 34.
18. One colleague has noted that a husband/wife imbalance which resists treatment

often is associated with a high incidence of automobile accidents.

19. The *qi*-wild pulse condition is a loss of functional contact between the *yin* and *yang* of specific organ systems indicated by a unique set of pulse qualities. If not resolved, it may lead to death. See Hammer (1990, pp. 315, 336–338).

20. The concept of "possession," as it occurs throughout several traditions of Chinese medicine, is applicable here. Often the patient will be so stuck in one form of emotional expression (the internal devils) that there is no room for any spontaneity or subtlety of expression. The practitioner is unable to make contact with any sane or clear influences at the patient's core.

21. Homann, 1976, p. 47.

22. Watson, 1964a, p. 49.

23. Graham, 1990, p. 26. Girardot (1983, p. 160) points out the emphasis in Daoism is on learning to return while still alive. *Gui* (鬼), "the dead," is a homophone of *gui* (歸), meaning "to return" or "one who has gone home."

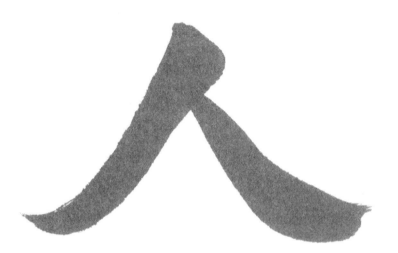

8

THE
FIVE
ELEMENTS

C HAPTERS 1 THROUGH 7 FOCUSED ON THE PROCESSES
that guide the course of human life from conception through
death. We discussed how each human life follows developmental stages
based on the inner workings of the *dao*. The numerical significance of
one, two, and three was emphasized as they correspond in the macrocosm to earth, *chongqi*, and heaven, and in the microcosm to the
primordial influences of *jing, qi,* and *shen*.

The fourth stage of *dao* represents either a return to primordial
unity or a fall from unity to the material universe of the "ten thousand
things." The number five allows us to navigate in the material world
and to discern how the influence of early heaven impacts the functioning of material reality. Chapters 8 through 10 explain how the
five-element system and the notion of constitutional type play a role in
recognizing the loss of, and facilitating the return to, original nature.
Chapter 11 examines the physiology of *qi* and blood from the perspective of the inner tradition.

Orienting to the Five-Element System

Five-element theory provides a qualitative standard of reference that allows us to characterize the functional dynamics inherent in any observable phenomena.[1] All observations are referenced to the standards—water, wood, fire, earth, and metal—as they describe the dynamic movements of *dao* inherent in any given situation. Based on the assessment of quality rather than structure, the five-element system is ideal for studying the nonmaterial aspects of being that exist in the domains of mind and spirit. Here we examine the theoretical basis of the five-element system as it pertains to the fulfillment of destiny.

The Five Transformations[2]

> During the Great Antiquity the sovereign pair, possessing the supreme power of the *dao*, placed it in the middle. Spirits yielded and transformations took place. The four sides were bathed in peace. Thereafter, heaven followed a regular motion and earth remained immobile; the progression [of seasons] took place without fail; waters flowed out without containment, providing both beginning and end for the ten thousand beings.[3]

Although several of the relations found in five-element theory (such as the five directions) are evidenced in records of the Shang dynasty (1766–1122 B.C.E.), the five-element system was not fully elaborated until about 350 B.C.E. by Zou Yen.[4] Note that the phrase *wuxing* (五行), commonly translated as "five elements," has been better translated by Porkert as the five "evolutive phases."[5] The term "elements" suggests a static fixed manifestation of life, yet water, wood, fire, earth, and metal were never conceived by the Chinese as elemental constituents of matter as atoms are in modern physics. The term *wuxing* rather denotes five dynamic movements that continually transform into each other as the seasons do.

The language used by the early Chinese to describe their world is one of simple poetic images rich in associative value. Water names the element associated with winter because of its tendency to freeze and become focused in that season. Wood names the element associated with spring because it grows rapidly at that time of year. Fire names the element associated with summer because of the increased heat during those months when the sun reaches its zenith. Earth names the element associated with late summer as the fields are abundant then with the fruit of earth's bounty. The imagery of the metal element is often the most difficult for new students to comprehend. Minerals are a natural expression of the metal element in nature. Minerals are of great value yet lie hidden within the earth and symbolize the essential, precious, and rarified aspects of life. Fall is the season when what is of value must be harvested while all else must be left to wither in the fields. Thus metal names the element associated with fall as the farmer's knife reaps the harvest of that season.

The laws governing nature's dynamic process of change were codified over thousands of years. The system of five transformations provides a qualitative standard of reference to which we may refer all observations regarding the functional dynamics of all phenomena.[6] The five-element model became an implicit part of virtually every discipline in ancient China. Considerations of the five elements are foundational in domains as diverse as military strategy, the martial arts, architecture, painting, poetry, politics, and medicine.

As our ancestor, the *dao's* implicit movement is present in all things to which it gives birth. In its movement away from and return to itself, the *dao* is centered on an axis, or "pole of emptiness" *(xuji: 虚極)*.[7] The four stages of movement and the central pivot (stage five) are present in later heaven as the four seasons and the five elements (see Figure 8.1 and Figures 8.2a and 8.2b).

Reconciliation of Five Elements and Four Seasons

The earth element corresponds to the number 5 in the Daoist enumeration of creation. The number 5 in Chinese *(wu:五)* is a picture of the earth (+) showing four directions and a center (yielding the number 5), located between heaven and earth (二), the primal *yin* and *yang*.

The scientists of ancient China struggled to formulate a "unified field theory" that would combine all the various numerical systems into an accurate calendar. In so doing, one of the major difficulties was in reconciling the existence of five elements but only four seasons.[8] Over time, three different solutions were arrived at. In the first scheme, the earth phase is divided into four eighteen-day segments with each placed at the end of one of the other seasons. Although the most popular solution to the problem, it was heavily criticized by Wang Fuzhi as "truncating a duck to augment a crane" or, in other words, forcing the issue.[9]

Movements of Dao Correlated with the Appropriate Stage of Dao					
Movement	Stage	Element	Season	Power	Number
Great	One	Water	Winter	Origin	1,6
Moving away	Two	Fire	Summer	Naming	2,7
Far away	Three	Wood	Spring	Distinction	3,8
Return	Four	Metal	Fall	Death/Return	4,9
Pivot	Five	Earth	Late summer	Integration	5,10

Figure 8.1
MOVEMENTS OF *DAO* CORRELATED WITH THE APPROPRIATE STAGE OF *DAO*

The movements and stages of dao, *which occur cosmologically in the domain of early heaven, are the implicit basis of all transformation experienced during life. These movements occur as the five elements in later heaven and denote the broad qualities of* dao *as it manifests in life. Each of the elements is associated with a power that typifies the quality of dynamic change evidenced when that element is influential. Water (one) is the origin of life and is identified with the seed of the inherited constitution. Fire (two) is associated with the activation of the infant's* shen *and therefore self-awareness. Wood (three) is associated with the distinctions made by the mind perceiving duality in the world. Metal (four), the fourth stage, governs the return of all things back to the unity of primordial* dao. *Earth (five) provides the center around which the seasons rotate and governs integrity through transitions. The numbers 1 through 5 denote the creation of the five elements in early heaven. The numbers 6 through 10 denote the order of creation of the elements in later heaven.*

Each of the five elements is associated with a season, color, sound, odor, emotion, and virtue. In recognizing which of these associations predominate an individual's self-expression, a practitioner may assess the relative balance of the five elements in each patient. The season associated with each element denotes the time of year during which the expression of a given element is particularly strong. These associations are discussed in further detail in Chapters 9 and 10.

In the second solution, earth is seen as the transition point around which the seasons change. This is represented in the five-element chart (Figure 8.2a) showing earth as the center or pivot point. The last effort to reconcile the numbers of 4 and 5 is seen in traditions that consider the earth element to be representative of a fifth season occurring between summer and fall and located between the fire and metal element on the *sheng* cycle (Figure 8.2b). All three ways of looking at this question have their useful attributes. In taking the essence from each, the earth element may be thought of as providing stability and centeredness during transitions.

The Five Elements and Humanity

Daoists viewed humans as microcosms of the universe, and the five-element system allows for the assessment of each individual's relationship to his or her own inner nature as well as to the surrounding world. Five-element theory describes the character and relationships of the identifiable functions comprising human nature. The associations of the five-element system allow us to qualitatively assess an individual's relative degree of functional balance through the interpretation of signs that emanate continually with every form of personal expression.

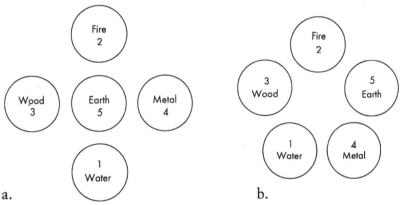

Figure 8.2
THE FIVE ELEMENTS

The five elements are depicted in two different configurations. In (a) the elements associated with the four seasons are shown cycling around the earth, which represents the primal axis as it exists in later heaven. Human beings, in aligning themselves with this central axis, may witness life as it transforms around them. This model therefore emphasizes the relative nature of all phenomena to the perspective of the observer.

In (b) the earth element has been moved to a location between fire and metal to create the sheng *cycle. The fifth season (late summer) was created in an attempt to reconcile the existence of five elements but only four seasons. Humanity is recognized as one of the primal forces in the triumvirate of heaven, human, and earth. In this scenario, earth is recognized not just as representing the neutral position of the observer, but as a dynamic force of nature that equally affects, and is affected by, the other four elements. Thus the awareness of the observer is recognized as vital in maintaining the balance of nature.*

The five-element tradition of Chinese medicine finds its theoretical basis in the transformations of *dao* enumerated in the *Dao De Jing* (discussed in Chapter 1). In the five-element system, each individual is believed to have a constitutional tendency to emulate the quality of expression of one season of the year more than others.[10] The natural qualities of this season define an individual's inherited weaknesses and strengths. Some associations of each element are listed in Figure 8.3.

In its most basic form, the tradition elaborates the five broad movements of *dao* into twelve "officials," the relative balance of which constitute the dynamic web of the *sheng* and *ke* cycles (Figure 8.4). The *sheng* cycle (creative cycle, *xiangsheng:*相生序) names the order in which the elements produce, or give birth to, each other. Hence the water element may be said to give birth to the wood element along the *sheng* cycle. This sequence is the natural order that the seasons create during the year. The *ke* cycle (control cycle, *xiangkexu:*相克序) gives the order in which the elements limit, or control, each other. Hence water may be said to control fire across the *ke* cycle. An example of this relationship between water and fire is that the potential present in any seed (water) always limits the maximum height (fire) a tree may attain given the best possible environment.

In a state of functional balance the elements produce and limit each other effortlessly. When *qi* stops flowing in its natural progression around the *sheng* cycle and becomes fixed in its expression, the elements begin to overcontrol each other across the *ke* cycle. Note that *qi,* which travels along the *ke* cycle and is termed "aggressive energy," may form the basis of serious pathology (e.g., cancer, heart disease, and mental illness).[11] The functional consequences of this condition correspond to the fifth stage of development as described by Liu Yiming (see Chapter 6). Liu tells us that at this stage the five elements become conditioned and begin to separate.

Figure 8.3
THE BASIC ASSOCIATIONS OF THE FIVE ELEMENTS

The Basic Associations of the Five Elements					
Element	Color	Sound	Odor	Emotion	Virtue
Water	Blue	Groan	Putrid	Fear	Wisdom
Wood	Green	Shout	Rancid	Anger	Benevolence
Fire	Red	Laugh	Scorched	Joy	Propriety
Earth	Yellow	Sing	Sweet	Sympathy	Integrity
Metal	White	Weep	Rotten	Grief	Righteousness

In addition to our elemental type, our constitution may be further assessed according to the dictates of a particular organ system. Each of these twelve functions are further elaborated into many discrete aspects of function, which are represented by and accessible through the acupuncture points on the function's related meridian. Further, any given function has within it the implicit presence of the other elements and functions (see Figure 8.4). This presence is found, most notably, in the five-element points and reunion points that are present on each meridian.[12]

The Five-Element Points and the Transfer of Virtue

The holographic nature of the five-element system is such that each of the twelve officials possesses unique functions, yet each one is implicit

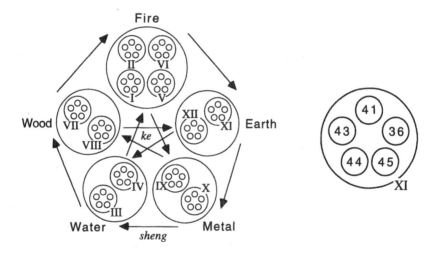

Figure 8.4
THE *SHENG* AND *KE* CYCLES

(a) The five elements are shown in their sheng *and* ke *cycle relationships. Each organ is denoted in the order of flow of* qi *according to the Chinese clock beginning with the heart (I). The elements create each other around the* sheng *cycle and control each other around the* ke *cycle. The elements are further divided into the twelve officials that comprise the* yin *and* yang *aspect of each element. Each official retains its own discrete function yet has within it the implicit representation of the whole five-element cycle. This representation exists as the five-element points that are associated with each meridian.*

(b) Here the five-element points associated with the stomach official are represented by their numerical position on the stomach meridian. Hence Stomach-44 is the water point, Stomach-43 is the wood point, and so forth.

within the functioning of the others. For example, the gallbladder empowers decision making, yet the facility of discernment is implicit within the sorting function of the small intestine or the stomach's function of integration. The five-element points associated with each meridian offer a way to empower any virtue associated with an official within any other official.

Each meridian possesses a horary point, which is the point with the same elemental nature as the meridian's associated element. For example, the liver is associated with the wood element, and therefore Liver-1, the wood point on the liver meridian, is also the horary point. Horary points strongly empower the specific virtues associated with each official. Hence Heart Protector-8, a fire point on a fire meridian, is particularly strong for empowering any specific virtue, such as openness or emotional warmth, associated with the heart protector official. This is particularly true if treatment occurs at the time of day and seasonal peak associated with each official. For example, Lung-8, if needled between 3 and 5 A.M. on the fall equinox, would be particularly potent at empowering the virtues and functions associated with the lung official. The relationship of the Chinese clock to the specific functions of each official are elaborated in Figure 8.5.

Think of a horary point as a "transmitting" point capable of empowering a specific virtue associated with an official within any other official if it is needled simultaneously with a "receiving" point on another meridian. A receiving point is that point on a meridian which possesses the same elemental nature as the transmitting point. For example, a virtue associated with the liver official is self-esteem as empowered by the vision of what is fundamental in one's life. As discussed in Chapter 13, an important point for empowering the virtue of self-esteem is the horary point Liver-1 ("great esteem"). If we wish to empower the virtue of self-esteem and deep vision within the heart protector official, the appropriate points to choose according to this method would be Liver-1 as the transmitting point and Heart Protector-9, the wood point on the heart protector meridian, as the receiving point. If we wanted to empower the virtue of planning within the stomach official, we would choose Liver-1 and pair it with Stomach-43, the wood point on the stomach meridian. Generally either the transmitting or receiving point is located on the patient's constitutional meridian.

Note that this method is not a way of transferring *qi* either by tonifying a deficiency or dispersing a relative excess. In the previous example, if liver is excess relative to the stomach, this treatment will not disperse the liver or tonify the stomach. Rather this method allows the practitioner to address the functional relationship of two officials simultaneously regardless of their *sheng* and *ke* cycle relationships and relative state of excess or deficiency. For example, a virtue associated with the lung official is receptivity. Patients who may have suffered a traumatic loss in a relationship may have closed their heart protector in a way that they are no longer receptive (a characteristic of metal) to intimacy (a characteristic of fire). According to this method the practitioner may choose to treat Lung-8 as the transmitting point and Heart Protector-5 as the receiving point. Both Lung-8 and Heart Protector-5 are the metal points on their respective meridians. This treatment could empower the lung's virtue of receptivity within the heart protector official.

A good exercise for the student of the five elements is to imagine any aspect of being associated with a given official and how it is present implicitly within the function of every other official. Using the model of transmitting and receiving points discussed here, a point combination may be generated to address any such functional imbalance between two officials.

The Chinese Clock

The Chinese clock designates a two-hour period of time during which the function of each official is most empowered by cosmological forces (see Figure 8.5). The functional low time of each official is twelve hours later. For instance, the high point of lung function is 3 to 5 A.M. and its low point is 3 to 5 P.M. The Chinese clock also designates the directional flow of *qi* through the officials. Hence *qi* flow may be thought of as beginning with the heart, proceeding to the small intestine, onto the bladder, and ultimately to the spleen, where it completes a full circle back to the heart—beginning a new cycle.

The Chinese clock may help a practitioner know if the expression of a particular function is either excess or deficient in nature. For example, theory predicts that a deficient condition would improve during an official's functional high point, whereas an excess condition might be expected to worsen at that time due to the relative increase in *qi* in the associated function.

Lastly, the Chinese clock may aid the practitioner in selecting horary points. If a horary point is chosen during its high or low point on the Chinese clock, it can provide an unusually strong tonification or sedation of that official's function. This is especially true when points are

The Chinese Clock			
Official	**Flow of qi**	**Time**	**Function**
Heart	I	11 A.M. -1 P.M.	Emperor; coordinates the whole
Small intestine	II	1 - 3 P.M.	Sorts pure from impure
Bladder	III	3 - 5 P.M.	Stores and utilizes reserves
Kidney	IV	5 - 7 P.M.	Stores inherited constitution
Heart protector	V	7 - 9 P.M.	Governs circulation, sexuality, and intimacy
Three heater	VI	9 -11 P.M.	Regulates thermostat, social relations
Gallbladder	VII	11 P.M. - 1 A.M.	Oversees discernment, decision making
Liver	VIII	1 - 3 A.M.	Makes plans
Lung	IX	3 - 5 A.M.	Connects to essence, receptivity
Large intestine	X	5 - 7 A.M.	Lets go of impurity
Stomach	XI	7 - 9 A.M.	Integrates the whole
Spleen	XII	9 - 11 A.M.	Distributes nourishment

Figure 8.5

THE CHINESE CLOCK

The officials in the order of qi flow according to the Chinese clock. The function contributed by each official is summarized as well.

used seasonally. Hence Tonifying Liver-1 at 3 A.M. on the vernal
equinox could provide a very strong tonification to the liver official,
particularly in a patient whose constitutional element is wood.

The Five Elements and Holism

The worldviews offered by the Chinese science of the five elements and
that of Western analytic science complement each other. See the discussion in the appendix. It is interesting to note, however, that a worldview
has arisen out of modern quantum physics which is strikingly similar to
that of five-element theory. The holographic paradigm is important to our
discussion because it may help orient you to the quality of thought
inherent in the practice of the five-element tradition. It did not arise independently in the West but has a historical connection to Daoist
enumeration and the philosophies discussed here. The mathematician
Gottfried Leibniz (1646–1716), discoverer of integral and differential

calculus, proposed a similar model in 1714.[13] His studies of the *Yijing* contributed to Leibniz's discovery of binary math, which is the system of information transmission used in computers and all digital electronics.

In Chapter 1 we saw that the *Dao De Jing* describes the *dao* as a unity in which all things are implicit in each other. This unity is unknowable by the human mind, which can only comprehend individual things and perceives the interpenetration of all things as chaos. This description of reality precisely conforms to the structure of a holographic image (Figure 8.6).

How a Hologram Is Constructed

Holography is a lenseless form of photography that uses laser beams as a light source. A hologram is made by capturing the interference pattern of a wave field of light on a photographic plate. When the plate (the hologram) is illuminated by a coherent light source (one in which all frequencies are identical, for example a laser), the original image that created the interference pattern is regenerated in three dimensions. Because no focusing lens is used, the pattern on the plate appears as a meaningless array of swirls. Of great interest is the fact that illumination of any portion of the plate will produce the whole of the original image, although in less detail than if the entire plate is used. Hence every part of the hologram is needed to reproduce the complete image.

A parallel of this principle in biological systems is that every cell in the body contains in its DNA a template of the entire organism. However, cells from different organs and tissues perform different functions and all must be present for the integrity of the organism to be maintained. This same principle is maintained in the *sheng* and *ke* cycle relationships of the five elements and twelve officials as they are depicted in Figure 8.5. Each of the officials maintains its unique function while containing an implicit image of all the five elements.

In five-element theory it is impossible to discuss one function without eventually discussing all of them. For example, the small intestine in sorting the pure from impure implicitly relies on the decision-making function of the gallbladder. In accordance with the holographic theory, all functions must be present for life to continue, and each function retains its own identity while containing information about the whole.

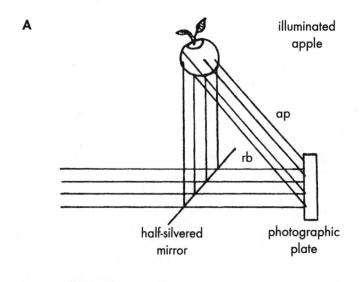

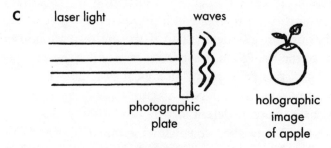

Figure 8.6
HOLOGRAPHY

A. *Light from a laser is passed through a half-silvered mirror. Part of the beam illuminates the apple while the other part travels directly to the photographic plate. When the light reflected off the apple (ap) interacts with the reference beam (rb), an interference pattern is created and recorded on the photographic plate.*

B. *The interference pattern appears as a meaningless array of swirls on the plate (the hologram), yet contains an implicitly ordered representation of the apple.*

C. *If a laser is used to illuminate the hologram, a wavefront is created that is similar to the one originally coming off the apple. To an observer, the apple appears in full detail and in three dimensions. If only a small portion of the hologram is illuminated, the whole image of the apple still appears, but in less detail and from fewer angles.*

Holographic Theory

Physicist David Bohm has proposed that the universe itself is constructed on the same principles as a hologram. He tells us that the equations of quantum mechanics predict there is more energy in one cubic centimeter of space than is contained in matter in the known universe. To Bohm, "matter is like a small ripple on this tremendous ocean of energy, having some relative stability, and being manifest." Bohm's description of the emergence of matter is quite similar to the Chinese view of primordial being arising as the *yuanqi* out of the vast ocean of *dao*.

In Figure 8.6, the image of the apple is enfolded into the "implicate" order of the swirls on the holographic plate. According to holographic theory, just as the hologram contains an unmanifest, although implicitly ordered image of the apple, material reality evolves from an underlying implicate order. This order is enfolded in nature in the form of electromagnetic waves, sound waves, electron beams, and all other wave forms of movement. Colliding with each other, these waves produce holographs constructed by the brain, which interprets them as material reality. The waves of the implicate order are "carried" on the vast ocean of underlying energy that Bohm has termed the "holomovement."

Five-element theory may be considered a map of the holomovement. It allows us to assess the implicate order of *dao* as it manifests explicitly in each individual. This is done by gathering data through the four examinations (to see, hear, ask, and feel) and integrating it to assess each individual's dynamic pattern of functioning.

How is it that five-element theory allows us to know the implicate realm by studying the explicate? Consider the following example. Imagine the vast ocean of energy described by Bohm. Into this ocean we throw two rocks. Assume rock A is an individual's inherited constitution and rock B the sum total of his or her life experience (environmental influences). The rocks will produce concentric circles emanating outward that will eventually overlap.

The crests and troughs of overlapping waves will produce an interference pattern similar to the swirls on the holographic plate. The holograph generated will be that of the underlying event (the rocks tossed into the lake, or life process of the individual), which is now invisible to us except for the waves. If a photograph is taken from directly above at time T-1, it may look like Figure 8.7.

The wave pattern in Figure 8.7 represents the momentary functional dynamic of the person we are examining. Notice that the

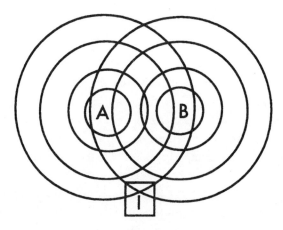

Figure 8.7
WAVES

examination of any overlapping region (i.e., region I) will give us information about the entire underlying event, because only that event could have resulted in this specific wave interaction. The event we wish to know about is this individual's constitutional type as viewed through the momentary combination of all inherited and environmental influences. Our constitutional element is the foundation that shapes every possible manifestation of our being during life. The way we learn about a patient's constitution is through the interpretation of manifest signs such as the patient's color, sound, odor, and emotion. The hologram of the five elements is implicit (implicate) in the manifest (explicate) signs that emanate continually from each person.

The amount of information we are able to glean from a given sign is limited only by our powers of observation and the adequacy of the system of interpretation we are using. Every region of overlap in Figure 8.7 gives us information about the whole. The more regions we study, the better we know the underlying event. Hence constitution is knowable in an instant from the perception of any clinical sign, because the qualities of individual constitutional type permeate every aspect of being continually. However, the degree to which different clinical indicators confirm each other is the degree to which an integrated diagnosis can be formulated.

Each official has a tendency to express itself more in certain parts of our behavior, personality, and physiology than in others. (Otherwise, a system based on the differentiation of signs, such as five-element theory, would not be possible.) However, the function of every official (the whole) must be present in some proportion in every atom (the individual parts) constituting a human being. For instance, the qualities present on the left distal pulse position represent heart function, but implicit in whatever qualities are present in that position are all the functions of the five elements and twelve officials.

The waves continually emanating (Figure 8.7) may be likened to the explicate realm of the holomovement. Photographs taken from above at different times will yield different pictures of a patient's functional balance, physical symptomatology, and life story. Yet each picture will provide us with information about the same underlying event, which is the patient's constitutional type. In this sense, time does not exist in the holomovement. Signs that appear simultaneously are related and useful in diagnosis. This is true regardless of their separation in space. For instance, signs occurring concurrently on the tongue, abdomen, and foot may confirm each other because the twelve functions permeate them all.

Karl Pribram states, "In the absence of space-time coordinates, the usual causality upon which most scientific explanation depends must also be suspended. Complementaries, synchronicities, symmetries, and dualities must be called upon as explanatory principles."[14] This is precisely reflected in Chinese medicine, which deals with standards of reference based on the complementarity of *yin* and *yang*, the synchronicity of the signs it interprets, and the symmetry of the five elements and twelve officials. As we see in Chapter 9, the concept of constitutional type is the ever present cause that allows the practitioner to assess the quality of each patient's destiny.

Summary

Five-element theory is a purely relational system of thought that allows us to qualify the functional relationships which exist in any given moment and in any observable phenomena. Reference to the five elements allows us to experience the implicit nature of *dao* as it supports the instantaneous presence of each thing to which it gives birth. The basic associations of the five elements presented in this chapter are only a beginning point of inquiry for the serious student. Color, sound, odor, emotion, season, time, and number are the foundation of reference in the five-element system. The student endeavors to recognize the quality of all arising phenomena referenced to these basic associations until, eventually, one is intuitively aware of the inner workings of *dao* moment to moment both within the treatment room and without.

Questions

The five-element system allows for the consideration of a human beings relationship to nature both within and without.

1. In your own tradition of practice, what tools enable you to consider the role played by the *quality* of a patient's inherited constitution in contributing to his or her relative balance of health or illness?

NOTES

1. See Porkert, 1982, p. 44.
2. Here I provide a brief review of five-element theory that may serve as an introduction for readers not familiar with this system of thought. For a more comprehensive introduction to this material, see Connelly, 1994.
3. Larre et al., 1986, pp. 95–96.
4. Kaptchuk, 1983, p. 345.
5. Porkert, 1982, p. 2.
6. See Porkert, 1982, p. 44.
7. Chen, 1989, p. 94.
8. Henderson, 1984, p. 181.
9. Ibid.
10. The concept of the five-element constitutional types is presented in Chapter 64 of the *Ling Shu* and later here in Chapters 9–11.
11. This concept can be traced to the 53rd and 54th difficult issue in the *Nanjing* (see Unschuld, 1986, pp. 485–494).
12. A reunion point is an acupuncture point at which the functions of several officials may be addressed simultaneously. For instance, Liver-13 ("chapter gate") may be used for simultaneously treating both the liver and the spleen officials.
13. In his text *La Monadologie* (Monadology), Leibniz proposes that all of creation consists of basic building blocks he calls monads. All individual substances, or monads, are dimensionless points that contain all of their properties—past, present, and future—and, indeed, the entire world.
14. Pribram, p. 34; in Wilber, 1982.

9

CONSTITUTIONAL
TYPE

Man receives the decree of heaven (ming),
and therefore is loftier (than other) creatures.
– DONG CHONGSHU[1]

HEAVEN, IN CONFERRING DESTINY ON HUMANS, HAS
cast us as mediators between heaven and earth, making us one
of the three primal powers in the universe. Although heaven may will a
unique nature for each of us, it is not certain that each individual will be
true to this nature and manifest destiny. Just as the *dao* loses its original
nature of unity to give birth to the "ten thousand things," so too do we
humans fall from our original nature as we gain self-consciousness. The
concept of constitutional type provides practitioners of the inner tradition with a window deep into their patients' being that helps illuminate
both the nature of their destiny and what blocks its expression.

Constitutional type is one of the features that distinguishes Chinese
medicine's complement to the practice of Western medicine. Inherent
in the concept are the very deepest traditions of Chinese philosophical
and spiritual thought as well as the worldview of the more modern
holographic paradigm. In this chapter I trace the origins of constitutional type and discuss its relevance to Chinese medicine as a modern
science of the human condition. I show how constitutional type pro-

vides a framework for both assessing the quality of humans' destiny and guiding them back toward the full self-expression that is synonymous with health.

My discussion of constitutional type is influenced by the concept of "causative factor" taught by J.R. Worsley and the Traditional Acupuncture Institute. However, I consider the term "causative factor" to be misleading because the traditional Chinese concept of causality is so different from that used in the analytical sciences. I suggest that "constitutional type" is a more accurate term as I use it throughout this text. The concept of constitutional type elaborates the concept of causative factor, inasmuch as I pair the constitutional types with specific qualities of destiny associated with the five elemental virtues. Much of my discussion of constitutional type reflects my own thoughts and does not reflect the teaching of the Worsley school.

Constitution: The Theme and Thread of Life

> *Holding on to the* dao *of old,*
> *So as to steer in the world of now.*
> *To be able to know the beginning of old,*
> *It is to know the thread of* dao.
> – DAO DE JING [2]

The different stages in the evolution of *dao* are not separated in time and space but rather occur simultaneously in each moment. The *dao* as unity is always present at the heart of each thing, and, in each moment, it continually falls from, and spontaneously returns to, its original nature. This rhythm is both the heartbeat and breath of life. The motion of the *dao*, eternally moving away from and returning to itself, is the ever-present cause that lies at the heart of all creation.[3] By centering our "self" and shutting off the senses, we are able to return immediately to the truth that lies in heaven's heart. Meditation is the symbolic act of closing the seven holes in our head and returning the primordial influence of *dao* to our life.[4]

The *dao* as the primary cause is not a "cause" in the sense used by modern science, however, which views time as linear and thus claims a cause must always precede an effect. Chinese medicine, in contrast, proceeds by synthesizing a picture out of all the information present in a given moment. Cause is not seen as a past event but rather as that which ties together and generates every event. Clinically, this "cause" is the patient's constitutional type, which "colors" the spontaneous expression of *dao* as it unfolds in each individual's life, contributing simultaneously both the nature and the nurture of the individual. This cause may be described as each person's reason for being. In this sense the term "cause" may be viewed as that "cause" for which we work in life. It is the purpose *(zhi)* that lies in each human heart, placed there by heaven at conception. Acting in a way that is consistent with our innermost purpose constitutes the fulfillment of destiny.

Every novel, from the first word to the last, has a central theme around which the plot is organized. In a similar fashion, the events of human life are organized around a theme that ties the moment of conception to the moment of death. This is the thread of individual destiny that weaves together the "fabric" of each human life and lies at the heart of each individual's constitution.[5] The theme around which our life unfolds is organized in a way that is both knowable and therapeutically useful to the practitioner of the internal tradition. The concept of constitutional type allows the practitioner to know the nature of the thread of *dao* as it is uniquely present in each patient. This is not to say that the practitioner knows the precise destiny of each individual. That corresponds to the eternal *dao,* which always eludes our knowing. This principle is addressed by the *Dao De Jing,* Chapter 14, which tells us that the *dao* may be looked at but not seen, listened to but not heard, and grabbed yet never caught. A system such as the five elements affords us a glimpse into another's true nature and destiny, yet this is not to be equated with fully knowing the destiny of another. We may know the quality of a patient's inborn nature but the ultimate truth of their being cannot be arrived at, for that is known only to heaven.

Rather, constitutional type provides a framework for looking ever onward toward that "light" which burns in each person's depth so long as life exists. We are reminded by Han Feizi (280 B.C.E.) that "[t]he enlightened ruler holds fast to the beginning in order to understand the wellspring of all beings."[6]

Just as the central theme of a story never changes from the first word to the last, so too does individual constitution remain the same throughout life. Although the theme may never change, the plot may be transformed from one of disharmony to one of harmony. This transformation is the aim of the traditional practitioner. The pristine purity of *dao,* always present at the patient's core, must be the aim with the placement of every acupuncture needle and the prescription of every herb.

The Sheng *and* Ke *Cycles*

Think of the twelve functional relationships that constitute the dynamic web of the *sheng* and *ke* cycles as a chain. The patient's constitutional type is the weakest link in that chain. Therapeutically, if everything is done to strengthen the other eleven links, it is analogous to focusing therapy on only the symptomatic expressions of, and compensations for, the underlying weakness. If the weakest link is not addressed, then, despite other actions, nothing has been done to strengthen the chain. By first addressing the weakest functional link as the focus of treatment, the other functions may stop compensating for its aberrant behavior. Treatment must be addressed toward the whole, but with an emphasis on the patient's constitutional element, which is the common thread of imbalance that touches each function.

The diagnosis of constitutional type must not be allowed to overly define the patient in the eyes of the practitioner, as is often the case with the diagnostic categories of Western medicine. Patients are not just treated on the meridians that correspond to their constitutional type. Rather, their constitutions, as a basic elemental imbalance, serve as the focus in relation to which everything is treated. A person theoretically has only one constitutional type during life, but it may be masked by certain traumatic life events that generate an elemental overlay which must be resolved before the constitutional type can be addressed directly. For example, rheumatic fever during childhood may so affect the liver that the imbalance resulting from the illness may make a person appear constitutionally wood. After a course of treatment, this "overlay" will often resolve, revealing a picture of the underlying element that is closer to the patient's essence.

I consider the question of whether or not constitutional type can change to be unanswerable. I believe that, ultimately, a given practitioner can never actually diagnose a patient, but is limited to diagnosing the relationship that lies between him or herself and the patient. Different practitioners may generate different diagnoses, each being able to reach the patient in his or her own unique way. Hence an absolutely correct diagnosis is not possible, since the "correct" diagnosis is one which yields a treatment that is the most efficient at balancing the patient in the moment. As soon as a therapeutic action is taken it can never be known if, in that instant now past, another action would have worked better.

Constitutional Diagnosis as Family Therapy

Family therapy addresses the functional dynamics of a group rather than focusing intervention on a given individual who exhibits the most obvious behavioral problems. For example, a child may be underperforming in school and beginning to be a discipline problem. Rather than focusing intervention on the symptom and disciplining the child, it might prove more fruitful to examine the functional dynamics of the entire family. Should it be determined that the mother is an alcoholic, focusing therapy on her drinking problem might improve the child's well-being more than any intervention aimed directly at the child. To focus treatment on the child's symptoms would only result in a long gradual decline in the child's situation with greater disciplines being needed and eventual involvement in the legal system. But therapy that addresses the mother's behavior will touch the root cause of the imbalance.

This example illustrates the mother/child relationship, which is of great importance in the five-element tradition. It states that when symptomatology is seen in a given element, it is frequently the element which precedes it on the *sheng* cycle that is the root cause of the imbalance and often corresponds to the patient's constitutional type. The notion of constitutional type allows the practitioner of the inner tradition to see past symptoms toward the primary cause of all imbalances, which is the constitutionally destined tendency of each individual to forget the true self and to neglect the fulfillment of life's purpose.

The twelve officials may be conceived as constituting a family of interrelated functions. So long as each family member does his or her assigned job efficiently, harmony in the personal household of being is maintained. However, as soon as one member fails to perform adequately, the entire balance on which peace in the home depends becomes compromised. The practitioner's task is to determine which official stopped working first and is therefore the root source of all imbalances and symptoms. Every other clinical sign and symptom in every aspect of being is understood to be a secondary compensation for the failure of the constitutionally weak official to perform its function.

Consider a home in which twelve individuals live, each possessing a particular responsibility for running the household. One person is in charge of taking out the trash (large intestine), one cooks the food (stomach), one makes the plans (liver), one coordinates all activities (heart), and so forth. Life progresses smoothly until one day the large intestine, rushing to an appointment, neglects to pick up an empty soft drink can from the table and deposit it in the trash. Noticing that the large intestine has failed to perform its function, the stomach, busily cooking at the stove, obliges by taking a moment to walk to the table and deposit the can in the garbage where it belongs. The stomach is only too happy to do this because it likes the large intestine and, after all, it is only one can.

The moment the stomach expends its *qi* to support the poor function of the large intestine, a dysfunctional relationship is established that will eventually undermine the balance of the entire household. The time spent throwing away the solitary can is not spent by the stomach fulfilling its own function of cooking. Further, because another official performed the large intestine's job, the large intestine itself was disempowered, and in fact reinforced, not to fulfill its function appropriately in the future.

Noticing the following day that the can had been thrown away, the large intestine rushes out of the house and leaves a bag of garbage in the kitchen. The stomach realizes there will not be room in the trash for refuse after the next meal and so once again obliges by putting the trash out at the curb. This scenario progresses until eventually the large intestine is not performing its function at all. The stomach is now exhausted from both having to cook and take out the trash and, in disgust at having to cater to everyone else, stops cooking entirely. Now everyone in the home becomes distressed and the heart, in charge of coordinating all activities, calls a family meeting. Everyone is hungry and outraged at the stomach for failing to perform its function of cooking, and the large intestine sits quietly in the corner. The gallbladder demands justice and screams unrelentingly at the poor stomach.

An outside observer seeking to remedy this situation might be inclined to focus intervention on the member in the room who is screaming the loudest, in this case the gallbladder. Extending this analogy to the realm of medicine would entail treating the physical symptom that the person complains about the most (for example, treating the headache generated by the gallbladder's shouting in response to the current stress). A more astute observer might discern that all shouting in the room is directed at the stomach and infer that by aiming therapy at that organ, peace will be restored. We could consider this situation analogous to treating an underlying symptom that is thought to generate the primary complaint. For example, we might treat a person's headaches by addressing the digestion if we thought poor digestion was contributing to the genesis of the symptom.

The notion of constitutional type allows the most subtle practitioner to see past the current situation and all secondary compensations back toward the root of the problem. By supporting the function of the large intestine, the official that stopped working first, the stomach will be supported to once again begin cooking, and every other official will be empowered to cease compensating for the underlying primary imbalance. In this way not only will the patient's headaches subside, but improvement will be seen in every functional domain of life as well.

Diagnosis by Color, Sound, Odor, Emotion, and Pulse

Anybody who looks and knows it is to be called a spirit;
anybody who listens and knows it is to be called a sage;
anybody who asks and knows it is to be called an artisan;
anybody who feels the vessels and knows it is to be called
a skilled workman.
— NANJING[7]

The sixty-first difficult issue in the *Nanjing* compares the abilities of those who diagnose by looking (color) to that of the spirits *(shen)*, by sound to that of the sages, by asking to that of the artisans, and by pulse to the ability of the skilled worker. I take this as a hierarchy indicating that even using physical indicators such as the pulse is not as "deep" (revealing of spirit) a diagnostic method as the others mentioned. Just to look at the patient and know the diagnosis (destiny) is thus the highest form of practice.

In the five-element tradition, the determination of constitutional type is premised on the most subtle and rapidly changing (fast) wave forms that emanate from the patient's being. These are the patient's color, sound, odor, and emotion (CSOE). That these wave forms change so quickly reflects their synchronicity with the momentary functional state of the patient. The process of being in communication with these signs during diagnosis and treatment affords the practitioner the deepest possible contact with the patient's dynamic state of functioning.

The way an individual attaches meaning to life becomes embodied in every aspect of his or her being and is decipherable using the associations in the five-element system. By noticing every spoken word and subtle gesture and the patterns of behavior and attitude they reveal, the practitioner may weave a personal tapestry from the patient's presentation of color, sound, odor, and emotion that corresponds to the constitutional theme of the person's life.

Diagnosing by CSOE ensures that the practitioner is perceiving the whole of the patient using the entire sensory apparatus. The practitioner becomes a finely tuned instrument for reception of data as he or she is able to discern finer and finer shades of human expression. The practitioner's intuitive capabilities are empowered as he or she is able to more readily assimilate diagnostic information. In cultivating the awareness of these subtle cues we are called to remove all obstacles between our own hearts and minds that impede the accurate perception of reality. Hence the process of practicing in this way is actually a path that may lead to the rectification of the practitioner's own heart.

Color

The color associated with each element is most clearly seen in the area of the lateral canthus next to each eye. Generally, colors are perceived as a reflection or radiation from the skin, although they may comprise the actual color of the skin as well. Although each element is said to have its associated color, red for fire, green for wood, and so forth, the colors present as a spectrum of shades depending on a variety of individual factors. Each color is presented differently depending on whether a person's constitution is governed by the *yin* or *yang* official associated with his or her constitutional element. Colors associated with *yang* officials tend to be brighter and more vibrant in nature, whereas those associated with *yin* officials tend to be deeper. The colors associated with water, wood, earth, and metal are notable by their presence. However, the color associated with fire also presents as an ashen color or "lack of red." Lack of red is often noticeable in patients who have heart disease, indicating that the fire which supports the function of the heart and circulatory system has burnt out.

Sound

Each element is typified by a certain quality of speech. These sounds are notable by either their presence or absence in relation to the overall content of a person's speech.

Groaning is the sound associated with the water element. It imparts a gravely quality to the voice and may be likened to the sound of sheets of ice rubbing against each other as they thaw and freeze.

Shouting or lack-of-shout are the sounds associated with the wood element. The shouting voice rises from a quiet volume to a loud volume. The lack-of-shout voice does the opposite, often falling in volume to a whisper over the course of a sentence.

The sounds associated with fire are laugh and lack-of-laugh. The laughing sound imparts the quality of laughter to the patient's voice regardless of the nature of what is being discussed. The lack-of-laugh sound imparts an actual crying quality to the voice.

The sound associated with earth is singing or lack-of-singing. Singing may be heard in the voice as a regular modulation of tone that occurs regularly between low and high frequencies. The singing tone can sound like a southern or English accent. The lack-of-singing quality sounds monotonous and is as unvaried as the dull buzz of insects during late summer.

The sound associated with metal is weeping, a breathy and mournful. sound that reminds me of the wind rustling through the leaves in fall.

Odor

It is relatively easy to smell the odors when they are associated with chronic organ pathology or during an acute infection. However, these same odors are present years before pathology manifests in a given organ.

The odor associated with the water element is putrid. The putrid smell is caustic like ammonia and has its most physical basis in the uric acid found in the bladder and kidneys.

Rancid, the odor associated with wood, is similar to the smell of rancid oil. The physical basis of the odor is the gallbladder bile and the oil of the liver.

The odor associated with fire is scorched, which is similar to the smell of sulphur present when a match has burned out. The physical basis of this smell is heat emanating from the circulatory system.

The odor associated with earth is fragrant, which is a sweet smell that reminds me of scented soaps. The physical basis of this odor originates from the by-products of fermentation in the digestive system.

The odor associated with metal is rotten, which originates from feces that are stagnant in the large intestine.

Emotion

Each of the five elements is associated with the habitual presence or absence of a specific emotion. At the moment the child begins to interpret life, the emotion of his or her constitutional type surges through and is forever paired with the pain of separation from true self. Whenever the given emotion is present in either self or in another, the individual is driven into habitual behavior in an unconscious attempt to avoid pain. Therefore, whenever the emotion associated with their constitutional type arises, it is displayed inappropriately, manifesting in either an excessive or deficient manner.

Each of the emotions is distinguished by its habitual presence, or absence, when patients are responding to emotionally charged material generated either by their own thoughts internally or by another person. For example, a person who is wood constitutionally will habitually display the emotion anger inappropriately. In its excess display, anger may manifest as belligerence in life over what appear to be inconsequential details. In its deficient display, lack of anger may manifest as timidity or a willingness to compromise foundational principles in the face of life's challenges. For a list of some excess and deficient behaviors that correspond with habitually disordered emotions, see Figure 9.3. The dynamics of each element's emotion are discussed in more detail in Chapter 10.

In my clinical experience I have identified five emotional states that represent the "toxic" counterparts of the otherwise healthy emotions already identified in the practice of Chinese medicine. These toxic emotions both result from, as well as perpetuate, extreme habitual reaction to the presence of otherwise healthy emotional states. As discussed previously, each of the elements is associated with the presence of a given emotion. The healthy and toxic emotions are listed in Figure 9.1.

Each of these pathological emotional states is associated with a deviant type of behavior as well as an outward display of the toxic emotional state. Here I present examples for each of the elements.

Reacting to the presence of the emotion fear with fear itself, the paranoid person projects distrust externally and is therefore secretive. Lying by omission, secretive people manipulate personal relationships by never quite revealing their intentions. They use their hidden resources in an attempt to overwhelm and intimidate others with their pathological will.

Angry over "being made" to feel the emotion anger, resentful people act passive aggressively. They avoid direct confrontation and manipulate their world by trapping others into compliance with their plans and decisions. The suppression of anger leads to mounting internal pressure, which manifests as seething.

Having lost the joy of relationships, fire types may become brokenhearted and bitter. Bitterness over perceived betrayal may lead to lying as they wear a false face in the world and are no longer able to trust enough to let another close. Sarcasm and teasing are the resulting

Toxic Emotional States				
Element	Emotion	Toxic	Behavior	Display
Water	Fear	Paranoia	Secrecy	Intimidating
Wood	Anger	Resentment	Passive aggression	Seething
Fire	Joy	Bitterness	Lying	Sarcastic/Teasing
Earth	Sympathy	Disgust	Ingratiation	Complaining
Metal	Grief	Disdain	Pontification	Snide

Figure 9.1

TOXIC EMOTIONAL STATES

In health, individuals are able to feel each emotion without habitually reacting to its presence. It is not that healthy water constitutional types do not feel fear, but rather that they do not unconsciously react to the presence of that emotion. Fear does not dictate their actions in the world. When we habitually respond to the presence of a given emotion with that same emotion itself, then over time the emotions feed on each other and transform into their toxic counterparts. Therefore, fear of fear becomes paranoia, anger over our anger becomes resentment, sadness as a reaction to our sadness becomes bitterness, needing sympathy because we have so much sympathy leads to disgust, and grief over our grief leads to disdain.

forms of communication that may serve to prevent others from becoming too close. Both behaviors indicate that the essence of the heart is not being communicated clearly to the outside world.

Out of a reaction to feeling sympathy, earth types become ingratiating, catering to others' needs endlessly. Excessive sympathy leads to the craving of sympathy for the terrible plight of having to take care of everything and everyone. They become disgusted, having "had it up to here" (pointing to Stomach-9), literally not being able to swallow. They communicate disgust by constantly complaining about the neediness of others.

Metal constitutional types may react to the presence of the emotion grief with grief itself. Possessing the unique ability to find the fatal flaw in everything, metal types may come to disdain what is regarded as lowly. Talking down to everyone, metal types pontificate to the unworthy. What is impure within the self is expressed outwardly as being snide.

These toxic emotional states all result from the compounding of emotions upon themselves. Such states may all be felt in the *yang* complementary positions of the pulse as tight, biting, and often slippery qualities. These very same qualities often indicate the presence of an acute infection. However, when they are present chronically, they may indicate that like an infection, the emotions themselves have become toxic. Very often the presence of these pulse qualities and related emotions and behaviors suggests the presence of "aggressive energy" (pathological *qi*) that may form the basis of serious illnesses such as cancer.

According to the teachings of the Traditional Acupuncture Institute, Columbia, Maryland, aggressive energy is *qi* that attacks officials following the *ke* cycle. This is in contradistinction to healthy *qi* that travels in the *sheng* cycle. Its presence is indicative of functional toxicity, which, if left untreated, can form the basis of serious illness. Aggressive energy is "drained" through superficial needling of the *yin shu* points. If present, aggressive energy often manifests as a dark red circle on the skin around the acupuncture needle in the *shu* point corresponding to the affected organ. The needles are generally retained until the redness disappears, indicating the aggressive energy has been drained.

I also find the *luo* points (Figure 9.2) on the *yang* meridians particularly useful for "draining" the *qi* that perpetuates these negative emotional states. The *luo* points may vent the suppressed *qi* to the outside world and thereby deflate the internal pressure that feeds habitual nature. The *xi*-cleft points on the *yang* meridians may be used in conjuction with the *luo* points to help move the stagnation which supports the pathological expression of these emotional states. With this tension removed, the habit may be broken long enough for patients to gain perspective on their situation and to stop making it worse by perpetuating it with negative thoughts and behavior.

Pulse

Unlike color, sound, odor, and emotion, which are wave forms that can be sensed at a distance, the pulse is the most subtle and rapidly changing wave form that can be accessed by physically touching the body. The amount of information gleaned from the pulse is limited only by the ability of the practitioner and the sophistication of the system being used. Nonetheless, because pulse information is conveyed through physical touch, I feel that it is skewed toward providing information about relatively more physical levels of being than the other diagnostic methods mentioned.

All ill health results from a suppression of the true self, and pulse

Luo Points		
Meridian	**Luo Point Number and Name**	**Xi-Cleft Point Number and Name**
Bladder	58 ("fly and scatter")	63 ("golden gate")
Gallbladder	37 ("bright and clear")	36 ("outer mound")
Small intestine	7 ("upright branch")	6 ("nourishing the old")
Three heater	5 ("outer frontier gate")	7 ("assembly of ancestors")
Stomach	40 ("abundant splendor")	34 ("beam mound")
Large intestine	6 ("side passage")	7 ("warm current")

Figure 9.2
LUO POINTS

The luo points on the yang *meridians may be thought of as pressure valves that help to vent functional consequences of self-perpetuating emotional states trapped in the interior. Note that the names of these points all impart a sense of clearing stagnation and opening to the exterior. The* xi-cleft *points help to move the stagnation upon which these dysfunctional emotional states are predicated.*

diagnosis may help to determine precisely how this suppression is present as functional and ultimately physical pathology. Pulse diagnosis plays an important role in prescribing herbal formulas, selecting acupuncture points, and assessing the progress of treatment. Although I do not depend on the pulse to determine constitutional type, I do find that it is the single most important diagnostic method for confirming my diagnoses for CSOE. Precisely because pulse diagnosis relies on physical touch, I find that it, in effect, "grounds" my assessment. Pulse diagnosis also contributes in large part to my understanding of the patient's eight-principle physiology. The eight-principle system is used to assess a patient's physiology according to patterns of imbalance which are referenced to a system of eight criteria rather than the five elements and twelve officials. These "eight guiding criteria" are used to qualify an imbalance according to whether it is relatively *yin* or *yang*, internal or external, excess or deficient, and hot or cold. While the five-element system informs us of how one's spirit and consciousness influence the physical substrate of the body, the eight-principle system informs us of how inherited and acquired physical aspects of being impact consciousness.

Constitutional Diagnosis and Prevention:
Which Way Does the Wind Blow?

I am often asked how constitutional diagnosis allows me to predict the past, present, and future of my patient's health so accurately. The following metaphor may serve to explain my orientation toward Chinese medicine as a preventive form of therapy.

Imagine that we are at the beach on a quiet day. We may notice that all the trees are leaning to the east. If I were to ask you what way the wind generally blows there, you would be able to state with some certainty that it blows from west to east. If I ask you what direction the tree will eventually fall, you can tell me that too with a high degree of accuracy. If I plant a tree and ask you which way it will bend in twenty years, you can also predict with a high degree of accuracy that it will be leaning east.

Like the wind blowing through the trees, the quality of *qi* flowing through each human being has a direction of influence which may be assessed according to the patient's constitutional type. Given every diagnostic observation that can be made in the moment, it becomes possible to predict likely clinical outcomes if nothing is done to change the person's path. In time, the direction of our patterns of dysfunction influence the body the way the wind bent the tree at the beach. If a patient comes to treatment early enough, acupuncture may, in effect, be used to change the direction and quality of that "wind" *(qi)*. Hence the tree may bend back to a straight and upright position. However, eventually the tree may have bent so far, there is not time in that tree's life to bend back the other way, no matter how hard we try. Functional pathology may eventually become embodied to a degree that physical symptomatology cannot be compensated for or corrected. But the direction of the wind may be changed in a moment. That is, although physical embodiment of illness can no longer be altered, a person's experience of life and relationship to pain can change in an instant.

I believe that people can gain insight even moments before death that may lead them to fulfill their destiny. Hence the inner tradition of Chinese medicine is greatly effective in conditions that cannot be reversed clinically, such as terminal illnesses and insulin-dependent diabetes. Regardless of the physical severity of a disease, the quality of an individual's life is always capable of improvement.

Constitution: The Nature of Virtue

A man's faults all conform to his type of mind.
Observe his faults and you may know his virtues.
– CONFUCIUS[8]

Throughout this text, we emphasize the number three as corresponding to the primordial nature of *dao* and the true, deep nature of each individual. However, this stage in the enumeration of being corresponding to early heaven (inherited constitution) does not allow us to know and diagnose the world of later heaven (acquired constitution).[9] The number five, which corresponds to the five transformations *(wuxing),* is the first stage in the evolution of *dao* that is clinically useful in forming an integrated constitutional diagnosis.

Each person embodies the quality of expression that is present during one season more than the others. This "element" is the patient's constitutional type and provides a framework for organizing observations of how the patient has come to embody his or her interpretation of life in every aspect of being. Constitutional type may be thought of as the tint on the window through which people observe life, and their interpretation of the meaning of everything they see and experience is filtered through it and colored by it. The concept of constitutional type allows us to see into the depths of our patients, through the accretions of their acquired experience in later heaven and back toward their source. It allows the practitioner to determine the specific way that each individual embodies the meaning he or she attributes to life. It both allows the practitioner to understand how the patient has lost touch with true self and gives a framework for determining the steps that need to be taken to restore original nature.

At its core, each of the five elements has a quality of destiny that encompasses the process of life transformation for individuals manifesting the corresponding constitutional type. This process involves transforming the unbalanced emotional expression consistent with a constitutional type back into its corresponding virtue (see Figure 9.3).[10] For example, if we consider a patient to be fire constitutionally, then we may be sure that, given any major stress in life, the patient will interpret what is happening according to the associations of his or her constitutional element, in this case fire. As the habitual presence or lack of a given emotion increases, there is a corresponding erosion of the virtue associated with that constitutional type. Hence Liu Yiming asserts, "The five internal organs (kidney, liver, heart, spleen, lung), having form and substance, are inns for the conditioned five elements, not the gardens of virtues of the primal five elements."[11]

In monitoring a patient's progress in treatment, the practitioner must focus on transforming the primary disordered emotion and resulting habitual behavior back into their corresponding virtue. For example, if the patient responds habitually to avoid the emotion fear, then the behaviors of recklessness or conservativeness may be displayed. If the patient can remain in the presence of the emotion fear and not let it dictate actions, then the corresponding virtue of wisdom is empowered. The skilled practitioner is able to test the patient's emotions both during the intake and throughout the course of treatment in order to determine if they are functioning more appropriately over time. A positive shift in the patient's emotive state toward the emergence of a given virtue always indicates that healing is occurring on the deepest level as the primordial *qi* reasserts its influence in the patient's life.

The virtue that lies at the heart of each element is a natural expression of some pristine aspect of being which perfectly reflects the harmony of primordial *dao*. This virtue is the spiritual and behavioral corollary of *jing, yuanqi,* and *shen* as the guiding influences in life. By identifying the patient's constitutional type we are able to access those qualities of his or her constitutional endowment which hold the greatest potential to guide healing and evolution from within.

After having lost touch with original nature, the created self begins to assert its influence and govern our life. In time, the virtues associated with the elements are obscured by acquired conditioning, and our behavior becomes increasingly motivated by the habitual functioning of the mind, which struggles ceaselessly to avoid pain and to fulfill its desires. Inevitably, physical symptoms may occur to compensate for the underlying imbalance as our distortions of reality become increasingly embodied as illness. From the point of view of the inner tradition, these symptoms are always regarded as a sign pointing deeper into the spiritual life and belief system of the individual.

Constitution and the Creation of Meaning

When I was in sixth grade, my teacher, unknown to the rest of the class, had arranged for a student to run into the room and shoot him three times with a cap gun in the middle of a lesson. The teacher fell to the floor and lay there motionless. After the excitement diminished my teacher jumped up smiling and informed us that we had fifteen minutes to compose an essay about exactly what events had transpired.

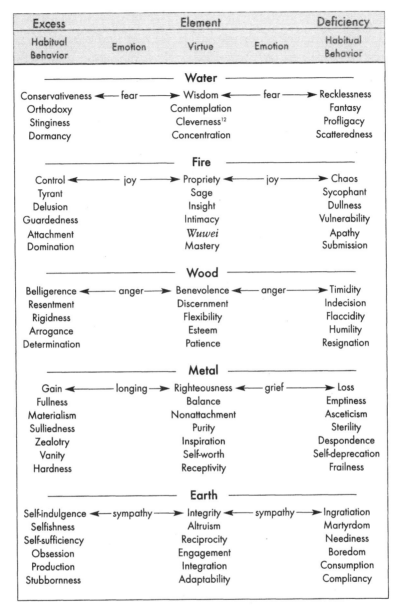

| Excess | | Element | | Deficiency |
Habitual Behavior	Emotion	Virtue	Emotion	Habitual Behavior

Water

Conservativeness	←— fear —→	Wisdom ←—	fear —→	Recklessness
Orthodoxy		Contemplation		Fantasy
Stinginess		Cleverness[12]		Profligacy
Dormancy		Concentration		Scatteredness

Fire

Control	←— joy —→	Propriety ←—	joy —→	Chaos
Tyrant		Sage		Sycophant
Delusion		Insight		Dullness
Guardedness		Intimacy		Vulnerability
Attachment		*Wuwei*		Apathy
Domination		Mastery		Submission

Wood

Belligerence	←— anger —→	Benevolence ←—	anger —→	Timidity
Resentment		Discernment		Indecision
Rigidness		Flexibility		Flaccidity
Arrogance		Esteem		Humility
Determination		Patience		Resignation

Metal

Gain	←— longing —→	Righteousness ←—	grief —→	Loss
Fullness		Balance		Emptiness
Materialism		Nonattachment		Asceticism
Sulliedness		Purity		Sterility
Zealotry		Inspiration		Despondence
Vanity		Self-worth		Self-deprecation
Hardness		Receptivity		Frailness

Earth

Self-indulgence	←— sympathy —→	Integrity ←—	sympathy —→	Ingratiation
Selfishness		Altruism		Martyrdom
Self-sufficiency		Reciprocity		Neediness
Obsession		Engagement		Boredom
Production		Integration		Consumption
Stubbornness		Adaptability		Compliancy

Figure 9.3

THE TRANSFORMATION OF VIRTUE

The virtues encompassed within the five elements (water, fire, wood, metal, and earth) are listed along with the personal attributes or virtues (wisdom, propriety, benevolence, righteousness, and integrity) that emerge when the destiny of a specific constitutional type is being fulfilled. As a given virtue erodes, an habitually occurring behavior arises depending on the presence of an excessive or diminished emotion (fear, joy, anger, longing, sympathy). Along with each of the virtues ascribed to the elements in the Bai Hu Dong, *I have listed other virtues I associate with each element.*

Each student in the class was then asked in turn to stand and read aloud their summary of the events. It became immediately clear that everyone in class had seen something different. Rather than report the facts of what had happened, everyone ascribed some unique motivation to the teacher and to the "assassin," attributing a personal meaning to the events at hand. Each student had made up a story that was uniquely and personally meaningful.

In fact, no event in life has any meaning implicit within it. We saw earlier that it is the human attempt to create meaning which causes the *dao* to lose its primordial nature and to give rise to the ten thousand things. During Liu Yiming's fifth stage of losing touch with original nature, the five elements separate and constitutional imbalances assert themselves. A life-defining event of such magnitude has occurred that the checks and balances of the *sheng* and *ke* cycles are not able to spontaneously restore functional harmony. Humans create meaning in the face of such an event out of an unconscious attempt to avoid the pain, confusion, and shock felt in that moment when true self is lost. In reality, even such a life-defining event contains no implicit meaning. The meanings ascribed by each human being to the defining moments of life are entirely self-generated and determined in quality a priori by constitutional predilections. The notion of constitutional type is a tool that allows the practitioner to comprehend how a patient has attributed meaning to life and embodied that meaning as both health and pathology.

Next I examine the role of constitutional type in determining the quality of our attribution of meaning in life and its consequences for health and illness. During this discussion I present a clinical example of how the principles of constitutional type can operate in shaping the development of a person's life. This "case study" is offered to elaborate the role played by constitution in the diagnosis and treatment of how the patient's attribution of meaning in life becomes embodied as pathology. The patient in this example came for treatment in his early forties. The infant and the sage may both be considered to live safely at home in harmony with the eternal *dao*. I therefore refer to the male figure in my example, whose constitutional type is metal, as the "traveler," for in losing original nature he has left his home.[13]

The Fall

Consider a young boy sitting at the dining room table with his parents. Prior to this moment the child has functioned in a relatively balanced state governed in large part by his primordial endowment.

Those close to him would describe his character as openly receptive and inspired. He is the gem at the heart of his family's life, treasured by all. In an instant his father stands up, and, banging his fist on the table, declares, "I've had enough." The father then proceeds to walk out the door and drives away, an incident culminating in the divorce of that child's parents. This certainly would be a traumatic event in any young life. However, the meaning ascribed to this event, as well as any subsequent embodiment of pathology, will be unique in every single case depending on constitutional variables. Each person will see this event through a window colored by his or her constitutional predisposition.

In the scenario just described, a child whose constitution is metal would be flooded with grief as his father struck the table and left his family home. His interpretation of the event might lead him to believe that nothing in life of value can be held on to and that, if he had been sufficiently valued by his father, his parents would never have divorced.[14] The quest to reestablish his self-worth becomes an unconscious motivation that presents itself in every aspect of life.

The moment the child or young adult compensates for the shock of the pain being felt by ascribing meaning to life is the moment the created self is born. Projecting the pain of the event both internally and externally, the individual comes to believe a fundamental truth about both his or her own nature and the nature of life itself. People proceed through life gathering evidence to support their thesis that they, and life, are a certain way. The nature of this thesis is determined entirely by the associations of their constitutional type. The thesis represents a distortion of one or more inborn virtues that are constitutionally determined and now lie dormant in their heart of hearts.

In the preceding scenario, the traveler's thesis that "nothing of value can be held on to in life" is an external projection of his own inner loss of the virtue of self-worth. As a metal constitutional type, the tint on the window through which he views the world is white (the color associated with metal), and every event in life viewed from this perspective is interpreted as substantiating his thesis.

As he grows older, life provides our traveler with ample evidence that everything he has ever valued has been lost. Increasingly driven in life, he has grown apart from his lover and sacrificed both his relationship and health, struggling in vain to establish his self-worth through accomplishment in his profession. Each successive loss substantiates his thesis and fuels his habitual drive to find value externally in the world. The reality, however, is that he has appended the meaning of loss to the significant events of his life as he has unconsciously followed the dictates of his internal programming. Had he been fire constitutionally, he might have viewed the very same events as proving a life thesis that intimacy is not safe. The meaning of life is not implicit in any event, but rather in the person who is experiencing it.

Constitutional type is a double-edged sword that defines both our weakest characteristics and greatest strengths. By definition, our constitutional official is the weakest link in our dynamic chain of functioning. As a compensation for this underlying weakness, a corresponding strength is developed in certain domains of life. However, behaviors based on both the weakness (deficiency) and strength (excess) are displayed inappropriately because they are fueled by motivations that are habitually driven. Only actions that flow from and empower the virtues of each constitution are consistent with the fulfillment of destiny. For example, the traveler in our story suffers from a lack of self-worth. This inability to find value within himself may be compensated for by habitually trying to find the best in everything and everyone externally in life. Hence our traveler's search for value has led him to a career as a gemologist with a reputation for precision in his work and an uncompromising taste in selecting the finest stones for his customers. Internally, as he struggles to grasp the best from the past and future, however, the habitual emotions of grief and longing become manifest. His actions in life, dictated by a habitual response to the presence of these emotions, manifest as excess or deficient behaviors such as vanity or self-deprecation. Some of the excess and deficient behaviors associated with each of the constitutional types are shown in Figure 9.3.

When we are deeply immersed in habitual behavior, life becomes unfulfilling as our minds continually dictate our actions in an attempt to avoid pain. As soon as any desire is attained, satisfaction is experienced for only moments before the force of our habits reassert themselves. For example, our traveler who is driven to find value in life continually strives to possess objects of increasing worth. This search may involve the acquisition of cars, jewelry, an attractive lover, or nonmaterial things such as a better relationship. When what he longs for is attained, he experiences only temporary satisfaction at having fulfilled his quest. However his habitual nature quickly reasserts itself. Ironically, he soon finds the fatal flaw inherent in the prized object, and thus a new search begins for something of increased value. Each constitutional type is associated with a fundamental irony that lies at the center of each habitually driven life. The ironies associated with each constitutional type are discussed in Chapter 10.

If our traveler is free to create meaning in life, then why does he habitually create meanings that hurt him by perpetuating separation from true self? Negative meanings are perpetuated because to consider any other meaning would imply he is wrong about his life thesis. To be wrong about his thesis means he is left not knowing what the event that he attributes his creation to actually meant. This quandary is synonymous with the death of his created self. The death of his self-image is unconsciously identified with the pain initially experienced in life at the moment when his original nature was lost. *Our force of habitual functioning in every domain of life is entirely propagated to keep us from experiencing this pain.*

Heaven continually sends our traveler challenges in life, the nature of which can only be solved through reconnection to the virtue shut off in his heart of hearts. Until he regains possession of his virtue, heaven will continue to provide him with opportunities to learn his life lesson—that the nature of value which is never lost in life lies within. However, every opportunity for learning in life will be lost unless the influence of the habitual influences that drives his separation from true self can be eliminated. The entire thrust of the inner tradition is to empower the patient's awareness by harmonizing the functional imbalances upon which ignorance of the true self is predicated. The concept of constitutional type provides the practitioner with a framework for recognizing the quality of acquired *qi* that does not conform to true self and for guiding patients back home to their inner virtue.

The nature of the meanings created in response to life's challenges determines the relative state of each individual's health. As children, our thesis, synonymous with our compensation for the loss of original nature, may serve the purpose of protecting young psyches and spirits that are too fragile to assimilate such great pain. Events in life are rarely as devastating to an individual's well-being as the meanings ascribed to them and the embodiment of those meanings as pathology over the long term. The events of life happen neither for or against us—life is literally what we make of it. As we grow older, the tools are hopefully gained in life that allow us to perceive the reality of past and current situations without the need to further inflict pain on ourselves. That we persist in doing so is a result of our force of habit.

Hence our traveler mistakes his created world for reality and wanders through life lost in the delusion of his own interpretations. Every action is based on his unconscious motivation to avoid the pain on which his separation from true self is predicated. His childhood virtues of receptivity and inspiration have been forgotten long ago. These virtues have, in time, been twisted into the habituated behaviors

associated with his constitution (Figure 9.3). Cut off from his spiritual life, he has become a religious zealot longing for connection to God,
his heavenly father. Distanced from perceiving the balance between
loss and gain in life, he works increasingly hard to fill his internal
emptiness with material possessions. Cigarette smoke fills his lungs as
he seeks to avoid the habitual presence of the grief and emptiness that
reside there. With his immunity weakened, he suffers repeated lung
infections and his health becomes increasingly frail. Now the habitual
functioning upon which his separation from true self is predicated has
become embodied as physical pathology. Left on this course, our traveler will surely meet with ruin. As the primordial influences that
empower health and balance are obscured, illness will eventually manifest to the point that either his quality of life becomes permanently
compromised or life itself is lost. However, good fortune smiles on our
traveler and the winds of fate begin to change.[15]

After endless rounds of antibiotics, immunizations, and perhaps
even sinus surgery, our traveler has become weary of standard medical
treatments. During a particularly bad bout with pneumonia, our traveler reaches a turning point. Coughing, he reaches for a cigarette, and,
for one instant, hesitates. Sickened at the thought of another puff, he
decides that only by stopping smoking will he be able to combat his
chronic lung infections. Following a friend's advice he makes an
appointment to see a practitioner of acupuncture and herbal medicine.
By taking an action on his own behalf he has unconsciously taken his
first step in his journey toward the restoration of original nature.

The Return

Our traveler has come to acupuncture and herbal medicine to stop
smoking and to address the issue of his chronic lung infections. These
complaints, however, are just symptoms that have helped him get his
foot in the door. To the degree he willingly extends his hand to the
practitioner in partnership, he provides an invitation to be taken as
deeply as possible toward the restoration of true self.

Next I examine how constitutional type provides a framework for
healing in the inner tradition.

The Intake and Discernment of Constitution

To reiterate, like a novel, each human life possesses both a plot and a central theme. The plot of life constitutes what happens from the moment of conception to death. It is one's life story constructed of each individual event in life. Because we live in a society centered on a causal worldview, we tend to view our lives as the momentary result of some past event. If you ask us who we are, we define ourselves by what has happened to us. It is precisely this notion of self that Liu Yiming defines as illness when he tells us that in our spiritual quest we must "shed the dust of personal history."[16] If our definition of self is based on the past, then we are forever trapped, habitually responding to every new situation based on past experience.[17] The theme of our lives, synonymous with our reason for being, is continuously present in each moment. Personal freedom exists when we possess the awareness to respond to present circumstances, unencumbered by past experience, based on our commitment to manifesting virtue.

The process of conducting an intake often entails listening to a condensed version of each person's life story. Invariably, the practitioner listens as patients ascribe their present condition to some past cause that affected them and made them who they are today. The real cause of true personal identity, however, is as present in the moment as it was at the patient's conception. This is the primal cause of patients' lives, their unique endowment of *dao* whose quality is identified by their constitutional type. It is the practitioner's task to identify this theme and restore it to the patient's conscious awareness as a motivating force in life.

Arriving for his appointment, the practitioner notices how finely our traveler is dressed, his black pants and shirt offering a stark contrast to his pale white complexion. A silver ring and large bright diamond catch the practitioner's eye as the patient is invited to have a seat and the session begins. In relating the story of who he is, and what has happened to him, our traveler is able to provide abundant evidence that his thesis in life is correct. Beginning with the birth of his created self, he explains during the intake that he lost his father when his parents divorced, and his story proceeds through a litany of the other losses suffered in life: the death of a grandparent, loss of his intimate relationship, and numerous others including job opportunities and ultimately his health. Each time emotionally charged material is present during the interview, the practitioner notes changes in his color, sound, odor, and emotion. In the case of our traveler, these are white, weeping, rotten, and grief, respectively. The pervasiveness of these associations during every part of the intake confirms the practitioner's assessment that the themes of the metal element are the organizing framework of the patient's life and that metal is his constitutional type.

Unraveling the Thread: The Suggestive Process in Healing

If a patient's illness is predicated on erroneous interpretations in life, then helping guide him or her toward creating meaning in a way that empowers health is one of the practitioner's strongest therapeutic tools. A central task for the practitioner is to support patients in gaining awareness about the nature of their created stories. This is accomplished by using the associations and language of the five-element constitutional paradigm to draw connections for the patient among symptoms, belief systems, and habitual behaviors. The imagery of this language derives from the associations of the five-element system. It is present in the names and functions of acupuncture points and herbs that are chosen for their abilities to strengthen the primordial influences and to remove the mundane influences that drive habitual behavior and obscure connection to true self. As patients' awareness increases regarding the habitual nature of their behaviors, the perspective gained provides an emotional distance from the events at hand. This perspective empowers an increased awareness of the option to respond to events in a way that both springs from, and engenders, virtues synonymous with the restoration of *jing, yuanqi,* and *shen* as a guiding influence in life.

Ultimately, all interventions, whether they be acupuncture, herbs, or dietary advice, are merely suggestions made by the practitioner to some aspect of the patient's being that it function in a more balanced way. Consider, for example, a patient who suffers from a chronic muscle spasm in her shoulder. The condition may reflect an underlying mechanism where spasm in the muscle results in pain. In turn, the resulting pain causes the patient to tighten her muscle, which further restricts circulation in the area of the cramp. This pain-spasm-pain model describes a feedback loop between the patient's shoulder, her perception of pain, and her reaction to it. This feedback loop is, in effect, a habit with a neurological, psychological, and circulatory component.

Acupuncture may break this feedback loop by providing a new source of input into this system. But this input is nothing more than a "suggestion" that the muscle stop spasming. The acupuncture points treated have potential effects that they empower by activating specific qualities of function. The aspects of being supported by a point's function, whether it be to improve circulation to an area or empower emotional openness, are again only suggestions that the patient may or may not take. People are not machines and acupuncture points are not switches that "automatically" make things happen. Like a laser, all suggestions in therapy must be congruent in illuminating that aspect of personal expression which has been lost. The patient's constitutional type offers a framework for making suggestions that are particularly effective and meaningful.

Although the interview explicitly focuses on diagnosis and gaining rapport with the patient, it also offers the practitioner an opportunity to initiate the process of healing. After concluding the interview, the practitioner reinforces our traveler's belief that stopping smoking will help his lungs to heal and increase his immunity against further infections. Our traveler is informed that air constitutes the most subtle and essential aspect of life and that stopping smoking will help him feel more connected to what the ancient Chinese considered heavenly *qi*. This last statement thematically ties together the key issues in the traveler's life including his zealotry and longing for connection to heaven, poor self-worth, smoking, chronic lung infections, and his search for quality in life. The practitioner has used language that is an extension of the patient's own belief system to redirect his consciousness toward the nature of the dysfunctional relationships perpetuating his illness. Suggestions offered in this way are planted like seeds deep in the patient's heart of hearts. With sufficient reinforcement from herbal prescriptions, the acupuncture points, and the words of the practitioner received during each session, these suggestions will germinate and grow from within to eventually initiate cracks in the patient's fortified belief system on which his suppression of true self is predicated.

The therapeutic focus of the inner tradition involves helping patients gain awareness about the ways in which unconscious habits motivate their lives. Initially these may be relatively gross habits such as addiction to substances such as cigarettes, coffee, or alcohol. Successful treatment always proceeds to increasingly subtle levels of unconscious behavior based on the patient's belief systems, whose quality is constitutionally determined. Before leaving the office, our traveler agrees that, rather than just unconsciously reaching for a cigarette, he will try and be aware of his behavior and take several breaths before lighting up. It is also agreed that several times daily he will make the decision not to smoke a cigarette when he craves one. Beginning to focus his

awareness on his patterns of behavior will allow him to experience
some emotional distance from his habit. Our patient's habit is perpetuated by his resistance to being in the presence of his grief, which arises
when he is not engaging in the behavior of smoking. The window of
time where he is aware of his need to smoke, but not engaging in the
behavior, provides room for the primordial *qi* to begin and reassert its
influence in his life. As the process occurs, his awareness is drawn ever
so slowly back to the moment of lost self.

The initial stage of treatment may be thought of as bringing a patient
out of shock. This is accomplished by gently leading him to the conclusion that what he seeks in life is merely a self-created concept that is not
in reality obtainable. From the moment of the intake, the practitioner
has led the traveler to associate the issue of his self-worth, search for
quality and connection in life, and stopping smoking with his physical
complaint of chronic lung infections. He has also been advised to pay
attention every day to how often the issue of self-worth motivates his
thoughts and actions. All these issues are linked thematically as associations of his constitutional type. By focusing his attention on them, the
patient is provided the opportunity to unravel his knotted belief system
that perpetuates his separation from inner virtue.

Throughout his life, the traveler has mistakenly searched for value
outside of himself. He has externalized the inner virtue of self-worth in
his habitual quest for worldly gain. His habitual search for value externally in the world has left him unfulfilled as he has found that the value
of whatever he possesses continues to slip away and allude him. By
focusing on the nature of the constitutional relationships that drive
him, he is encouraged to direct his attention inwardly back toward the
virtue that lies buried under the accretions of a lifetime of acquired
conditioning. The truth that awaits him there is that the greatest value
in life is to be found in that which is least substantial. This is his connection to heaven without in the form of fresh air, and heaven within
in the form of inspiration. The only value that can be held on to in life
is our capacity to remain connected to the spirit of a thing once its
form has been lost.

As our traveler moves increasingly close to the moment of return to
his original nature, a dynamic tension is set up between the thrust of
his primordial endowment that strives to reassert itself and the conditioned influences that maintain his illusion of the created self.
Approaching the turning point is an extremely critical juncture because
the patient is most likely to discontinue treatment at this time. As the
primordial *qi* mounts in strength, it begins to stir up old thoughts and

memories that have laid buried within. These may present themselves in the patient's dreams and thought patterns, and the practitioner should pay careful attention to their significance.

Our traveler has responded well to his initial course of treatment. He has cut his smoking from two packs to half a pack each day, given up drinking coffee entirely, and experienced an overall increase of energy. However, when he arrives for the present session, his practitioner can sense the patient is uneasy. He reports feeling depressed and as if he is being followed by a cloud. Further, he voices concern that in the past he had cut down his smoking in an attempt to quit and always failed. Now that he is so close, he doubts his ability to finally let go of the habit. During the current session the practitioner is able to feel the dynamic tension between the patient's mundane acquired influences that struggle to maintain their grip and his primordial *qi* that is pushing from within to reassert its authority in motivating the traveler's life. This healing crisis signals the arrival of the turning point in the patient's treatment.

Sighing deeply, the traveler shifts in his chair and tells the practitioner that he recently had a dream about his father. "I was walking toward him through fog. Every time I was about to reach him, he would disappear into the mist. That's just like him, always leaving me." Here the primordial influences are represented by the theme of reconnection to his father, and the conditioned influences are represented by his thesis that the things he values in life will always elude him. The same dynamic present in this dream is present in his belief that stopping smoking will always allude him, which is another goal he is literally pursuing through a cloud of smoke. Symptomatically this theme is embodied as he tries in vain to breathe fresh air (heaven without) through the phlegm and cigarette smoke stuck in his lungs.

The practitioner sits straight up, and establishing direct eye contact with the patient says, "You know, regarding your father, there is an alternative that you never considered." Our traveler looks up and replies, "Oh, what's that?" Maintaining eye contact, in a quiet voice the practitioner tells him, "Perhaps it is not your father who left you, but rather you who left your father." There is a stillness in the treatment room as the primordial *qi* begins to move. The practitioner does not interrupt the silence, waiting instead for the traveler to respond.

Just as the shock of his father's leaving occurred in one moment and initiated the loss of our traveler's original nature, so too can original nature return instantly. A key therapeutic goal is to break the force of the habits that drives the traveler's interpretation and belief in his story.

The practitioner may facilitate this process by making suggestions to a patient in a way that he is not able to interpret what is said to him in accordance with any prior experience in life. To gain the perspective that his thesis is a self-created story places the traveler back in the presence of his original pain, unable to compensate in a way that removes him from his experience of it.

After a moment of silence the traveler speaks: "You know he sent me a gift for Christmas this year, and I never even thanked him. His birthday is next week and I haven't bought him anything." Having not cried in as long as he can remember, a tear comes to his eye. The practitioner suggests that the traveler lie down on the treatment table, and in silence begins to take his pulses. Here it is imperative that acupuncture points are chosen which add to the momentum of the primordial influences in restoring original nature. In this case the points chosen are Lung-8 ("meridian gutter"), Kidney-7 ("returning current"), Lung-2 ("cloud gate"), Kidney-24 ("spirit burial ground"), and Conception Vessel-17 ("primordial child").

Lung-8 and Kidney-7 are the metal points on their respective meridians. By needling these two points simultaneously, water and metal are joined in their *sheng* cycle relationship. Kidney-24 is needled to resurrect the *ling* receptive aspect of spirit in the patient's life. Lung-2 is chosen for its effects in clearing phlegm from the lungs, thus removing the "clouds" that obscure the patient's awareness of the sun (his heart). Conception Vessel-17 is chosen because it is the reunion point of the lungs and pericardium and may therefore touch the function of both officials simultaneously. In this treatment gold needles are retained in all points for ten minutes.

The selection of these points perfectly matches the constitutional themes and functional dynamic present in the moment. Upon inserting the final needle, the practitioner gently holds the traveler's hand as he checks the pulses. He leaves the traveler with one last thought: "You know, sometimes our beliefs prevent us from receiving the best that life has to offer. Your father did leave home when you were young, but who knows what value lies in that relationship for you now?" Letting go of the traveler's hand the practitioner walks to the treatment room door and turning back before leaving, gently reminds the traveler to "breathe."

The actual insertion of the needle becomes the focal event which pulls together every therapeutic suggestion made prior to that moment. By invoking the unsullied aspect of the patient's true self, forgotten so long ago, the practitioner may help restore the patient's memory of original nature. Once he has experienced a glimpse of the true self, it is difficult to turn away. The *dao*, with its foot in the door, surges forth like a mighty river as health and spontaneity are restored and our traveler returns home. I always consider it the best sign of effective treatment when the patient reports, "feeling better than I have in years," or "having my old self back." My experience is that this can often be expected in under ten treatments.

Finale

This treatment truly did mark the turning point in the patient's life. He returned to the next session declaring that, not only had he bought a present for his father's birthday, but he had actually made arrangements to visit his father for the first time in seventeen years. Within a month he successfully stopped smoking and has not had another cigarette in eight years. His lung function has improved dramatically and he rarely suffers now from more than the occasional cold. His marriage, which had been on the verge of divorce, is now thriving. After many years of not wanting a child, he seems to truly have found a great source of value and joy in life with the birth of his son.

Summary

Who an individual is in any moment is the result of all inherited and acquired influences. The diagnosis of constitutional type derives from a qualitative assessment of one's primordial endowment received from the moment of conception and prior to the first breath. These are the foundational influences that contain our potential for every possible manifestation in life. The quality of our constitutional endowment is the deepest possible view that a practitioner can attain of a patient. Knowing patients' constitutional type allows the practitioner to understand how patients have embodied their belief system as illness, the elemental qualities of function that will most efficiently support their healing, and a framework for guiding them back to health and well-being.

Other models of Chinese medicine such as the four divisions, six stages, six pathogens, and eight principles all have their place in a balanced approach to treatment. However, only a constitutional approach allows the practitioner to diagnose and revive the innate influences which are the foundation of life itself. Without assessing the qualities of a patient's constitutional type, it is impossible to arrive at an integrated diagnosis that empowers the discernment of what aspect of being is most important to address in a given patient at a given time. An assessment of the patient's constitutional type allows the practitioner comprehension of what constitutes truth in the patient's life. Truth, in a therapeutic context, is that which empowers the presence of one's virtue and thus the fulfillment of destiny. For the virtues are outward expressions signifying that the potential stored in *jing, yuanqi,* and *shen* are being manifested in life.

The foregoing discussion should not be taken to imply that the position of the practitioner should be that of a psychotherapist. Chinese medicine is truly holistic in nature, however, and the practitioner must possess the tools to reach each patient at his or her depth. Patients have constructed their "reality" through words, and words, therefore, are a potent tool for helping return them back to the reality stored in primordial being. It is not necessary that discussion take a significant time during each session. But it is vitally important that the practitioner's words are chosen with clear intention. It is the concept of constitutional type that empowers the practitioner to hit the mark of original nature with every therapeutic suggestion made.

Questions

1. Can you think of the earliest defining moment you had in life?

2. What happened?

3. What did you learn about life?

4. What did you learn about yourself?

5. What further proof do you have that you were correct?

6. What price do you pay for believing this is true?

7. If you were able to let go of this belief how would your life change?

8. What is the thing you complain about most in life?

9. Why don't you change it?

NOTES

1. Fung Yu-Lan, 1983, vol. 2, p. 30.
2. Chapter 14; in Chen, 1989, p. 89.
3. See Gebser, 1984.
4. Chapter 10 of the *Dao De Jing* discusses the merits of meditation. See Chen, 1989, p. 78.
5. The point Bladder-11 is named "great shuttle." The characters *jing* (經) and *luo* (絡) indicating the meridian system are etymologically related to the warp and woof of a loom. The function of Bladder-11 may be compared to the shuttle of a loom that weaves back together the fabric of life when it unravels. Note that Bladder-11 is a main point for stimulating the production of blood.
6. Watson, 1970, p. 16.
7. Unschuld, 1986, p. 539.
8. Fung Yu-Lan, 1983, vol. 1, p. 70.
9. For an illuminating discussion of the early and later heaven sequence in the *Yijing* and their relationship to Chinese medicine, see Eckman, 1987.
10. See discussion of the separation of the five elements in Chapter 6.
11. Liu Yiming; in Cleary, 1986a, p. 66.
12. In the sense of prudence.
13. See Liezi's discussion of the living as travelers on top of page 115. See also J. Klate (1985), "Spirit path," *Journal of Traditional Acupuncture* 8, no. 2: 50. Those not familiar with the qualities of each constitution might prefer to skip ahead and read the description of the metal element and constitutional type in Chapter 10 and then return here.
14. Value and self-worth are issues associated with the metal constitution.
15. The use of the word "fate" here implies that he has been going along unconsciously through life a victim of his own created beliefs and circumstances. Rather than being a victim of fate, he is about to fulfill his destiny.
16. Liu Yiming; in Cleary, 1986a, p. 110.
17. I am reminded of the saying "those who fail to learn from history are condemned to repeat it." From the standpoint of our discussion we might change this to say "those who learn from history are condemned to repeat it."

10

THE
ICONOGRAPHY OF
CONSTITUTION

T HE FIVE ELEMENTS—WATER, FIRE, WOOD, METAL, AND
earth—as they are embodied in the human being provide a qualitative map for how destiny expresses itself in the life of each
individual. Each element is associated with a quality of destiny that
encompasses the process of life transformation for individuals manifesting the corresponding constitutional type. This process involves the
transformation of the unbalanced emotional expression, consistent
with a constitutional type, back into its corresponding virtue.
Accompanying this transformation is the resolution of habituated
behavior back into actions that are consistent with the fulfillment of
destiny. Each elemental type has a *yin* and a *yang* aspect that constitutes the "officials," or organ systems, of Chinese medicine. Hence, in
addition to the general theme associated with an elemental type, constitution can be further elaborated according to the dictates of a
particular official.

In this chapter I present the constitutional types and the life issues
and qualities of destiny associated with them. The quality and themes

of each element are described first, and then the nature of each associated official is elaborated. I have emphasized those aspects of each that have been most relevant in my own clinical practice. Throughout this chapter I use the Confucian virtues as icons for the quality of spirit that emanates from those who manifest destiny and preserve original nature. I have given my own interpretation of the virtues in relation to what I believe is their inner nature consistent with the teachings of Daoism. Each description of constitution contains several simplified case studies. Rather than choosing cases based on their outcome, I have picked ones that best exemplify key patterns of imbalance associated with each constitution. For each case, I mention an acupuncture point combination that I consider archetypal of the functional dynamic of the patient in question.[1]

The Relationship Between Yin *and* Yang *Officials*

At the moment of conception, heaven places the *yuanqi* within. Until birth, our development is presided over by the *yuanqi*, which burns like a diamond in our depths. This period of time is presided over by early heaven because our life is guided only by inherited and no acquired influences. At birth, the moment of our first breath corresponds to the assertion of acquired *qi* and later heaven as a guiding influence. As the influence of the inherited endowment is obscured by the process of socialization, our *shen* allows us to form an active conduit from heaven without (our life circumstances) to heaven within (the *jing* and *yuanqi*). This alignment between the outside world and our inner domain is replicated in the functional relationship between each pair of *yin* and *yang* officials.

The *yin* and *yang* officials associated with each element are termed *zang* (臟) and *fu* (腑), respectively. The character *zang* referring to the *yin* organs is etymologically related to the character *zang* (臧) meaning to "hide, "conceal," or to "store."[2] The character *fu*, referring to the *yang* officials, is etymologically related to the character *fu* (府). It denotes a treasury or palace and refers to the residence of a higher official where public affairs are transacted.[3]

The *yin* official of each element corresponds to the deepest aspect of functioning within the individual. The *yang* official is the emissary of the *yin* official into the external world. For example, in the wood element, the *yin* official is the liver, and its paired *yang* official is the gallbladder. The liver's function is to hold the plan of our life internally, and the function of the gallbladder is to implement that plan in the world and to evaluate the degree to which external events coincide with the internal plan. The *yin* official is the template against which all events in the external world and all actions taken by the *yang* official are compared. The *yin* officials are the basis of the virtues provided by early heaven as our constitutional inheritance and manifested in the world according to our constitutional destiny. In health, the function of the *yang* officials is to initiate actions in the world that manifest these virtues and bring the events of life directly to the core of our inner being (the functional integrity supported by *mingmen*), uncolored by interpretations and accretions of mundanity acquired in life.

The function of the *yang* officials may be likened to that of a window between the inner and outer world of the individual whose purpose is twofold. It must convey with absolute fidelity the image of who we are on the inside—the virtue in our heart that radiates outward as *shen*—to the outside. The window must also convey affairs outside our self that radiate as heaven's *shen* to the inside. The function of the *yang* officials is passive in that absolute fidelity of both inner and outer images is maintained when the *yang* official fulfills its task by doing nothing *(wuwei)*. In health, the *yin* and *yang* officials associated with a given element coexist in a state of functional harmony. In such a state the function of the *yang* official is transparent and we see exclusively the virtues associated with the *yin* official flowing effortlessly into the world. This order mirrors the functional unity of our heart and mind.

Think of the *yang* officials as corresponding relatively more to the function of the mind, and the *yin* officials as corresponding relatively more to the function of the heart. The nature of this relationship is reflected in the origin and termination points of both *yin* and *yang* classes of meridians. All *yang* meridians either originate or terminate on the head next to the sensory orifices, indicating a close link to the mind and its tendency toward interpretation. All *yin* meridians either begin or end on the chest in the upper burner, the domain of the heart.

The heart, as defined here, is the inner world of the *yin* officials. It accesses the template for life, stored in the kidney *jing*, that represents our internal standards against which we measure the appropriateness of all our actions. The mind comprises the *yang* officials. Its function is to transmit external life to the interior and to acknowledge the essential nature of what is stored internally, on which it based all willed actions. In health, the functions of the heart and mind are unified: The workings of the mind are transparent and only the will of the heart shining effortlessly into the world may be discerned. Illness is predicated on a separation of the heart and mind. In essence, the concept of constitutional type allows the practitioner to discern specifically the quality (element) and location (*yin* and *yang* pair) of where this separation initially occurred and how it is perpetuating the dysfunctional state.

The heart must acknowledge truth both internally and externally and then evoke the mind to initiate actions consistent with truth by governing the *qi*. The ability to evoke is predicated relatively more on blood and *ling,* and the ability to act is predicated relatively more on *qi* and *shen.* Consider, for example, the relationship of the emperor (heart) to the minister (small intestine) and the general (liver) to his troops (gallbladder). The emperor's place is on the throne situated at the center of the nation. The general's scout (gallbladder) reports that hostile troops are gathering on the northern border, and the general decides on immediate military action. The general approaches the highest minister and aide to the heart (small intestine) and informs him of the gravity of the situation. The small intestine assesses the situation to be of such import that he grants the general an audience with the emperor in his inner chamber.

The general enters the inner chamber reverently and approaches the emperor, who sits composed upon the throne. "Your majesty, 15,000 hostile troops are gathering at the northern border. We have three options. What shall we do?" The emperor sits up straight on his throne, closes his eyes, and looks deep within himself to the wisdom contained in his kidney *jing.* In a moment he opens his eyes and bids the general to initiate a specific course of action. Without delay, the general leaves the imperial chamber to command his troops and thus carry out the emperor's wishes.

The function of the *yang* officials, gallbladder and small intestine, has been to gather as much data from the outside world as possible and to convey it accurately to the internal world of the liver and heart. These *yang* functions correspond to the analytical facilities of the mind and are based largely on expenditure of *qi* and radiance of *shen.* The ability of the *yin* officials to attract this information from the outside world and thus command the reverence of the two *yang* officials emanates from the capacities of *ling* and *yin* to evoke action. For in health, no mechanical constraints dictate the loyalty of his ministers. Rather, the emperor evokes their loyalty through his alignment with heaven and his innate ability to perform ritual effectively.

Having assimilated all relevant information from the external world, the emperor then must look deep inside himself and initiate a course of action that precisely corresponds to the reality of the situation. He accomplishes this by looking deeply within and penetrating the depths of his own *jing* with his *shen*. In this way external reality as conveyed accurately by his ministers may be compared to the truth of his own personal destiny stored in his depths. In commanding the general to implement a specific course of action, the emperor again is exercising his power of *ling*. He cannot physically *make* the general carry out specific actions; he can only evoke these actions through exercising his moral authority, which springs from his own inner cultivation of virtue. Similarly, the general's authority in commanding his troops is patterned on the emperor's virtue in commanding the nation. The natural order underlying the integrated function of these relationships results from the alignment of the emperor's *jing* and *shen*, which, in turn, are aligned between heaven and earth. This central alignment is then replicated throughout creation as each *yang* official is aligned with its corresponding *yin* official, all of which are aligned with the central axis of heart and kidney, itself aligned between heaven and earth.

The life issues of people of a certain elemental constitution differ, depending on whether their constitution corresponds to the *yin* or the *yang* organ. For example, if a person's constitutional type is wood, then vision in all aspects of being is sure to be a life issue. If she is liver constitutionally (corresponding to *yin*), her imbalance will tend to manifest as a deficiency in self-esteem—a failure of inner vision. If she is gallbladder constitutionally (corresponding to *yang*), she may focus more on external issues such as injustice in the world and perhaps view herself as being treated unfairly by others. This case illustrates an imbalance in vision that has been turned externally. The virtue of self-esteem is nourished by blood, whereas the ability to act in a benevolent way consistent with esteeming others is predicated on *qi*.

When the functional yoke between the *yin* and *yang* officials of an element is broken, both officials evidence complementary dysfunctions simultaneously. Therefore, an individual of a given elemental constitutional type tends to evidence imbalances of the element's associated *yin* and *yang* officials. The practitioner's ability to discern whether an individual's constitutional type belongs primarily to an element's *yin* or *yang* organ is determined ultimately by his or her overall sense of the person. This sense is guided by subtle shades of difference in the patient's color, sound, odor, emotions, and pulses, which are of primary diagnostic value, and other secondary indicators of the patient's elemental type, such as tongue and abdominal diagnosis.

The Constitutional Types

Next I describe the characteristics of each constitutional type. The elements and their associated officials are presented in order of their cosmological generation according to the *Dao De Jing:* water ("the great"), fire ("moving away"), wood ("far away"), metal ("the return"), and earth ("the axis"). The discussion of each element is cast in the language of the virtues, emotions, and behaviors contained in Figure 9.3.

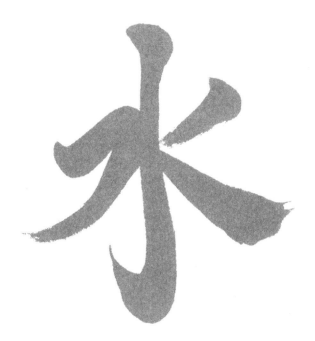

The highest good is like water,
Water is good at benefiting the ten thousand things,
And yet does not contend with them.
It dwells in places the multitudes detest,
Therefore, it is close to the dao.
– DAO DE JING [4]

WATER—THE GREAT

Chapter 25 of the *Dao De Jing* calls *dao* "great." The fundamental quality of *dao* as *yin* is indicated by its association with water throughout the *Dao De Jing,* the *Zhuangzi,* and other Daoist texts. The water element is the worldly manifestation of the first stage in the movement of *dao.*

Nature of Water

In assessing the qualities of each element within a human being, imagine how the expression of each element occurs in nature. For example, water may occur as a single translucent droplet, a fresh cleansing rain promoting new life in spring, a cool clear stream, a river overflowing its banks, a tidal wave overwhelming all that lies in its path, or as an entire ocean, deep, dark, and secretive. Using water in nature as an archetype, we may characterize the quality of any of the associations of the water element metaphorically.

For example, the environmental condition that injures the water element is cold. Therefore, an individual with driving ambition may be described as "cold" if he allows his assertion of willpower, like a tidal wave, to overwhelm the natural development of others. Cold may also prevent us from manifesting potential because the water element freezes similar to the way ice floes prevent the flowing of a stream in winter, the season associated with the water element.

The Nature of Cold

During the winter the earth becomes a seed. Dead on the surface, its potential is frozen deep within. The kidneys store the *jing,* which is the seed of the inherited constitution, containing the potential for all of life's varied manifestations. Cold may damage the healthy functioning of the water element by inhibiting the fires of *mingmen,* which fuel the kidney's transmission of inherited potential into the world.

The tendency of water to freeze during the winter is associated with the water element's powers of focus and concentration. Physiologically, the kidneys must concentrate the urine in the body so it may be excreted. Similarly, the will *(zhi),* which is the spirit of the kidney, must focus *shen* on the *jing* so wisdom *(zhi),* the virtue of the kidneys, is cultivated.

The psychospiritual correlate of the water element's tendency to concentrate lies in our capacity for reflection.

Habitual reaction to the emotion fear may inhibit the cultivation of virtue, leading to the conditioned behaviors of fantasy and orthodoxy. Orthodoxy represents a state in which evolution is hampered as our reaction to fear keeps us frozen and unable to accept change. Habitual fantasy also hampers evolution because the overactive mind and nervous system fail to concentrate our will adequately on our resources in a realistic way. As opposed to orthodoxy, which suppresses life's impulse for evolution in order to preserve the past in the moment, fantasy squanders resources in a vain attempt to bring a self-created future into the moment without doing the necessary work. In the face of the unknown, the virtue of wisdom empowers us to navigate in a way that is presided over by innate knowing. Wise people are able to allay their own fear through self-assurance by virtue of being in contact with the truth that arises from their depths and the flow of life's events externally. Self-assurance arrived at in this way manifests as the virtue of faith.

When fear obscures our connection to wisdom, the habituated mind begins to fantasize and attempts to fill in the missing pieces in life instead of relying on instinct. The solutions offered by the mind are motivated by fear and based on fantasy and not reality. Therefore they lead us to squander inner resources and rarely produce a potent result in the world. For the mind tends to generate either worst case or best case scenarios as it either perpetuates fear or tries in vain to quell it.

Virtue and Transformation: Fear into Wisdom

How is it that the kidneys correspond to wisdom? The kidneys are the essence of the [element water], and wisdom proceeds unceasingly without any doubt or uncertainty. Water likewise moves forward without uncertainty.
– BAI HU DONG[5]

The virtue associated with the water element is *zhi* (智), meaning wisdom. Some of the ways in which wisdom may harmonize the life issues of this constitutional type are listed in Figure 9.3. The heart *shen*, in illuminating our depths, can only ever penetrate to a certain limited depth. What lies beyond the depth of our awareness and intuition are the unknown aspects of life and self that reside in primordial realms of being and the subconscious. Fear is the emotion that arises in the face of the unknown. The sage through the clever utilization of resources and a focused will spends a lifetime cultivating wisdom. Wisdom is the virtue that empowers us to stand firmly in the face of the unknown and chart a steady course through uncertain waters. Wisdom empowers us to take the right action instinctively in a way that is presided over largely by the innate knowing in our primordial endowment which lies beyond the reach of conscious knowing. The sage in old age stares into the unknown, which toward the end of life presents inevitably as death. Wisdom empowers the sage to make this final journey in a conscious way that is not presided over by fear. Rather the sage aligns his or her will with the will of heaven, accepts the inevitable, and gracefully follows the flow of *dao* wherever it may lead.

As we move away from the virtues that define the heart of the water element toward life themes of either conservativeness or recklessness, fear manifests as either an excess or deficient emotion. Excessive fear manifesting as conservativeness may present as a habitual frozenness in life, preventing water constitution types from ever manifesting their deep potential. Lack of fear may lead them to recklessness by continually drawing on inner resources until their potential is squandered prematurely. In either instance, their ability to sustain the manifestation of potential may be compromised to the point that no action taken may have potent effects in the world.

An individual often manifests both excessive and deficient habitual behaviors in different domains of life. A person may manifest excessive fear that presents as an increased vigilance in situations which are non-threatening and deficient fear which leads him or her to partake in dangerous activities and squander personal resources. I am reminded of one patient with a severe imbalance of the kidney/heart axis associated with a Western medical diagnosis of manic depression. On the one hand, constant anxiety presented itself in the most trivial of situations. When buying a sweater he would stare at the rack for an hour, literally frozen with fear over the consequences of choosing the wrong sweater. On the other hand, his hobby was skydiving and he exhibited no fear at all when contemplating a jump out of a plane at 3,000 feet.

It is our false interpretations of life that initiate the separation between the *yin* and *yang* officials of our constitutional element. This separation is synonymous with separation between the specific aspects of heart and mind that are presided over by each element. In the water constitutional type, ignorance of life and self leads to the habitual presence of fear, which creates separation between the functions of the bladder and kidney officials. Fear associated with the kidney constitution tends to be relatively deep in nature and revolves around issues of life's purpose and personal destiny. Fear as it manifests through the bladder official is relatively more superficial and presents itself by attaching to any and every situation occurring in the moment. Agitation and free-floating anxiety are present like ripples on the surface of the ocean. The fear of the kidney type, by contrast, may be compared to that of a shark lurking in the depths.

The resolution of fear is wisdom. In its *yin* aspect, as associated with the kidney official, wisdom is a virtue that emerges as we gain awareness of the nature of the inner truth stored in our depths. In this sense, the function of the kidney is synonymous with the nature of our inherited constitutional potential. In its *yang* aspect, as expressed through the function of the bladder official, wisdom manifests as the clever utilization of life's resources as they occur internally in the kidneys and externally as postnatal *qi*. The cultivation of wisdom is contained in the image of the Daoist sage whose forehead is depicted as having grown larger than life. The kidney *jing* has traveled up the spine to the head, empowering the production of marrow (skull and brain) and indicating the transformation of potential into wisdom.

As treatment progresses, both excessive and deficient displays of fear will diminish, along with a reduction of aberrant behaviors such as stinginess or recklessness. Over time, the illnesses predicated on these habitual reactions should be mitigated as the virtue of wisdom steadily increases and individuals learn to cultivate and expend their life's resources appropriately. The dynamics of destiny and transformation as they pertain to the water element are evidenced in the case histories presented later.

The Rhythm of Water

The man of wisdom perceives calamity or good fortune
when it is still remote, and understands what is beneficial
or harmful when it is still early— . . .
Seeing a beginning he knows what its end will be.
– DONG CHONGSHU [6]

Each of the five elements has a rhythm to its expression that reflects a fundamental property of the endless cycling of *dao*. The rhythm of water possesses two beats that define the destiny of each human being. These moments of time reflect the conception and death of each thing that comes into existence. Life is turned on and off at its source like a stream that thaws and begins to flow in early spring and then ceases upon freezing again in winter. In between the points of conception and death, the flow of the water element must, through expenditure of the kidney's *jing*, lubricate all developmental processes in our being to assure that they unfold gracefully.

Dong Chongshu describes the vision of destiny empowered by the healthy presence of the water element, which represents the *dao* as the ultimate origin and destination of all things. The inherited constitution sets the limit on all that is capable of unfolding in our life from conception to death. The sage must be in contact with and acknowledge the quality and quantity of all available resources throughout life so these may be used wisely to empower the fulfillment of destiny.

The Spirit of Water

The *shen* of the kidney is *zhi* (will), a homophone with *zhi* (wisdom), the virtue corresponding to the water element. Each of the elements is associated with a spirit that is an emanation of the heart *shen*. It is the quality of an individual's will that determines whether life's resources are cultivated in a way which transforms fear into wisdom or squandered in a way that prevents the fulfillment of individual destiny.

The Life Thesis of Water

In the moment we lose original nature, a life theme is established that determines how we as individuals will interpret life and subsequently come to embody our interpretations as pathology. This theme is dictated by our constitutional type and corresponds in essence to a thesis about our inner nature and the nature of life itself. This thesis represents a distortion by our minds of one or more inborn virtues that lie buried in our hearts. The key life themes for the water constitution involve utilizing resources and bringing potential into the world in a way that cultivates the virtue of wisdom. If habitual reaction to the presence of fear obscures our access to wisdom, then our life theme is distorted into a thesis that compromises our balanced relationship to resources in every aspect of being. Money is the most externalized concrete example of a resource in life. Patients' relationship to money and financial security may serve as a metaphor for their relationship to the wise expenditure of reserves.

Our life's thesis may have as its theme either a quality of excess or deficiency. The archetypal life theme for water constitutional types that reflects excess may be stated as, "My inner purpose is so compelling that it must be manifested continually regardless of the consequences to anything or anyone that gets in its way." The archetypal life theme for water constitutional types that reflects deficiency may be stated as, "I am impotent to effect change in the world. What happens to me is a matter of fate."

Irony: Habitual Use of Will Is Exhausting

A fundamental irony in life is associated with each constitutional type. The irony associated with each element results from the tendency of our habitual reaction to the presence of a given emotion to reassert itself in a way that leaves us forever unfulfilled. For only the expression and embodiment of the virtues associated with our constitutional element are ultimately fulfilling in life.

The irony lying at the heart of the water element is that *true power comes from wisdom which results from the cultivation of resources.* Habitual reaction to the emotion fear drives the kidney and bladder officials to either over- or underutilize willpower in governing the expenditure of resources. If we are reckless with our resources, ambition may push us to exhaustion as we struggle to manifest potential in the world. With the completion of each new project, however, satisfaction is felt for only a short while before the controlling influence of our habitual fear reasserts itself, driving us to ever larger projects.

If we are conservative in the expenditure of potential, we may appear habitually frozen in the face of our fear, as nothing issues forth from our life. Every project started is only momentarily fulfilling before our habitual fear of exhausting our resources reasserts itself and any new initiative is called to a halt in midstream. Cultivating wisdom is the fulfillment of destiny for the water constitutional type. Only through the realization of this virtue can the water constitution reach a state of quiescence based on the cultivation of internal reserves of power.

Testing Emotions: Reassurance

In discerning the patient's constitution, the practitioner must assess the quality of function for each of the five elements. Key in this process is the technique of testing the patient's emotions. The principle here is that patients will act inappropriately to the presence of the emotion associated with their constitutional type every time it is made present. The practitioner therefore endeavors to embody each of the emotions in turn in order to note which one initiates habitual unconscious behavior on the part of the patient.

Water constitutional types habitually respond to the presence of the emotion fear. By offering reassurance and noting the quality of patients' reactions, the practitioner may assess the qualitative function of patients' water element. When water is in a functional state of balance, reassurance from the practitioner should help allay any fears that patients are displaying. However, a hallmark of the water constitution is that reaction to fear is the unconscious motivating force behind the habitual behavior. When offering patients reassurance, therefore, the practitioner will find patients' fears are only allayed briefly, if at all. A defining characteristic of the water constitution is that once reassurance is offered, it will be continually elicited by patients throughout the interview. No amount of reassurance can do more than temporarily allay the fears that unconsciously motivate those of the water constitutional type. For reassurance comes externally, and only the internal virtue of wisdom can rectify their relationship to fear.

On the other hand, patients may respond to fears expressed by the practitioner by being unable to acknowledge them. In this way, patients suppress their experience of the emotion fear. For example, during the intake, a patient may discuss how both parents had heart attacks in their early fifties. The practitioner, embodying the emotion fear, may ask the patient about her own developing high blood pressure. The patient may assure the practitioner that she is at no risk for heart attack because of having exercised vigorously for many years. But the practitioner may deduce that, in fact, fear is the unconscious motivating force behind the patient's exercise regimen and she is ignorant of the degree to which fear motivates her.

In the moment of engendering fear or offering reassurance, the practitioner must note changes in the patient's color, sound, odor, and emotion. The finding that these intensify, and the patient becomes blue, groaning, putrid, and expresses either fear or lack of fear is enough to confirm the patient is water constitutionally.[7] If this dynamic truly reflects the patient's constitutional type, it is expected to be present thematically throughout the patient's life and during the interview.

The Suggestive Process in Treatment[8]

In offering effective suggestions to a person in a therapeutic context, (1) phrase the suggestions in a language that naturally speaks to the patient, and (2) make the suggestion the logical extension of everything the patient already believes to be true.[9] I have always felt that the ability to characterize the functional dynamics of a therapeutic moment with a precise metaphor is one of the greatest tools possessed by the advanced practitioner. The five-element system offers a potent framework for offering suggestions to patients of each constitutional type. For each elemental type is by nature prone to taking suggestions if they are offered in a specific way.

The water type is motivated by fear, and suggestions that either allay fear or engender it are particularly effective therapeutically. The practitioner may empower the offering of any given therapeutic suggestion by creating a context for it by using language filled with the associations of the given element. For example, in motivating a patient whose constitution is governed by water to quit smoking, the practitioner might say, "This is merely a matter of asserting your will. I have no fear that you'll be successful in your attempt and I think this accomplishment will lay a good foundation for future health."

The Water Officials

The Inner Physiology of Kidney and Bladder

The kidney fuels the fires of *mingmen* with an individual's inherited endowment of *yuanyin* and *yuanyang*, a process mediated by acupuncture points Governor Vessel-4 ("gate of destiny") and Bladder-47 (52, "room of will"). These influences correspond to early heaven. The bladder brings acquired experience into *mingmen* via the eyes, which also radiate the expression of our inherited constitution into the world, a process mediated by acupuncture point Bladder-1 ("eyes bright").

The kidney's relationship to the storage and utilization of reserves is relatively concerned with the access to, and quality and quantity of, the inherited constitution. The relationship of the bladder to the storage and utilization of reserves is relatively more concerned with the quality and quantity of the acquired constitution. In this sense the relationship of the bladder and kidneys is similar to that of water and the well, rope, and bucket that contain and tap its resources. With regard to the inherited constitution, the resource of water in the well is kidney *jing,* and the well that contains the resource is the kidney. The bladder is the bucket lowered via a rope, representing the kidney's will, to tap the resources and bring them into the world. The kidney internally presides over the allocation of *jing* as a resource to be distributed to the other *yin* officials. With regard to the acquired constitution, the well represents the bladder, which stores the vital resources of rain (the essence of acquired fluids) to complement and supplement the kidney's reserve. Next we examine the qualities of the water element as they are expressed through the kidney and bladder officials.

Kidney

> *The kidneys are responsible for the creation of power.*
> *Skill and ability stem from them.*
> *– NEI JING SU WEN*[10]

The function of the kidney is to store our deep source of potential for all of life's manifestations as they exist in the *jing* and *yuanqi.* The kidney represents the wellspring of life. The quality of the treasures that lay within are determined initially at the moment of conception and represent all that we bring to this life from our inheritance and previous incarnations. These influences, present as *jing* and *yuanqi,* are to be conserved and utilized wisely over the course of our life as destiny unfolds. We cannot have too much of this endowment, and the general idea in all of life's endeavors is to draw only as much of this resource as necessary to effectively accomplish the task at hand. In effect, we must live substantially off the interest (acquired *qi*) of this trust while trying our best to conserve the principal (inherited *qi*).

Kidney *qi* may be deficient for one of several reasons. First, our source of inherited *qi* may be insubstantial from the moment of conception, signifying a weak inborn constitution. Second, we may have overused our will and thus expended our deep source of potential in the form of either kidney *yin, yang,* or *jing.* Finally, we may have been malnourished early in life and thus our store of acquired *qi* is so diminished that a disproportionate amount of inherited *qi* has been burned to compensate for our poor environment.

The life issues of those who are kidney constitutionally revolve around the general theme of utilizing resources appropriately. Wisdom, the virtue associated with the kidneys, empowers us to be in contact with the entire scope of our destiny from conception to death. We must know our capabilities relative to each endeavor and have a realistic picture of what will be called for at each step of life's journey. At the end of any given project, we must concentrate and reinvest the profit of our actions so our deep reserves are continually replenished. Hence an important function of the kidney is to strengthen our reserves through investing resources wisely. The kidney empowers the virtue of wisdom so that in the face of the unknown we are able to take correct action in the expenditure of resources by following our instincts rather than reacting to our fears. The cultivation of resources through reflection and the appropriate use of will is the kidney's contribution to the internal alchemy that leads to sagehood.

Archetypal Image: The Relationship of Cleverness and Wisdom

An image of the bladder and kidney officials in balance is the boxer who must fight a fifteen-round match. The fighter knows how long he must fight and his opponent's strengths and weaknesses as well as his own. He expends as much energy during each round as needed to hold his own, always keeping some in reserve and never letting his opponent know just what he is capable of. He assesses at each moment just how much force to use and always has a reserve of technique and stamina left for the final moments of the last round should the fight go that long. These abilities are governed by cleverness associated with the bladder in governing the expenditure of reserves. However, all these parameters may only be assessed to a given point, and the outcome of every match is uncertain. The kidney empowers the contender to flow with his instincts as the fight unfolds. Confronted with the unknown or, even knowing he is outmatched, he finds his execution of technique is never limited by fear. He remains unattached to the result of the match and focuses instead on cultivating wisdom through the exercise of his art.

When bladder and kidney function is unbalanced, habitual reaction to fear compromises the scenario just described. We may recklessly underestimate our opponent or our own abilities. Out of fear we may conserve too much energy and inhibit our technique or come out flailing, trying to overwhelm our opponent in the first round. Either way defeat is certain if we are motivated by fear and not the virtue of wisdom and the talent of cleverness.

A Lesson in Reserves: The Compulsive Gambler

When the kidneys are not functioning harmoniously, we are habitually led to squander any resource they have access to. I am reminded of the story of the beggar who encounters a genie in the marketplace.[11] The genie asks how much money would be enough to help the poor man, and the beggar quickly responds that 500 *yuan* would be sufficient. Within a few days, of course, the money is spent and the beggar is again sleeping in the marketplace.

Once again the genie returns and asks the beggar how much money would be sufficient to help him. This time the beggar takes a moment to reflect, and he answers 10,000 *yuan*. The beggar is able to buy a small house and hire several servants. In time, however, his financial deals go bad, and once again he finds himself in the market. When the genie reappears, the beggar now asks for 100,000 *yuan*, thinking that surely will be enough to last a lifetime. Now the beggar buys fancy clothes, marries, and has a family. With his money comes prestige, and he is appointed to a high-ranking position in the court. In time, however, his funds are again squandered through his excessive lifestyle and the financing of a failed campaign against a neighboring state. Upon once again seeing the genie walking toward him in the marketplace, the beggar this time turns and runs away.

As important as the quality of our inherited and acquired endowments, our ability to care for them and expend them wisely is even more important. Educating patients regarding the appropriate expenditure of reserves is one of the key therapeutic tasks in the inner tradition.

The Bladder Official

> *The Bladder is responsible for regions and cities.*
> *It stores the* Jinye *(Body Fluids).*
> – NEI JING SU WEN[12]

The function of the *yang* official associated with each element parallels that of the spirit associated with each *yin* official and serves as a conduit from the *yin* official into the external world. For example, the spirit of the kidney is will *(zhi)*. When the kidney and bladder officials exist in a state of harmony, the virtue of wisdom is seen to flourish in all domains of a patient's being. In this scenario the will forms a functional yoke between the internal world of the kidney's inherited resources and the acquired resources that come externally to us from later heaven. This conduit between the inner and outer world of the individual is precisely mirrored in the functional role of the bladder in mediating the utilization of the kidney's resources of *jing* and *yuanqi*.

Whereas the kidney defines the quality of our inherited constitution, the bladder official is in charge of storing acquired reserves and utilizing both inherited and acquired *jing* as resources in the external world. The attributes of the bladder in balance may be likened to those of an appropriately functioning reservoir. A reservoir needs to be able to contain resources without dissipating them and must expend exactly the correct amount of resource as dictated by the demands of the moment within the context of the overall project. The healthy function of the bladder official is to empower us to assess adequately both the quantity and quality of our reserves. Like the will, the bladder must also guide us to expend these reserves appropriately.

Fear of Death

In health, we are able to will action in response to danger appropriately. When the *yin* and *yang* officials of the water element exist in a dysfunctional relationship, fear is habitual even though no immediate threat is present. The imbalance of each of the *yang* constitutional types results in part from an inability to introspect because of habitual reaction to the presence of a given emotion. The separation of heart and mind perpetrated by our reaction to the emotion fear effectively prevents the bladder from looking inside to the wisdom stored in the kidney *jing*. Without the kidney's wisdom, the bladder is unable to assess the relevance of any immediately received threat. Therefore the bladder projects the unrealized nature of its fear externally into the world in a way that manifests as free-floating anxiety predicated on the overstimulation of the nervous system by the mind. The kidney, in contrast, is unable to communicate to the external world without the bladder. In the absence of external confirmation for its inner truths, the kidney may generate both secretive behavior and paranoia.

Ultimately, the greatest fear underlying all others is the fear of death. In the bladder this fear may present itself as habitual frenetic energy and the inclination never to rest, for the underlying fear that drives this constitution equates rest with death. In such a scenario, individuals may work constantly, dynamos of seemingly unending energy and motivation. However, the moment they sit down, for example to read, they fall asleep, having worn themselves out completely.

Archetypal Image

The relationship of the bladder constitutional type to inner reserves is like a person driving an automobile who notices her gas gauge reads empty while simultaneously seeing a sign indicating the next gas station is coming up in ten miles. Immediately, a dialogue starts rushing through her mind about whether her fuel reserves will carry her that far. Questions arise: (1) Is the gauge really on empty? (2) Does it go above or below empty as the car goes up- or downhill? (3) How far did I make it last time it was on empty? (4) Do I have enough money to pay for gas, towing, a telephone call? and (5) Why didn't I fill up the tank when I had the opportunity? These questions flood the driver's mind as she drives faster in direct proportion to her increasing fear and anxiety. To the outside observer, this automobile may appear to have a great deal of energy. After all, the car is racing along, and it's the driver's lead foot propelling it. All this activity, however, is predicated on deficit, not on a substantial base of reserves (kidney *qi, yin, yang,* and *jing*) that would grant our traveler the wisdom to drive more slowly and conserve her resources. This same scenario is played out whenever we have an urgent need to urinate and no opportunity to do so. Again, nervousness and anxiety prevail as our mind, lost in fantasy, can focus on little else. The nervousness and anxiety associated with the bladder official expresses itself through overstimulation of the nervous system in general.[13]

Water: Case Studies

Two Examples of the Bladder Constitutional Type

ANDRE: UNMANIFESTED POTENTIAL

Complaint: Shoulder and neck pain, resulting in limited mobility.

Background: Andre was a 32-year-old computer programmer, entirely self-taught. He was talented and clever in his approach to every project. Andre was well aware of this, and yet he felt frozen and afraid to pick a direction in life. He described his fear as similar to "being in a room with many doors." If he were to choose to walk through any one door, the opportunities presented by the others would be lost forever, so he felt paralyzed to move in any direction at all. This dynamic became so strong after becoming engaged to be married that he was seriously considering calling off the wedding.

Andre enjoyed the problem solving involved in computer programming, yet found the work unfulfilling. He continued in the job, however, out of a sense of responsibility to the spiritual community where he lived. In his presence, I had the impression that his mind and nervous system never ceased working. His psychic resources were continually called upon as his attention was drawn to everything around him.

Analysis: The limited mobility resulting from Andre's shoulder and neck pain may be viewed as a consequence of the impeded flow of *qi* through the meridian associated with the functioning of his bladder official. This symptom reflects his embodiment of paralysis as an expression of his own fear and anxiety about picking a direction in life. Andre's sense of orthodoxy about his responsibilities played itself out in an interesting way. Although he had chosen an alternative lifestyle by living in a "conscious" spiritual community, his sense of responsibility kept him trapped in a job that failed to tap his deeper potential. The overactivity of his nervous system is an example of a mind expending its resources, in this case in fantasizing, ultimately destroying mental concentration.

Treatment: The therapeutic issue here was to help Andre gain conscious awareness of the ways he allowed his fear to limit him. I suggested to him that, regardless of which door in life he chooses, he would always wind up in yet another room confronted with still more doors. That is the nature of life. In fact, it was his cleverness and ability that empowered him to find all of these options from which he then felt compelled to choose. He would continually create this dilemma of being frozen throughout his life until he was able to act freely and not in reaction to his fear. I pointed out that the agitation and anxiety brought up by impending decisions could be viewed as a warning, signaling his entry into a new depth of mastery of his potential.

In order to relax his nervous system and ease his anxiety, I prescribed an herbal formula called "Quiet Contemplative," which is based on the traditional formula called "Six-flavor Rhemmania."[14] This formula addresses constitutional imbalances in the water element. An archetypal selection of acupuncture points for Andre might include Bladder-66, Bladder-10, and Gallbladder-43. As the water point on the gallbladder meridian, Gallbladder-43 may help tap the resources inherent in the water, thus bringing them forth into life. The name of Gallbladder-43 may be translated as "valiant stream." This name gives the image of courage that may empower the manifestation of potential in the world. I am reminded of the inner strength and reserve that plants must tap as they break through the dirt in early spring and in this way bring hidden potential to light.

After treatment, Andre went on to marry and spend several years traveling around the world. Eventually, he committed to a career in computer programming, which he learned to practice without overtaxing his resources.

NEIL: ANXIETY LEADS TO DEPLETION OF RESOURCES

Complaints: Lower back pain, sciatica, occasional incontinence.

Background: Neil was a 52-year-old accountant who worked in excess of eighty hours each week in order to support his family. Although his income was quite good, he was habitually driven to increase his cash savings out of a nagging fear that in a calamity, his reserves would be insufficient. Ironically, the harder he worked, the more his own reserve of strength was depleted, more or less in direct proportion to the increase in his financial reserves. A great fan of the theater, he missed every performance he attended by falling asleep within fifteen minutes of the opening scene.

Analysis: The functional depletion of Neil's water element lay at the basis of his physical symptomatology. His career choice of accounting served as a perfect metaphor for his constant anxiety over his own monetary reserves. His symptomatology represented the embodiment of his anxiety about his own material resources in life. His bladder's inability to contain reserves, resulting in incontinence, reflected his own inability to regulate his resources adequately.

Treatment: A key aspect of Neil's treatment involved helping him gain conscious awareness of the way he frittered away his reserves daily. I compared him to a compulsive gambler who immediately spends any money coming into his possession so that, ultimately, no reserve of money is great enough to support him. I emphasized to Neil the importance of cultivating strength internally and how that would pay larger long-term dividends than constant overwork. Neil was saved from an early grave and serious illness by the good fortune of being able to afford an early retirement—a gamble that seldom pays off, as exemplified by the lead character in the play *Death of a Salesman,* who dies just after making the last payment on his mortgage. Rarely are we able to beat a debt incurred by unwisely squandering our life resources. Over time, Neil's problems with bladder control improved to the point that he experienced only occasional difficulty. Archetypal points for Neil included Bladder-36 (50) ("receive support"), Bladder-40 (54) ("equilibrium middle"), and Bladder-23 and 28, the *shu* points associated with the kidney and bladder officials, respectively.

Two Examples of the Kidney Constitutional Type

LYNDEL: AMBITION RUN WILD

Complaint: Lower back pain.

Background: Lyndel was a 58-year-old real estate developer and entrepreneur. His good heart was evidenced in his forceful and deep laugh. His voice was typified by a deep groaning, like ice floes creaking as they freeze and thaw. The strength of Lyndel's boundless potential was evident in his exceedingly strong, pounding pulse, which was full and overflowing in all positions. Lyndel was quite successful in business, and his ambition knew no bounds. His activities manifested as uncontrolled growth in all directions, and he would overwhelm anyone who got in the way of his development projects. Although his projects all evidenced a degree of class and style, he acquired far more real estate and took on far more projects than he could manage. He eventually became mired in lawsuits, which he saw as a tremendous block to manifesting his potential and vision. He was singularly unable to rest for a moment, always consumed with one project or another. Even while sinking in lawsuits, he continued to plan even greater ventures. Lyndel was diagnosed with malignant melanoma, yet, like Confucian philosopher Zhuxi (Chu Hsi) (1130–1200 C.E.), his mind and will continued to drain his resources even though his body was failing. He attributed his illness to years of having been a "sun worshiper."

Analysis: Lyndel's lower back pain resulted from long-term overuse of his will and ambition, which constitute the spirit of the kidney official. His mind habitually drained his resources as he struggled unceasingly to manifest his potential in the world in material ways. His malignant melanoma was an embodiment of the uncontrolled growth that resulted from the habitual overuse of his will. His habit of exposing himself to the sun mirrored perfectly the functional dynamic of his fire element (heart *shen*), burning so brightly that it evaporated his water element (kidneys).

Treatment: My general strategy was to balance the connection between Lyndel's mind, will, and resources by working on the functional relationship between his heart and kidneys, the seat of his resources. I also persisted in trying to establish a healthier connection between his water and wood, so his liver would not be continually inundated and overwhelmed by his ambition. After one such treatment, consisting of the acupuncture points Kidney-1, Liver-8, and Heart-9, he passed a kidney stone within twenty-four hours. After the removal of this very real block, the pounding on his pulses diminished somewhat and he appeared more relaxed. Ultimately, however, Lyndel's imbalance had physically manifested to a degree that was impossible to reverse. Even as he lay dying, he told me that, were he cured, he would live his life in exactly the same way, even if it meant recreating his illness.

SCOTT: RESURRECTION OF HEART SPIRIT

Complaint: Depression.

Background: Scott was the first patient who came to me for treatment during my clinical training. At the time, he was 34 years old, and he had recently moved to Washington, D.C., after living for seven years as an anthropologist in a community of Kali worshippers in the jungle of British Guiana. During this time, he had become close to the community and particularly close to its spiritual teacher. After moving to the city, he felt depressed and empty, having left his spiritual home. Scott was quite intelligent, yet he seemed drained of vitality. He was the classic picture of kidney deficiency, expressed through depletion of the *shen* and *ling* spirits empowered by the kidney points in the upper burner.[15] Scott had dark circles under his eyes, and his upper chest was caved in, giving an impression of weakness, and his appearance was generally disheveled. I sensed he possessed deep spiritual resources but lacked the means to access them. It was as if his well was full, but he lacked the strength to dip down and hoist the bucket to the surface.

Analysis: The spirit of the kidneys *(zhi),* which manifests as will, had weakened, and Scott's stature suffered correspondingly. Although he possessed wisdom, his belief that its source lay externally in his spiritual community effectively denied him access to his own inner strength. After concluding the interview, I emphasized that his access to spirit existed internally and should not be confused with external symbols of his spirituality. He was taken aback and commented that these were the last words his teacher had spoken to him at their parting.[16]

Treatment: The appearance that Scott's power and effectiveness had been turned off at their source suggested a relative imbalance of the *ling* and *shen* spirits. My general treatment strategy was to rebalance his *shen* and *ling* spirits by treating the kidney points in the upper burner. Over several sessions I needled Kidney-23, Kidney-24, Kidney-25, and Kidney-26 as well as Bladder-11 and Bladder-52 (-47). After one such treatment (Kidney-24, "spirit burial ground"), I informed Scott that a national anthropological convention was being held in Washington and encouraged him to attend. I even called him several hours before it was scheduled to begin to impress on him that it was important to start actively pursuing his interests again. Upon walking into the lobby of the hotel, he found his spiritual teacher from Guiana standing in front of him!

This type of synchronicity happens frequently in the most effective treatments. It demonstrates the power of *ling* at work. I could not through force of will have made Scott's teacher appear, yet through effective performance of ritual miracles may occur. This encounter marked the turning point of his healing, as his spiritual power reawakened, flooding all aspects of his being. With each ensuing treatment, he seemed to carry himself more elegantly and to appear as if his reserves of life and spirit had been turned on at their very source. Eventually, Scott went on to marry and have a child. Today, ten years later, he has achieved his goal, so distant then, of a tenured position at the university of his choice.

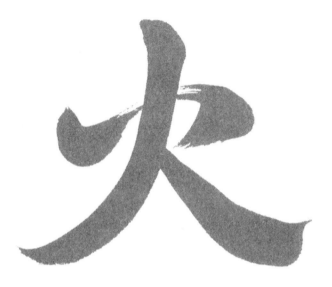

How can one wish to hold for long the light of the setting sun?
— CONFUCIUS[17]

FIRE—MOVING AWAY

As the North Star rises out of the ocean of *dao* to create the dual poles of heaven and earth, so too does *shen* arise out of *jing* to recreate this polarity within each human being. The emergence of the fire element is the second stage of development as each human being recapitulates the ontogeny of *dao*. At the moment of receiving a personal name, our heart *shen* is activated. As self-awareness begins to dawn, we "move away" from the primordial influences contained in the kidney and water element. The emergence of and identification with the personal self may be likened to the sun at its height on the summer solstice. The fire element in nature is at its peak, illuminating the ten thousand individual manifestations of *dao* in the world. Yet the sun is only at its height for a fleeting moment. *Yang* immediately begins to wane and the influence of *yin* and winter begin to descend. As the bright light of summer fades, it is human nature to cling to life's varied manifestations.

In life, as the influence of fire wanes, the initial separation of *yin* and *yang*, water and fire, may increase as we cling to our identification with the false self. At the height of self-awareness, however, we may catch a glimpse of the original self that has been lost. At this moment, we may seek to transcend the personal self and return to the universal self, *dao*. This surrender is often the first step in restoring original nature. In this section I examine the general nature of the fire element and then elaborate how these themes are expressed through the function of the fire officials.

The Nature of Fire

All movement and life in our solar system is oriented toward the sun, the ultimate embodiment of fire. Even a microbe living in a cave at the bottom of the ocean depends on the sun for its life and sustenance. As the life-giving center, the sun may be likened to the controlling influence of the emperor who sits at the heart of the nation. In balance, the fire element gently supports life as a hearth warms a home. However, the fire element within a given individual may present in either an excessive or deficient manner.

If fire is excessive in nature, the sun may scorch and parch the earth, creating a barren desert where life is a struggle for survival. Similarly, individuals with excess fire may appear to be overly hot, their struggle for survival manifesting as an excessive need for control in all aspects of being. Heat in nature accelerates processes and causes expansion. Hence excessive fire may contribute to the acceleration of any physiological process, which may manifest as a quickened pulse, eating too quickly, or any process that is proceeding at a faster than healthy rate. Heat trapped in the heart may be the physiological correlate of unexpressed desires. In an attempt to dissipate this heat the heart may overwork, contributing to high blood pressure. A heart and circulatory system (heart protector) so expanded may lead to "burnout" in the form of a heart attack or stroke. Expansiveness may also present as a lack of boundaries in relationships, as the fire element "burns" those significant others when boundaries are crossed inappropriately.

If the sun does not shine for prolonged periods, cold and dampness characterize the landscape. If the fire element is deficient within, cold predominates as physiological processes begin to slow and contract. This may manifest as an overly slow pulse, poor digestion reflecting the inability of the stomach to "cook" food, or slowness of thought. Contraction may present as an inability to maintain relationships as personal fire is withdrawn in an attempt to protect the self from the pain of disappointment.

The Virtue of Fire

How is it that the heart corresponds to propriety?
The heart is the essence of [the element] fire.
[The quarter of fire is] the south, where the exalted yin *holds a superior position, while the lowly* yin *holds an inferior position. Propriety maintains social differences between the exalted and the lowly. Therefore the heart resembles fire, being red in color.*
– BAI HU DONG [18]

The virtue corresponding to fire is *li* (禮), which has been translated variously as "propriety," "ritual," and "ceremony." The character *li* has three components. On the left is radical 113, *shi* (礻), signifying the moon, stars, and sun as they radiate our destiny from heaven. On the right is the character *li* (豊), depicting two plant shoots (丰) that represent vitality and abundance, over the character *dou* (豆), indicating a sacrificial vessel.[19] The virtue of propriety is evidenced by our capacity to be in the right place, at the right time, doing the right thing. Ritual and ceremony may be considered the inner and outer aspects of the virtue propriety. Internally, the ability to perform ritual effectively emanates from the integrated functioning of every facility presided over by the twelve officials. The central axis of this integration is the interpenetration of the heart (fire) and kidney (water) officials (see Figure 10.2a). The fire element, in illuminating the depths of the water element, reveals the nature of the inner truths that serve as the foundation for all insight and correct action in life. This is the inner alchemy that empowers each human being to become an effective agent of change in the world.

In Confucianism, the virtue of ceremony is comprised of adherence to a social order that dictates the proper relationship of all beings to each other. However, we may consider the inner aspects of ceremony to be the practice of any discipline that empowers the effective performance of ritual. The perfection of any discipline, whether it be martial arts, calligraphy, music, or pulse diagnosis, empowers the momentary presence and focus of the heart. With mastery, the virtue inherent in any art form becomes generalized and is eventually expressed in every action. For example, the practice of calligraphy may empower the virtues of grace, flow, and a natural appreciation of aesthetics that manifest in every domain of physiological, emotional, and spiritual function both internally and in the nature of our movement through life.

In ancient China, a purpose of ritual was to summon benevolent spirits and ask them to bestow favor on self, family, village, or nation. This aspect of ritual is disempowering to the degree that we imagine the source of our potency to effect change in the world as exisiting outside of ourselves. The appropriate use of ritual as embodied in the disciplines discussed here is the cultivation of insight and presence empowered by the healthy functioning of the heart *shen* as it manifests through the fire officials. This is well expressed by Confucius's view of ritual, as summarized by Fingarette, who states, "Spirit is no longer an external being influenced by the ceremony; it is that which is expressed and comes most alive in the ceremony."[20]

Virtue and Transformation: Chaos into Propriety

Joy *(le)* is the emotion associated with the fire element. The character *le* (樂) has the meaning of both music and joy, which are often discussed together in the Confucian analects.[21] According to Confucius, the purpose of ritual *(li)* and music is to permit human desire and emotion to be expressed in a healthy fashion without excess.[22] The presence of the emotion joy *(le)* immediately engenders its opposite, which is lack of joy *(bule:*不樂*)* or sorrow—hence Confucius's commentary on the *Yijing* hexagram for fire ("the clinging"), cited at the head of this section (moving away/fire).

The struggle to maintain, or inability to express, joy are the key emotive states that drive people who are fire constitutionally. Habitual reaction to the emotions of joy or sorrow leads them away from the virtue of propriety toward life themes centered around an excessive need for either control or chaos (see Figure 9.3). Reaction to past sorrow may lead them to keep their hearts habitually closed in an attempt to avoid disappointment and pain. In this case individuals may appear as joyless tyrants who struggle for control in all domains of life. A general principle of physics is that the more tightly an atom is confined, the more it vibrates and thus generates heat. Similarly, the tighter the heart is held as they attempt to maintain control, the more heat and pressure are generated as the heart fails to express its purpose. In this scenario, *yin, ling,* and *jing* are consumed as the heart fire rages. Habitual reaction to sadness may also lead to the excessive quest for joy. This may manifest as the tendency to cling to whatever engenders feelings of happiness in life. Here they evidence a lack of self-control, ultimately exhausting their store of heart *qi* and *yang* in the hedonistic pursuit of pleasure. Chaos ensues as the patient's heart fails to provide a stable center capable of accessing the potential wisdom stored in the *jing*.

As treatment progresses, both excessive and deficient displays of joy will diminish, along with a reduction in aberrant behaviors such as the need for excessive control or submission. Over time, the illnesses predicated on these habitual reactions should be mitigated as the virtue of propriety steadily increases. The dynamics of destiny and transformation are evidenced in the case studies presented later.

The Rhythm of Fire

Fire governs the moment-to-moment presence in life that is reflected in the steady beating of the heart. Any deviation in the rhythm, rate, or intensity of the pulse speaks directly to the quality of our momentary presence governed by the fire element. Historically, a pulse that was either too rapid or too slow was thought to reflect the presence of either heat or cold, respectively. However, people in affluent cultures today are not subjected to such harsh environmental conditions as they were in the past. Unless there is compelling evidence to the contrary, any deviation of the pulse rate from normal must be considered a result of either a physical (e.g., car accident) or emotional (perceived betrayal such as rape, incest, or divorce) shock that impacted the integrated functioning of the fire officials.

The Spirit of Fire

The spirit of the fire element is the heart's *shen,* which itself is the basis of the spirit residing in each of the other *yin* officials. The quality of brightness in the eyes is evidence of the heart spirit radiating into the world.

The Life Thesis of Fire

The state of identifying with the created self is one of delusion. The key life themes for fire constitution types involve transforming attachment to the desires of the imagined self into the ability to surrender to the acknowledgment of the truth that lies in their inner heart. If habitual reaction to the presence of joy or sadness obscures access to the virtue of propriety, their life theme is distorted into a thesis that compromises the ability to be in synch in every aspect of being. In this scenario, identification with the created self leads them to miss every relevant cue that emanates from heaven both internally as an expression of *yuanqi* and *jing* and externally as their life events. Rather than proceed according to the insight afforded by the heart, their actions are presided over entirely by the mind's attempt to seize control, prolong pleasure, and avoid pain.

The archetypal life theme for fire constitutional types that reflects excess may be stated as, "My insight is so profound that I must actively control every aspect of my life as well as the lives of those around me." The theme that reflects deficiency may be stated as, "Control is an illusion in a chaotic world. I must surrender to my desires and the desires of others in order to be happy."

Irony: Do Nothing

The irony at the heart of the fire element is that *true control comes from doing nothing.* This is exemplified in the Chinese concept of *wuwei* (無為), or inaction. For several thousand years the emperor had a sign over his throne bearing these characters as a reminder that the best course of action is often to aid life by encouraging it to unfold on its own. Habitual reaction to the emotions joy and sadness drives the fire officials to maintain either excessive or deficient levels of control in the exercise of their respective functions. Thus the heart of fire constitutional types is ultimately unfulfilled as each new relationship is only momentarily satisfying before they are compelled to a new level of either dominance or submission.

Testing Emotions: Companionship

The quality of a patient's fire element may be assessed by either offering companionship and initiating connection with the patient or by withdrawing emotional warmth. This may be accomplished by a gesture as simple as smiling at the patient and noting his or her response. People who are fire constitutionally habitually respond to the presence of joy or sadness by either initiating excessive contact or by withdrawing their own emotional warmth in a way that helps them feel safe. For example, a patient whose fire is deficient may make poor contact during a handshake and quickly retreat in an attempt to avoid contact. Conversely, the patient with excess fire may shake the practitioner's hand vigorously, failing to let go when it is withdrawn.

When fire is in a functional state of balance, the patient's display of either joy or sadness should appropriately reflect the emotional content of the material being discussed during the intake. When fire is out of balance, the color, sound, odor, and emotion associated with fire present themselves inappropriately whenever the patient is discussing emotionally charged material. For example, a patient may display laughter and inappropriate joy when discussing a painful event such as a divorce. Or the quality of a patient's laugh may sound like crying when discussing a joyful event such as a recent engagement.

The degree to which we assess the display of an element is inappropriate is the degree to which it suppresses balanced functioning in the moment. For example, it is quite possible that even twenty years after the end of an intimate relationship a patient may appear momentarily sad when discussing it. If the integrated functioning of the fire element is intact, the patient will gently move through the sadness and on to whatever material follows during the process of the intake. To the degree there is separation between the heart and mind of the fire constitution, the patient will become stuck in the display of either sorrow or joy. Patients' inability to move easily through the momentary display of these emotions during the intake is also reflected in the finding that their disappointment with romance twenty years ago still limits the degree to which they can experience healthy intimacy.

Compassion on the part of the practitioner may manifest in attempting to realign patients with the insight and intuition that emanates from their own hearts. I define compassion here as an act that relieves suffering. In the short term, insight provided by the practitioner may initiate feelings of emotional pain in patients as they experience sorrow trapped in their hearts. However in the long term such insight may realign the heart-kidney axis of patients in a way that empowers insight and intuition. The restoration of these virtues is paramount if original nature is to be restored. A hallmark of those of the fire constitution is that reaction to joy or sadness is the unconscious motivating force underlying habitual behavior. The person has long ago rejected the inner knowing of the heart in order to pursue the mind's desires and avoid pain in life.

Upon initially offering patients compassion and insight, the practitioner will find their pursuit of joy or flight from sorrow is allayed only briefly, if at all. When compassion is offered to fire constitutional types, there will be one of two results. Compassion may be rejected as the patient's mind seeks to take control and dominate the situation. In this scenario patients seek to avoid connection with their hearts by controlling the interview and, by extension, the therapeutic process. I am reminded of a patient who was very ill with a degenerative neurological condition. Soon after beginning the interview, she informed me that all men suffer from a defect of character she would rather not discuss. Upon hearing this I laughed and smiling, asked her if she realized I was a man. Her response was to laugh in return and say it wasn't a problem because all her healers had been men. In reality, she was telling me her mind felt safe with me in treatment because she would let nothing I do touch her heart in a way that promoted healing.

Or the patient may continually elicit compassion throughout the interview in an attempt to initiate intimacy inappropriately with the practitioner through self-revelation. No amount of external compassion can do more than temporarily allay the search for joy, or flight from sorrow, that unconsciously motivates the fire constitution. Only through connection to the internal virtues of insight and propriety that empower compassion for the self can the separation between heart and mind be rectified.

The Role of Suggestion

Imbalance of the fire element is typified by the patient's inappropriate relationship to the issue of control. Initially, the practitioner must either overtly take complete control in directing the course of treatment or seemingly yield it completely, letting patients perceive they are controlling the course of events. Using the language of the fire element is the best way to motivate people by aligning them with the insight of their own hearts. For example, in motivating a patient whose constitution is fire to quit smoking, the practitioner must offer the suggestion in one of two ways. If the patient displays an excessive need for control, the practitioner might say, "You will know the precise moment when you are best able to quit. It will be wonderful to really see you retake control of your life." Or the practitioner may need to direct the course of treatment exactly. In this case the practitioner might say, "I will know precisely when you will be able to quit smoking effectively. For the first four sessions you will smoke no more than one pack a day and then we will reassess your progress." As patients' health improves, they will govern their lives more appropriately and therefore relinquish some control or take more control in their process of healing. The therapeutic relationship will increasingly become a partnership as the power differential diminishes.

Fire and Intimacy

The healthy experience of intimacy with others is based on knowing what lies in our own heart. Ultimately, the organ functions that contribute to our experience of intimacy are paramount to the integrity of each human being. The officials associated with the fire element are of particular importance in regulating the appropriate function of intimacy in human beings. One of the key functions of the fire officials is to define and mediate the functioning of several levels of boundary between our true self (heart) and the outside world. Next I discuss the inner nature of the fire officials as they relate to establishing personal boundaries, with emphasis on the human experience of intimacy with self and others.

The Fire Officials

Heart

> The heart holds the office of lord and sovereign. The radi-
> ance of the spirits (shenming) stems from it.
> – NEI JING SU WEN[23]

In the inner tradition of Chinese medicine, the circulation of *qi*
among the twelve meridians begins with the heart official. This reflects
an orientation that ultimately seeks to help patients each access the
insight empowered by their own hearts. In terms of a personal boundary, the heart is both the origin of the capacity for connection as well
as the ultimate goal of connection. The main function of the heart as
sovereign is to acknowledge momentary reality as it occurs, unimpeded by the mind's interpretation of events. A well-functioning heart
empowers us to respond freely and spontaneously to each new situation in life. Hence the sage accepts each new situation as heaven's
attempt to cultivate the seed it has planted within at the moment of
conception. Internally, the heart allows us to acknowledge our true
nature as stored in the *yuanqi* and *jing*. In this way the heart provides
the capacity to be intimate with oneself. All illness may be considered
indicative of having lost touch with the truth in one's "heart of hearts."
For a depiction of the relationship between the heart and mind, see
Figure 10.1.

A Further Discussion of Heart and Mind

> Illumination is the energy of open awareness in the
> palace of fire (the heart); it is the spirit of humans, the
> master of mind. When the mind is open it is aware; the
> original spirit is in charge of affairs, and illumination
> is managed properly. One can thereby balance yang.
> When the mind is unruly, it wanders; the discriminatory
> consciousness handles affairs, and illumination is not
> properly directed. This is sufficient to damage yang.
> Therefore fire is beneficial to correctness and development.
> – LIU YIMING[24]

When I was learning Chinese medicine, my teachers would often
make statements such as "The heart and mind are one." In teaching us

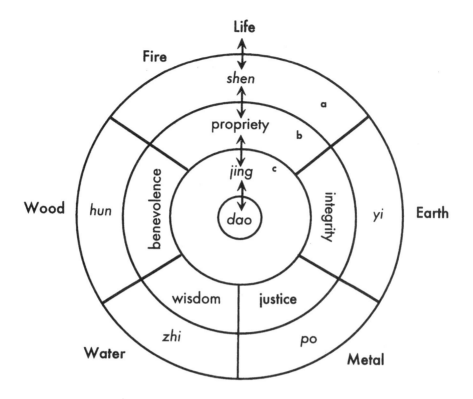

Figure 10.1
HEART AND MIND

This figure depicts the relationship between the mind, the heart, and primordial dao. The mind (a) is portrayed as a relatively "outer" level of being whose functioning comprises the yang *officials as they relate to the sensory orifices. It is the illusion of material existence conveyed through the senses that distances humanity from original nature. The* yang *aspect of each element is identified with the* shen, *that aspect of self capable of introspection and conveying the essence of the heart into the external world. The heart (b) represents a relatively inner level of functioning comprised of the heart official itself, as well as all the other* yin *officials. The* yin *officials provide access to the* yuanqi *and* jing *of each element, which is the potential source for each individual's manifestation of virtue in life. The heart spirit (shen) itself has risen ontologically out of the individual's true deep nature as present in the kidney* jing *(c). This nature, planted by heaven at conception, may be said to be the truth that lies in one's "heart of hearts." It is the kidney* jing *that provides our connection back to the primordial* dao. *The* yang *officials are conduits between the outer and inner worlds of the individual. The double arrows indicate that the functions of the mind and heart must be aligned with* dao *so reality, both internally as original nature and externally as life's events, may be accurately perceived.*

diagnosis it was emphasized that the practitioner must discern which level of body, mind, or spirit is the genesis of dysfunction in each patient. These two statements, which often followed in the same breath, always seemed to me to be at odds. The first presupposes a unity and the second a separation between the physical and nonphysical aspects of being. I didn't understand why a duality posed by the words *heart* and *mind* would be used to describe a concept predicated on unity. Next I elaborate the notion of heart and mind from the perspective of the Chinese language and the thesis of this text.

The character *xin* (心) depicts a heart with three beats.[25] In describing the function of the heart, the *Nei Jing Su Wen* tells us that the "radiance of the spirits" (*shenming*) stems from it. In health, the spirit rests quietly in the heart, a state evidenced in the brightness of the eyes. In modern times, the term *shenming* has been generally interpreted to signify the mind. This interpretation represents a break with the traditional notions of spirit as that which animates the body. It also represents a shift toward the atheistic and materialistic view of Western science that avoids discussing spirit and sees the mind as an emanation of the nervous system.

The Chinese characters for psychology are *shenxue* (神學), meaning literally "study of the spirit," and the characters for the nervous system are *shenjing* (神經), meaning literally "lines that conduct *shen*." In fact, the ancient Chinese had no word that corresponds directly to the Western concept of mind. From the preceding it is clear that illnesses we perceive as propagated by dysfunctional emotional states are in fact predicated on a disordered relationship between the heart and the spirit. From the standpoint of the ancient Chinese, the entire gamut of habitual patterns referred to in this text are based on a disordered spirit that is unable to rest tranquilly in our heart.

In this text my use of the word *mind* occurs in two contexts. In health, I use *mind* to refer to that aspect of spirit which is able to penetrate into our depths and the depths of life externally to discern truth. To a degree this process involves the procurement, analysis, and integration of sensory data. In this sense I have compared the function of the mind to the *yang* officials that serve as an interface between the internal world of the *yin* officials and the external world perceived by the sensory apparatus. I also use the term *mind* to refer to the aberrant operation of this analytic facility when separation between the *yin* and *yang* officials allows it to rule our life instead of serving it. Although I use the term *mind*, you must remain aware that a disordered mind is predicated on a disturbed spirit.

When the core of our being functions harmoniously, the heart and mind function as one. Harmonious function of this relationship, however, is apparently the exception rather than the rule. Hence it is frequently possible to distinguish between the functions of the heart and mind. The heart empowers the capacity to acknowledge the nature of life both internally and externally as it changes from moment to moment. The mind is the faculty of data analysis and, when harmony prevails, initiates action, via the will *(zhi)*, based on the truth we find in the heart. The heart cannot will what it feels and is only able to acknowledge truth. Actions based on the heart are undertaken because the individual has no choice but to accept reality as it occurs in the moment. Following our heart is often most difficult in the short term, yet pays the biggest dividends in the long run. Actions based on the heart lead to personal integrity and empower the virtue *(de)* of intuition. Hence the heart must rule and the mind must follow. Ultimately, the heart is nourished by the momentary presence born out of commitment to all actions that empower the fulfillment of individual destiny.

But the habituated mind feels constrained in the moment and seeks forever to escape it by fantasizing about the past or future.[26] The mind always justifies its actions in an attempt to be reasonable. Whenever the patient is justifying a course of action, we may be sure the mind is in control. The mind, reflecting the conditioned nature, most often picks that action which makes us most comfortable in the moment. Actions based on avoiding what makes us uncomfortable in the moment always pay the smallest dividends in the long term because they lead us away from the heart and true self. Therapeutically, the traditional practitioner must help guide patients to know when they are following their minds versus when they are following their hearts.

In my view, the separation of heart and mind denotes a tearing apart of the fundamental fabric of life, indicating a dire separation of *yin* and *yang*. The essence of the spiritual path in the inner tradition is that all concepts and beliefs which create separation between our mind and heart must be methodically rooted out. Only when our mind is able to spontaneously acknowledge and act on the truth within our heart is healing complete. We could say this experience of intimacy with and connection to our true self is the first step in fulfilling individual destiny.

Virtue and Spirit: The Heart/Kidney Axis

By extending *shen* into *jing*, the heart empowers the virtue of insight into our depths. This insight empowers connection to our primordial influences and the wisdom contained therein. In balance there is a direct continuum between these two. As our heart reaches the limit to which conscious awareness of self and other can penetrate in life, the kidney begins to empower innate unconscious knowing that manifests as faith. The heart/kidney axis is the central axis of spiritual stability and power to which all other human facilities must align. This axis is replicated throughout the *yin* and *yang* relationships of all the other officials (Figures 10.2a and 10.2b).

An attribute of the holographic nature of the functional relationships of the *sheng* and *ke* cycles is that when separation occurs between the *jing* and *shen* of an element, it is reflected in the disordered function of every other element. For example, if the liver and gallbladder lose communication in a wood constitutional type, the *shen/jing* axis of communication is compromised in the other four elements and ultimately undermines the functional relationship of the heart/kidney axis itself. By restoring the natural communication between the *yin* and *yang* officials of a patient's constitution, the practitioner touches the depth of all separation in the patient's being.

Treating the source and *luo* points together on the patient's constitutional element is one of the strongest treatments for reasserting the balance between the *jing* and *shen* of each elemental pair. For example, treating Liver-3 and Gallbladder-37 will direct the aspects of mind governed by the gallbladder back inward toward the virtue of the liver. Conversely, treating Gallbladder-40 and Liver-5 will allow the virtue of the liver to radiate toward the outer world.

Heart Spirits: Ling *and* Shen

> Once shen *attains the one, it is efficacious* (ling).
> – DAO DE JING [27]

The *yin* and *yang* of heart spirit are present as the *ling* and *shen*, respectively. The harmony of the *ling* and *shen* spirits empowers the emperor to rule through the doctrine of inaction *(wuwei)*. The *shen* is the radiant spirit that shines through the eyes, indicating the quality of fire in *mingmen*. The *shen* is the impulse that emanates from the balanced *xin* to illuminate the *jing* and manifest our potential. *Shen* is the spirit empowering our momentary presence and focus. If our *shen* has been injured, we may evidence an ashen complexion and dullness in the eyes, with an attendant loss of ability to sustain contact. The integrity and focus of the *shen* in part depends on the functional integrity of the other fire officials and the other officials in general.

The *ling* is the highest emanation of the *jing* and the *yin* of heart spirit. It empowers us to be effective in the world. With our destiny fulfilled, the *ling* emerges to grant us the magical power of the sage. We may perform rituals effectively and petition heaven for change outside our self. If the *ling* is damaged, we may appear spiritually impotent in all realms of life. An important part of the healing process often involves returning to our sense of potency, empowered by the *ling* spirit.[28] It is essential to help patients experience themselves, once again, as effective forces in the world. An individual with a heart whose *ling* spirit is unbalanced may be unsynchronized in all realms of life. When the *yin* and *yang* of heart spirit are balanced, things proceed "as if they were done by no one." Confucius refers indirectly to this quality of *ling* and heart spirit when he says that Shun, the great sage king, "merely placed himself gravely and reverently with his face due south; that was all,"[29] for "with correct comportment, no commands are necessary, yet affairs proceed."[30]

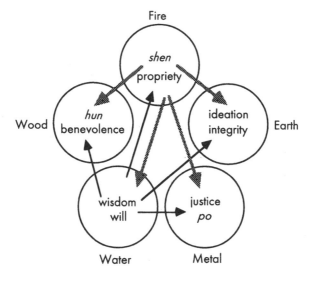

Figure 10.2(a)
THE HEART/KIDNEY AXIS

The shen *rises out of the kidney* jing *and ascends to its throne in the palace of the heart. The* shen *then radiates to each of the other elements as the emperor is present in each of his ministers. Hence the heart provides* shen *to each of the other* yin *officials. This relationship is depicted by the shaded arrows. The kidney provides* jing, *which is the basis of virtue in life to each of the other* yin *officials. This relationship is depicted by the solid arrows. The heart/kidney axis is the only direct line of communication between heart* shen *and kidney* jing.

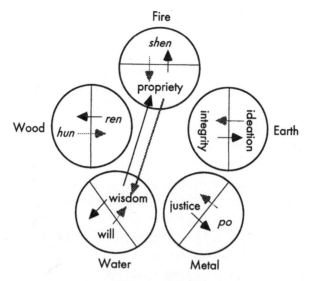

Figure 10.2(b)

The heart/kidney axis is replicated within each pair of yin *and* yang *officials as the* shen *and* jing *of each pair of officials interact. The relative nature of* shen *is yang, and the relative nature of* jing *is yin. The radiance of each element's spirit may be likened to the workings of the mind in probing our depths and in conveying our virtue to the outside world. Inasmuch as this is so, the* shen *of each element may be associated with the mental-level functioning of the* yang *official in each elemental pair. The* jing, *which is the basis of each element's virtue, is associated with the* yin *official in each pair. It is the action of each* yang *official in focusing the* shen *upon the* jing *that allows us to manifest our specific elemental virtue in life.*

Control: The Archetypal Theme of the Heart

With the highest [kind of rulers], those below simply know they exist.
With those one step down—they love and praise them.
With those one further step down—they fear them.
And with those at the bottom—they ridicule and insult them.
When trust (xin) is insufficient, there will be no trust [in return].

– DAO DE JING[31]

Here the *Dao De Jing* lists the quality of rule of various sovereigns in descending order of desirability. The best emperor is the one whose existence is merely known by the people and whose activities are hidden. The population does not notice the ruler directly but observes that all is right with the world. The next, lower level, is the emperor everybody loves. Although it is true the leader is loved, his subjects are continually aware of his presence. Hence we might say strings are attached to his love for them and it is not unconditional (the citizens' heart strings are being gently tugged as their leader maintains control). The next lowest ruler starts passing laws to maintain control, and people fear him. The lowest ruler is the joyless tyrant who governs by force and maintains control with an iron grip. The passage here from the *Dao De Jing* can be taken metaphorically to describe the genesis of heart disease. Hence issues of control are paramount for people with a heart imbalance, and heart palpitations, stuttering, insomnia, chest pain, and general confusion may be evidenced as the heart struggles for control.

The *Dao De Jing* informs us that the enlightened ruler employs each of his ministers according to their particular abilities.[32] A conductor must pull the best performance from each musician while assuring that each part is played at precisely the right moment. So too must the heart conduct the overall functioning of the twelve officials.

As we lose touch with our own heart, the capacity for intimacy with self and others dwindles. We now serve the habitually reactive mind and ignore the heart's innate wisdom as the path to ruin is trod one step at a time. Separated from the heart, all minds eventually become joyless tyrants, and all attempts to serve them are in vain. Unity between the heart and mind must be restored if therapy is to be effective and healing complete. Hence a foremost concern at the beginning of any effective therapy must be to stabilize the function of the patient's heart.

The Nature of Lying

Who we really are corresponds to the nature placed within at conception, contained within the primordial endowment stored in the kidneys. With the gaining of personal name, we move away from these influences that lie in the darkness and depths of self. In moving away we proceed toward the light of the fire element that illuminates our personal face in the world as distinct from the ten thousand other beings. Our heart *shen* provides the means to reconnect to the true self stored in our depths. However, access to this truth is lost to the degree that identification with the created self compromises the functional integrity of the fire officials.

To the degree they have lost touch with true nature, it becomes difficult for fire constitutional types to convey their heart essence accurately to the outside world. They in effect proceed through life wearing a mask, believing it to be their true face. This mask is an external projection of their internal process of continually lying to self about who they really are. With trust compromised as a consequence of past disappointment and perceived betrayal, the habituated mind may perpetrate acts of deliberate miscommunication in a dysfunction-al attempt to protect the heart. In this scenario, lying becomes a way of avoiding connection and intimacy. Lying may occur subtly as they withhold communication about their true nature or less subtly as they deliberately mislead another about their intentions.

Particular aspects of being are governed by a given element, yet each element is capable of manifesting them in a unique way. For example, lying is a fire attribute, yet each element lies in a distinct way. The water element tends to be secretive and lies by omission. The fire ele-ment lies by wearing a false face in the world. The wood element, in an attempt to always be right, lies by perpetrating the myth that the end justifies the means. The metal element lies by misrepresenting the value of things. And the earth element lies by being ingratiating rather than sincere.

An excellent exercise for the student of the five elements is to discern as many aspects of being as possible and to determine (1) which ele-ment governs that aspect of being, and (2) the unique ways in which it is expressed through the other elements.

The Nature of Commitment

The heart rules the blood and the constancy of its beat reflects its commitment to fulfilling its role as sovereign ruler. Any irregularity in the pulse may reflect the heart's faltering commitment and struggle to maintain control. Hence the quality of a person's commitment may be seen as reflecting the quality of the heart's intention. Confusion regard-ing the notion of commitment is a key imbalance predicated on betrayal of our heart's purpose. With trust in our own insight eroded, we may fail to trust our own heart's capacity to live up to its ideals. Our mind becomes overwhelmed at the notion of commitment in all domains of life and particularly in regard to intimate relationships. Even if we are in a satisfying relationship, the mind may continually lead us to avoid the momentary presence required for true intimacy to emerge. Intimacy, the one thing for which the heart longs, poses the greatest threat to the mind in its attempt to avoid pain. For the basis of intimacy with others is afforded by that connection to our own heart, which the mind is denying.

In attempting to reunite heart and mind, I have found it effective to "reframe" this dilemma by asking patients to describe their interpreta-tion of the concept of commitment. Most often the response is similar to this: "Commitment means you will always stay in the relationship no matter what." I reframe commitment as "the ability to be 100 percent present while we are engaged in a particular activity." Commitment need not mean we will forever remain in a relationship regardless of circumstance. It can merely indicate the willingness to be fully present while in the relationship. After all, relationships can always be ended.

Fear about being able to keep our commitments frequently emanates from the underlying fear of momentary presence. When patients grasp this concept, I then assign them the "homework" of being conscious of all the ways they avoid being present in their daily life. Patients' process of inquiry into the nature of commitment may play a major role in helping their hearts to heal.

Irony: True Control Is Effortless

The heart is the foundational function of the fire element, and the irony which lies thematically at the center of the heart constitution is identical to that described earlier as generally being true for all the fire officials: *True control comes from doing nothing.* The habituated mind in its attempt to create a condition of safety for the heart struggles unceasingly to either maintain or abdicate control in life. In so doing, it either overly constrains or fails to focus the heart in a way that prevents it from ever connecting to true self. Hence, as long as the mind dictates our course of action, the heart remains unfulfilled. The irony is that only in the surrender of the mind can the heart reestablish its authority and again govern through its innate wisdom.

Summary

The heart as emperor lives well protected at the center of the nation in the purple forbidden city.[33] No injury must come to the heart, and as long as the heart's function is intact, there is always hope of healing.[34] The heart is so important that it is the only official with three other functions to protect it.

Next I examine the function of the other fire officials—small intestine, heart protector, and triple heater—as they relate to the establishment of a boundary, the protection of the heart, and the appropriate function of intimacy in human beings.

Small Intestine

The small intestine is responsible for receiving and making things thrive. Transformed substances stem from it.
– NEI JING SU WEN[35]

The small intestine is the heart's closest minister and the conduit both from the heart into the world and from the world into the heart. The functioning of the small intestine mediates the clarity with which we are able to perceive and communicate the truth and penetrating insight *(shenming)* stored within our heart and the hearts of others. It is rare to be granted a private audience with the emperor and, at best, we are received by the highest minister. The emperor must be concerned with only the most important details in running the kingdom, and it is up to his minister to sort out what messages are appropriate to relay to the imperial chamber. Conversely, it is the function of the minister to communicate the essence of the emperor's wishes to the nation at large. The small intestine, the heart's closest minister, must, without distortion, convey the heart's decree *(ming)* to the other officials as well as to the outside world. These principles mirror the small intestine's physiological function. Hence the small intestine sorts out what essence, in the form of amino acids, will be absorbed from food into the blood and transported to the heart, and what constitutes waste to be sent onward to the large intestine for elimination.

A paramount responsibility of the small intestine is to ensure that communication between heart and mind, and heart and the outside world, occurs in a way that cultivates virtue. The integrity of the small intestine's function is vital if mind and heart are to communicate clearly. Any deviation in the function of the small intestine significantly perpetuates habituated behavior. As the mind increasingly distorts momentary reality, the spontaneous function of *mingmen* is gradually extinguished.

Small Intestine Imbalance

If the function of the small intestine is compromised, confusion is the result, as we misinterpret both our own intention and the intentions of others. Now the heart can no longer communicate its insight, and the mind begins giving and receiving mixed messages. Bitterness, the flavor associated with fire, is also the emotional correlate of the toxicity that results physiologically if the small intestine does not perform its function of sorting properly. Sexual "perversion" may be interpreted as the result of the small intestine not being able to receive or transmit heart essence appropriately.[36] I define "perversion" here as forcing intimacy on an unwilling party.[37] Sarcasm may also be considered to reflect emotional bitterness and the small intestine's inability to convey heart essence appropriately.

Because a primary function of the small intestine is "listening" to the heart, patients with severe small intestine imbalance often evidence a complete inability to hear what the practitioner is saying. The patient's mind so colors life that interpretation of what is said and what occurs bear no relation to reality. In fact, the patient's interpretation of what is said is often diametrically opposed to the actual communication. Another hallmark of small intestine imbalance is that the patient may have a predominant sense of not being heard by others. Patients may be convinced that others do not understand them, not realizing it is a result of their own unclear communication.

In effect, the small intestine is a lens that focuses the intention of the heart. The confusion that typifies small intestine imbalance may appear as a type of dissociation. This dissociation results from the small intestine failing to focus the expression of the heart spirit *(shen)* appropriately. Balancing the relationship between the heart and small intestine is often an important step in stabilizing the fire officials and, therefore, our entire functional dynamic.

The Virtue of Listening

The Chinese alchemical text "Secret of the Golden Flower" *(Tai Yi Jin Hua Zong Zhi,* eighteenth century*)* describes the role of listening in aiding the heart's spirit to penetrate into the interior (depths of self). It paraphrases a legendary text, the *Danshu* (Book of the Elixir), and states,

> The hen can hatch her eggs because the heart is always listening. The hen can hatch her eggs because of the energy of heat. But the energy of the heat can only warm the shells; it cannot penetrate into the interior. Therefore she conducts this energy inward with her heart. This she does with her hearing. In this way she concentrates her whole heart. When the heart penetrates, the energy penetrates, and the chick receives the energy of the heat and begins to live. Therefore a hen, even at times when she leaves her eggs, always has the attitude of listening with bent ear. Thus the concentration of the spirit is not interrupted.[38]

This example serves as a metaphor for the way the function of the small intestine's capacity for attentive listening may empower the function of the heart. The elaborate ritual of the hen caring for her eggs is based on attentive listening. It is the concentration of our *shen* that brings intention into the world in a way that fulfills destiny. If habitual reaction to the emotions of sorrow or joy perpetuate a dysfunctional relationship between the heart and small intestine, the heart *shen* will not be focused in a way that promotes connection to life's purpose.

The Small Intestine and Heat

In illness, the small intestine cannot sort out the difference between the wishes of the heart and the desires of the mind. If the small intestine fails to convey accurately the heart's wishes into the world, these may accumulate in the heart, resulting in both heat and internal pressure. Bitterness, sarcasm, and perversion as alluded to earlier are the psychospiritual correlates of this heat being dissipated. Physiological heat from the small intestine that enters the blood may exit through the skin as toxicity, presenting as boils or open sores (e.g., shingles).

Thesis: I'm Confused/You're Confused

The key life themes for the small intestine constitution involve communication in a manner presided over by the virtue of propriety. Effective performance of ritual dictates saying the right thing at the right time. If habitual reaction to the presence of joy or sorrow obscures access to the heart's insight, then our life theme is distorted into a thesis based on faulty communication. In this case the balanced relationship between speaking and listening is compromised in every domain of life.

The archetypal life theme for the small intestine constitutional type may be stated as, "Nobody hears me. Try as I might to explain myself, I am always misunderstood." The converse of this theme would rarely be stated because individuals possessing this imbalance generally insist they have heard and understood what was said. Keeping this in mind, the converse theme may be stated as, "Nobody speaks clearly to me. Try as I might, I always seem to misunderstand what others are saying."

Irony: Listen to Be Heard

The irony at the heart of the life of the small intestine constitutional type is that *the basis of true communication is listening*. The ability to speak clearly is based on our ability to access, through listening, our own inner truth. In illness, the mind of the small intestine constitution is turned outward away from the standard of truth present in our heart and the hearts of others. It is therefore only able to communicate its habitual desires and in the end distorts all that is heard and spoken.

Habitual reaction to the emotions joy and sorrow drives the small intestine official to either excessive or deficient sorting when under stress. In this scenario patients often give the impression they are not listening to what you are saying. Rather, they are listening to what they are thinking about what you are saying. In its extreme, excessive sorting may present as stuttering, which hinders precise communication of the heart's commands. The inability of small intestine constitution types to listen or speak clearly is often a defensive mechanism of the mind vainly attempting to protect the heart from pain associated with intimacy. With each communication, satisfaction is felt for only a short while before feelings of not being heard reassert themselves, driving them to initiate further contact in an attempt to get their point across.

Communication in a way that rectifies the heart is the fulfillment of destiny for small intestine constitutional types. Only through the realization of this virtue can they ever experience true connection with self and others.

Heart Protector and Triple Heater

One of the unique contributions of Chinese medicine to our understanding of human function is the concept of the heart protector and triple heater officials. These two functions are unique among the officials because they are the only ones not correlated with individual organs. Think of the heart protector and triple heater as the guard stations protecting the imperial city and the borders of the country, respectively. This functional relationship is imaged in the names of the acupuncture points Heart Protector-6 ("inner frontier gate") and Triple Heater-5 ("outer frontier gate"). The inner nature of these points is discussed in Chapter 13. These officials play a unique role in regulating human intimacy.

Heart Protector

*The heart protector has the charge of resident as well as
envoy. Elation and joy stem from it.*
– NEI JING SU WEN[39]

Just as the emperor lives at the center of the purple forbidden city, so too can the heart be conceived as living at the center of the body surrounded by a protective network comprising, most immediately, the functions of the other fire officials. The small intestine may be conceived as the minister who guards the emperor's inner quarters, and the heart protector is like the keeper of the drawbridge who regulates passage both into and out of the capital. The heart protector is concerned with discerning the appropriate cues for lowering the boundary that limits access both into, and out of, the inner frontier which is the domain of the heart.

A chief characteristic of the heart protector is that it "receives" blows aimed at the heart. Ultimately, the heart itself must remain pure if life is to proceed in a balanced fashion. Most imbalances, both symptomatic and functional, ascribed to the heart in actuality represent compromised function of the heart protector. The heart protector plays a key role in many of the functional imbalances related to intimacy. These are discussed jointly with imbalances of the triple heater.

Triple Heater

> *The triple heater is responsible for*
> *the opening up of passages and irrigation.*
> *The regulation of the fluids stems from it.*
> – NEI JING SU WEN[40]

The "outermost" official of the fire element is the triple heater. The triple heater is like the emissary of the emperor stationed at the nation's borders. Whereas the heart protector represents the walls around the castle, the triple heater functions like the great wall at the periphery of the nation. Like a customs guard at a border station, the triple heater must discern who will be allowed to enter and to leave the kingdom of one's heart. In this sense, the triple heater contributes to the body's outermost defensive mechanisms *(weiqi:衛氣)*. It is paramount that potentially damaging insults to the heart are stopped at the outer layer of defense. Once the threat of "invasion" has reached the castle gates, a good part of the damage may already be done. By providing good reconnaissance from the periphery of our surroundings, the triple heater may empower the heart to stem trouble intuitively before it establishes itself.

Physiologically, the triple heater may be thought of as the body's thermostat that maintains homeostasis by regulating the distribution of fire *(yang)* and water *(yin)* throughout all aspects of being. A good thermostat maintains equilibrium between internal and external environments. In order to fulfill this function, the triple heater must maintain constant connection with every relevant aspect of our surroundings. Thus the triple heater is responsible for the gathering and assimilation of the environmental cues the heart needs in order to rule effectively.

Compared to the heart protector, the triple heater governs the more social aspects of fire, and gathers and assimilates subtle cues in the environment relevant to the regulation of intimacy. Intimacy is a dynamic function that, in health, must operate according to the same principles as a well-functioning thermostat. The gates regulating access to our inner kingdom must operate spontaneously—without conscious thought. Just as the body's internal temperature must be held at 98.6° F as the external temperature changes, so too should the gates providing access to our inner being open and close appropriately. The spontaneous function of these gates must stem from the heart, from the center of which the virtues of intuition and propriety emerge. As we see later, this spontaneity is lost as the heart protector and triple heater lose functional equilibrium.

Imbalance of the Heart Protector and Triple Heater

The healthy function of intimacy depends in large part on the harmonious balance between the heart protector and triple heater. I focus here on the dynamics of heart protector and triple heater imbalance as they form a functional yoke. A virtue of fire is that it empowers the quality of maturity. Often those who have had their hearts protected by the heart protector appear very young and perhaps emotionally immature. These individuals often are late bloomers in life who evidence a very quick maturation once the balance of these two officials is restored in treatment. In this scenario, the heart protector as a defensive measure has shut off access to the inner kingdom, and the childlike essence, retained in the heart, has remained intact. Early in life, this is a chief aspect of the heart protector's appropriate functioning in protecting the heart. However, later in life, individuals may be unaware of the ways an inappropriately protected heart, predicated on past emotional pain, may limit their experience of joy and intimacy. A patient whose heart protector is habitually closed may exhibit either a lack or excess of fire. The closer the heart is confined, the more it vibrates and the more heat is generated. This heat may be present as a wide range of dysfunctions in all aspects of personal expression. Emotionally and behaviorally, patients may evidence a tendency toward mania, including signs of hypersexuality. Eventually, however, even the most intense blaze must die out. We may be shut off from sexuality with heart fire so closed down that "coldness" is evidenced on all levels of personal expression. This "frigidity" may present as an inability to achieve orgasm.[41]

Physically, the triple heater may be involved any time there is an excess or deficiency of heat anywhere in the body. Individuals with a triple heater imbalance may have difficulty differentiating between social and intimate relationships, often falling in and out of relationships quickly. They may feel comfortable in groups but be truly afraid of intimate contact on a one-to-one level.

Any deviation in the functions of the heart protector and triple heater may compromise the heart's intention with a corresponding loss of spontaneity in intimate relationships. Often the line between social and intimate relationships becomes blurred, and we begin to continually send and receive mixed messages. Separated from the heart's intuitive wisdom, we now choose relationships based on the mind's analysis of data. The heart protector and triple warmer no longer function spontaneously and subconsciously but open and close according to the dictates of the habitually driven mind. Ultimately, confusion emerges around what signs constitute sufficient evidence for trust. This dynamic is at the root of several dysfunctional patterns that result from betrayal of intimacy.

Betrayal of Trust: The Thesis of Heart Protector and Triple Heater

The innate capacity of the heart to govern in a healthy fashion is compromised in life by betrayal of the heart's openness and insight. The mind, unable to assimilate the pain resulting from betrayal of the heart's purpose, often grabs control in an effort to feel secure.

Patterns of functional imbalance resulting from betrayal specifically affect the direct lines of communication between the heart (emperor) and his ministers.[42] As betrayal breaks bonds of trust between us and the outside world, trust is simultaneously eroded internally between our heart and mind. The emperor loses faith in his ministers as well as they in him. Our mind, no longer able to trust the heart's innate wisdom, seizes control of the will (zhi) and begins to dictate policy based on the faculty of reason and the analysis of data.

After any betrayal, the appropriate functioning of our faculty of trust may be compromised. I define "trust" here as the facility to take appropriate action based on our acknowledgment of the "safety" of a relationship in which we are involved—safety being the context in which our heart may thrive. As a way of compensating for the injury of betrayal, trust may be eroded in one of two key ways described later. Neither of these scenarios is mutually exclusive, as they both involve the dynamic functioning of the heart protector and triple warmer pair.

The Heart Protector's Thesis: Intimacy Is Not Safe

A dysfunctional heart protector makes it impossible to truly acknowledge the nature of the relationship we are having based on its own merits. The mind's commitment to avoiding pain in relationships colors our interpretation of every nuance of intimate connection. Having suffered the pain of past disappointments, the mind of heart protector constitutional types generates a thesis that intimacy is not safe. In an attempt to shield the heart from the pain of further blows, the heart protector closes the gate that provides access to the inner self. However, although new pain may be kept from the heart, pain already experienced by the heart is kept trapped within. The mind's investment in not feeling pain makes this gate increasingly harder to open. A hallmark of this imbalance is that relationships are often characterized by fear and confusion. Whenever their hearts open to receive intimacy, the *qi* from the new relationship enters the heart simultaneously with the letting go of the old emotional pain that has been stored there. Unable to distinguish between the old pain we feel and the joy of the new relationship, they project past pain onto the present. The pain felt is interpreted as indicating that the current relationship is not safe, and the gate to intimacy is once again closed as they push their partner away.

The Triple Heater's Thesis: I Must Follow My Heart

In the habitual pursuit of pleasure, the triple heater may lead fire constitutional types to initiate constant contact with others. In this scenario, they may feel compelled to trust, in a vain attempt to prove that life is indeed "safe." A typical pattern may manifest as a habit of continually rushing into relationships; it is as though they have thrown open the castle gate to rush out to the "outer frontier," but then catch hold of themselves. Feeling "exposed," they beat a hasty retreat as, once again, the castle door slams closed and their partner is pushed away.[43] Often people in this position justify their dysfunction by claiming they must continually "follow their heart." However, their heart is not involved in this process as they try in vain to satisfy their mind's addiction to the exhilaration that comes in the initial stages of new relationships. Try as they may, they never seem to get past the "social" outer fire of the triple heater to reach a deeper level of heart intimacy. Thus this pattern often evidences frequent inappropriate sexuality as a way of actually avoiding intimacy.

In either of these situations they may evidence a tendency to choose relationships in which there is no chance of real intimacy. They may eventually choose a relationship and cling to it even in the face of physical and emotional abuse, believing it is easier to stay in this harmful situation than to leave and open up to another person. The abuse received may validate their mind's thesis that intimacy is not safe and, thus, justify their life thesis.

The Virtue of Trust

The first scenario just discussed is typified by a refusal to trust. The mind is constantly vigilant in "protecting" the inner frontier. Fire constitutional types are constantly looking for cues to discern they are safe, and any internal message of pain is interpreted as a lack of safety. In the second instance, they attempt to follow the passions of the mind blindly, mistaking them for the heart's inner truth. Trust is a virtue that emerges in the healthy balance between the heart and mind.[44] We must be able to acknowledge the reality of a relationship based on the truth that lies in our heart, as well as take a look at what is "coming across the drawbridge." Only when our heart and mind act in unison may we achieve true intimacy based on trust.

Irony: Heart Protector—Strength and Openness

The irony that lies thematically at the center of the life of the heart protector constitution is that *true intimacy is empowered by strength*. Habitually driven to avoid pain, the mind of the heart protector strives to the point of weariness in its attempt to avoid the pain it associates with intimacy. Internally, the heart protector keeps painful events from consciousness, and externally the habitual mind either shuns connection with others or leads us into relationships where there is no real chance of intimate connection. The habituated mind tells us we are being strong by either avoiding or pursuing relationships with others. Behavior predicated on ignorance, however, always leads our heart to a state of being unfulfilled. Ironically, whether engaged in relationship or not, our sorrow grows for lack of the meaningful connection that nourishes the heart. True strength implies the ability to remain in the presence of pain resulting from both past and present relationships without letting it dictate our course of action. Only in finding the courage to rectify the relationship between our heart and mind can the destiny of heart protector ever be truly fulfilled.

Triple Warmer: The Flying Tiger

The irony that lies thematically at the center of the life of the triple heater constitution is that *the nature of connection does not wholly depend on self*. Ideally, the triple heater regulates external connection to the world in a way that is governed by the virtue of propriety. Like a well-functioning thermostat, the triple heater must make sure there is a corresponding change inside for every change outside in life. Habitually driven to avoid pain, the dysfunctional triple warmer initiates either excessive or deficient levels of external contact. In a display of excess, the triple heater may lead fire constitutional types to appear as "flying tigers," initiating contact with everything and everyone.[45] Their blazing fire may "burn" others as they overstep boundaries, attempting to make connection. In this scenario they may have many friends socially but few intimate relationships. If the triple heater is deficient, then they may fail to make contact and therefore misread external cues regarding the relative openness encountered in others or safety in initiating relationship with them.

Just as a person's life has a theme from conception to death, so too does each relationship have a theme from beginning to end. In fact, the quality of our connection is determined a priori by our own nature and the nature of that which we are connecting to. When the triple warmer functions properly we are not concerned with establishing or avoiding connection with others but with merely acknowledging the nature of connection that is already there. Only through connecting to our own heart and the hearts of others can the triple warmer establish the alignment between heaven internally and externally that leads to fulfillment.

The Heart, Heart Protector, and Memory

A key defensive mechanism of the heart and heart protector is regulating the memory of painful events. Often victims of sexual or physical abuse may not have memories of the event that took place for many years afterward, if at all. Two scenarios that pertain to the heart *shen* and heart protector blood may explain this phenomena.

Scattered Heart *Shen*

The first case represents a failure to store the painful event in a "concrete" way.[46] This may happen because the patient was too young to have developed a long-term memory, as in the case of preverbal abuse. Another possibility is that, as a defensive mechanism, the individual dissociated while the event was taking place. The memory of the event does not exist because, as described previously, the victim became numb at the time of the trauma and literally "was not present" during the event. However, the functional imprint of the event, which presents as "scattered heart spirit," is still present in all manner of personal expression. Evidence of this etiology is the tendency to go numb and dissociate when confronted by the practitioner during a treatment session. Similarly, a pattern of dissociation during sexual experiences may also be present. Often this dissociative pattern is typified by rolling of the eyes up in the head, rapid flickering of the eyelids, an irregular pulse, and pulse signs that indicate the "*qi* is wild."[47]

The Battered Heart Protector: Congealed Blood

The second scenario associated with lost memory is based on the failure of the mind to recover information that has been stored. The heart protector, unable to assimilate the pain of perceived betrayal or abuse, may shut off the harmful event in a way that prevents the damaging memory from entering consciousness. In effect, this lost information is separated from self in the same way a tumor may be viewed as encapsulated toxicity and pain. This separation from self is a function of the heart protector affecting the spiritual aspect of the function of blood. Hence failure to retrieve information may be primarily a congealed blood pattern.

If an individual's mind is turned exclusively "outward" in an attempt to avoid painful emotional issues, the progression of congealed blood may continue unchecked. In women, this may lead eventually to tumors, particularly in the reproductive and sexual organs and in the breast area over the betrayed heart. Convinced that life is not safe, they may alienate aspects of self-expression which are perceived as creating vulnerability. This alienation may ultimately affect the quality and flow of blood as governed by the heart protector, eventually leading to congealed blood patterns.

Fire: Case Studies

Example of the Heart Constitutional Type

MICHAEL: A BROKEN HEART HEALS THROUGH DEVOTION

Complaints: Diabetes, fatigue.

Background: Michael was a 35-year-old male. Thin and wiry, his upper chest appeared weak and caved in, suggesting a great emptiness there. A brilliant musician, he had found an outlet for his creativity in his music, which was inspirational and devotional in nature. The main trauma in Michael's life occurred when he was 16 and witnessed his father's attempt to kill his mother. This event and the ensuing divorce may literally have broken his heart.

A great struggle in Michael's life involved the relative balance between how much time he devoted to his music versus his other responsibilities as husband and father. Just talking about the allocation of his time to his various commitments made him feel as if he was having a heart attack. In all realms of his life, he struggled to balance his needs with those of his family. Michael's chosen form of exercise was running.

Analysis: Children have two immediately available forms of protection from emotional trauma. One is to close their heart so no further pain can come to them. The other is to erect an impenetrable wall around themselves by shutting down their respiratory rhythm, which, in health, empowers receptivity. These processes occurred in Michael because of the trauma he experienced at age 16, as evidenced by the weakness in his upper burner. Inspiration strengthens the lungs and devotion strengthens the heart. The musical skill that Michael had cultivated may be seen as a way to compensate and an attempt to heal the weakness of the organs in his upper burner. However, his feeling of constraints on time often kept him from being truly nourished by these aspects of life that he loved. The heart is the internal keeper of time and ultimately nourished by conscious awareness and presence in each moment. Michael's diabetes, a symptom based on an inability of cells to receive nourishment, is a perfect metaphor for the way in which Michael shut down the organ functions in his upper burner as a child. The central therapeutic challenge for Michael was to allow himself to be effortlessly present, soaking up the nourishment available in each activity he chose to undertake. Ultimately, this is a virtue of the heart that emerges when the heart is functioning in a balanced way. But a moment-by-moment choice by Michael to be present, rather than "running" from his pain, will empower the connection between his spleen and heart official, which in turn will provide the nourishment needed to support his heart function.

Treatment: The focus of treatment was to strengthen Michael's heart and to educate him about patterns of behavior and belief that undermined his heart's function and depleted its *qi.* I suggested he stop running immediately, as this is a form of overexercise that weakens the heart by draining heart *qi* and stressing the circulatory system. Herbs were prescribed to synchronize the rhythm of the heart and lungs and to ease any shock to the circulatory system.[48] The herbal formula Astragalus and Zizziphus (Yang Xin Tang) was selected to strengthen the heart, and the formula Rhemannia and Gypsum (Yu Nu Jian) was selected to cool the stomach fire that contributed to his diabetic condition.

After establishing functional harmony between Michael's heart and lungs, the focus of treatment turned toward strengthening his heart *qi* and opening up the connection between the spleen and heart officials. The emphasis of the acupuncture treatment lay in opening up the exit and entry blocks in the upper burner. Chief among these is the point combination of Spleen-21 ("great enveloping") and Heart-1 ("utmost source"), the exit and entry points of the spleen and heart officials, respectively. This point combination is archetypal for Michael inasmuch as it captures his underlying functional dynamics.

Example of the Small Intestine Constitutional Type

HELEN: CONFUSION AND LISTENING

Complaints: Carpal tunnel syndrome, chronic bladder infections.

Background: Helen was a 47-year-old female who worked as an employer/employee liaison at a large company. She complained of pain radiating from her right elbow into her wrist along the small intestine meridian with numbness in her right hand. Further, she had a history of chronic bladder infections, which were typified by burning urination. Raised by a stepmother she described as "dominating," Helen was sexually abused by physicians on two different occasions, the first when she was 16.[49] Further, she reported that her older brother had teased her incessantly throughout her childhood.

Helen exhibited extreme bitterness toward the medical profession and cried dramatically whenever discussing these events. Although she considered herself a lesbian, she surprised me one day by confessing she was attracted to me. After virtually every treatment, Helen would call me to clear up some aspect of our communication during that session. On many occasions, she would call me in tears with her feelings hurt, convinced I had in some way undermined her in treatment. Other times, she said she needed to check the instructions for taking an herbal formula, even though these had been clearly written out for her. After one session, Helen returned to report that what I had stated to her during the previous session had forever changed her life. When I asked her to repeat what I had said, it became evident she had abstracted a meaning that was diametrically opposed to the nature of my communication!

Analysis: Helen's arm pain can be considered the embodiment of the confusion that results from her small intestine's inability to create clarity in her life. The theme of being dominated in her life was present in both her relationship with her mother and brother and with the medical profession. Domination is defined here as an imposition on the heart by another's will. Teasing often has the effect of confusing the heart function by placing stress on the small intestine's capacity to sort out the nature and meaning of communications.

The healthy regulation of intimacy is an extension of the balanced functioning of the fire officials. Helen unconsciously attempted to perpetuate the theme of confusion and domination found elsewhere in her life by attempting to initiate an intimate relationship with me. Her confusion about her sexual orientation and appropriate boundaries was also evidenced by her attempt to initiate a relationship with her practitioner. For Helen, this confusion rose from the unbalanced function of her small intestine official, an organ that, in balance, empowers the ability to sort out messages arising from one's heart and the hearts of others.

Helen's small intestine imbalance was also evidenced by her constant need to call after each session and clear the air over what she considered to be ambiguous communication. The ability to perceive reality accurately through the facility of "listening" falls into the functional domain of the small intestine, and her inability to hear correctly what was being communicated to her also suggested a small intestine imbalance.

Helen's bladder infections were a result of heat accumulating in her heart and affecting her bladder function by way of the small intestine. The heat in her heart was an embodiment of undelivered communications that lay trapped there because of her small intestine's inability to channel the heart's will appropriately.

Lastly, Helen's job choice was fascinating in that it embodied the very functions utilized by the small intestine official, which must empower communication between the heart (the employer) and the other officials (the employees). This is an excellent example of how the nature of our chosen work may reflect the fundamental issue of our constitutional imbalance. We may develop an apparent strength in one aspect of life that compensates for a deficit in the same ability elsewhere. Further, we tend to "choose" situations in both work and relationships that challenge us to resolve our fundamental issue. For the only solution to meeting the challenges that arrive in such situations is to embody the very virtue with which we have lost touch.

Treatment: The central issue in treating Helen rested in empowering her conscious awareness of the virtue of listening. Further, it was crucial that she gain awareness of the ways she perpetuated confusion in her life and of the theme of domination in her relationships. I suggested to Helen an image of her heart as a thousand silk threads that had become entangled. I asked her to meditate each day on the image of her untying these knots one at a time and listening to her heart as each strand came free. I prescribed two Chinese herbal formulas. Heavenly Emperor's Pill to Mend the Heart (Tian Wang Bu Xin Wan) balances the function of the kidney and heart officials. Its herbs nourish the heart and "open" the heart orifice.[50] The herbal formula Rhemannia and Akebia (Dao Qi San) has the effect of helping drain excess heat accumulating in the heart by way of the small intestine and bladder. Archetypal points for Helen include Gallbladder-41, paired with Small Intestine-3. This point combination may empower the clarity and decisiveness of wood within the small intestine official. Points Small Intestine-6, -7, and -11 proved invaluable in her treatment as well. Small Intestine-6 ("nourishing the old") moves stagnation in the small intestine official, which in Helen's case corresponded to the accumulation of past pain and bitterness from perceived betrayals. Small Intestine-7 ("upright branch") may aid this process by allowing such stagnation to exit the small intestine official to the outside. Lastly, Small Intestine-11 ("heavenly ancestor") empowers the function of sorting in deep levels of spirit.

Example of the Heart Protector Constitutional Type

NATALIE: POETIC JUSTICE

Complaint: Emotional instability.

Background: Natalie was a 34-year-old woman who initially consulted me out of concern for her emotional and spiritual well-being. She was caught in a downward spiral of alcoholism and abusive relationships. Already twice divorced, Natalie tended to be attracted to complex people. Soon after beginning treatment, she became involved with a writer who was quite intellectual but addicted to marijuana. Shortly after this relationship began, Natalie discovered the man had lied to her about his sexual activity, and she had contracted an infection of human papilloma virus (HPV) from him. Fueled by the emotional pain associated with the infection and her betrayal, her habitual drive to right the injustices of the world surfaced and focused on organizing a national campaign to educate people about the virus.

Natalie gave the distinct impression of an individual with a huge knot tied in her heart, which prevented her mind and heart from communicating clearly. Her poetry was the only aspect of her life that allowed her to tap directly into her heart's will and purpose. In her initial visits, she repeated to me again and again her fear of dying and feeling her life force "drying up" inside. Natalie seemed somewhat twisted in her verbal expression and often complained about "feeling toxic" in all aspects of being. She was literally being poisoned by the accretions of her own unsorted past heartbreak and pain.

Analysis: Although Natalie is a heart protector constitutional type, she exhibits an habitual drive to correct injustice, which is more typical of the gallbladder constitutional type. This exemplifies how any issue or behavior may manifest as a secondary compensation for the primary underlying imbalance, which, in this case, resides in the function of the heart protector.

Upon commencing treatment, I asked Natalie to commit to a six-month period of celibacy and abstinence from relationships with men. This downtime would help her heart stabilize and give her a chance to gain perspective on her habitual patterns in relationships. In this way, she might reestablish a relationship with herself. The notion of celibacy was terrifying to her, but she agreed to try. But soon after making this commitment, Natalie initiated her relationship with the writer.

The nature of this new relationship allowed her mind to engage with the complexities of his intellect while her heart suffered for lack of any true connection. When I confronted Natalie about her commitment to a period outside of a relationship, she responded that she had to follow her heart. Her heart, however, was not involved in this process, as she sought merely to satisfy the habitual desires of her mind. Her heart protector's dysfunctional attempt to keep her from emotional pain manifested as a habit of continually choosing relationships with no chance for healthy intimacy. Holding her heart closed so tightly resulted in an accumulation of past pain trapped there. This ultimately undermined the function of her small intestine, which led to her feelings of "toxicity."

Natalie's poetry represented an attempt to reach the goodness in her heart and dispel the bitterness of her painful relationships. That she had this one area of life where her heart could freely express itself suggested a good prognosis. It is important for the practitioner to observe the ways in life that the patient is in contact with his or her primordial *qi*, for this may afford ways to access and cultivate this innate reserve.

Natalie's HPV infection was a manifestation of her own habitual tendency to twist purity (her heart's desire to love and be loved) into impurity (illness). Her fervor in campaigning for awareness of the HPV virus bordered on mania and ensured a quick burnout. Indeed, she was unable to sustain the fire of intention needed for such a massive project, and she abandoned it. Her burning desire to fight injustice represented a habitual drive, one which effectively kept her operating out of her intellect (gallbladder) instead of out of her heart. However, the functional force underlying her resulting anger, properly channeled with acupuncture and suggestion, helped open her heart by burning off the accretions of past pain resulting from "betrayal."

Treatment: In treatment, I guided Natalie through the process of taking responsibility for the events in her life. We discussed how she might resolve them in a way that would promote access to her heart. After again committing to a period of relationship abstinence, Natalie spent months focusing on untying the functional knots present between her heart and mind. For Natalie, the image of untying the knots directly addressed the function of the heart protector, which provides an unobstructed path to the heart. Shortly after the end of her six-month period of celibacy, Natalie experienced "love at first sight" with her writing instructor. They married within weeks and started a family immediately. At age 38, Natalie gave birth to a beautiful baby girl. With new clarity afforded by the balanced function of her fire officials, Natalie evidenced the virtue of immediate communication with her own heart essence and the heart of another.

Natalie's statement about feeling as though her "life force is drying up" speaks directly to the inner nature of upper kidney points Kidney-23, -24, and -25.[51] A turning point came for her with the treatment of acupuncture points Liver-1 ("great esteem") and Heart Protector-9 ("rushing into the middle"), paired with Heart Protector-1 ("heavenly pond") and Conception Vessel-17 ("primordial child"). The combination of Liver-1 and Heart Protector-9 may help focus the vision afforded by the liver as it exists functionally within the heart protector official. Heart Protector-1 is the "window of heaven" point associated with the heart protector official and may afford deep insight into the nature of safety and intimacy. Conception Vessel-17 may help return the childlike essence of the heart to consciousness.

Example of the Triple Burner Constitutional Type

BONNIE: TRIPLE BURNER—THE ENTERTAINER

Complaint: Heart palpitations.
Background: I first met Bonnie when she was brought to one of my

seminars as a new patient to be evaluated in front of the class. Even though she knew she was to be diagnosed before a group of twenty people, Bonnie entered the lecture room wearing a black leather miniskirt, high heels, and a tight leather top. This "intimate" clothing would have been more appropriate for a night out dancing than for a clinical session. As she entered the room, she joked and, with a loud laugh, proceeded to entertain the class.

Bonnie immediately established control of the situation and felt quite comfortable as she took a seat in front of the class with the students laughing with her. However, as we proceeded into the interview, her countenance quickly changed. I began the interview by asking about her family's health. Detecting the withdrawal of her fire when she mentioned her brother, I asked if they were close. She commented that she was not particularly close to her brother for reasons she was not certain about. She immediately became uncomfortable and clearly felt exposed in front of the class. She flushed red, and it was clear to me that her heart was palpitating. At this point, the interview quickly wound down as it was apparent she did not feel comfortable enough to continue. However, with fewer than five questions, the diagnosis of her constitutional type was complete. In this short time, an archetypal imbalance of the heart protector and triple burner had been fully expressed.

Analysis: Bonnie's use of humor with the students in the clinic exemplifies one way the external fire of the triple burner constitutional type may present itself. In this case, Bonnie used her ability to entertain as a way to maintain control and establish a superficial boundary between the group and herself. Conversely, her revealing clothing permitted strangers to be inappropriately close in a way that created vulnerability on Bonnie's behalf. Her heart palpitations were an embodiment of her struggle to maintain the appropriate balance between vulnerability and control.

Bonnie's embarrassment and other signs of fire imbalance exhibited when queried about her brother were highly suggestive. They led me to suspect her relationship with him could be a determining factor in perpetuating the habitual patterns and beliefs associated with the functional basis of her heart palpitations.

Treatment: Interestingly, some weeks after the class, Bonnie approached me for treatment. After eight sessions of treatment on the fire officials, Bonnie recovered clear memories of an incestuous relationship with her brother. This memory was later corroborated by both her brother and sister. Upon regaining this memory, Bonnie felt too exposed and unsafe to work through this material with a male practitioner. She left my practice, but went on to process this emotional material in treatment with a female therapist.

I initially prescribed the herbal compound Meridian Passage for Bonnie to clear the effects of the suspected betrayal and to stimulate her memories of the event should my hypothesis about her history of sexual abuse be correct (as it was).[52] Acupuncture points archetypal for Bonnie include the couplet Heart Protector-6 ("inner frontier gate") and Triple Burner-5 ("outer frontier gate") and the exit/entry combination of Kidney-22 and Heart Protector-1.

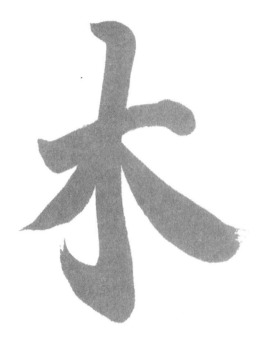

If you look at them from the point of view of their differences then there is the liver and the gall, Ju and Yue. But if you look at them from the point of view of their sameness, then the ten thousand things are all one.

– ZHUANGZI[54]

After receiving their personal names, children begin to judge their world. With discernments of right and wrong, good and bad, should and should not, children are led away from the unity that lies in their hearts. For the heart is only able to discern the truth that lies at the heart of each moment; it is not able to make decisions based on the evaluation of data. The mind, in contrast, the judge and evaluator of data, is only able to perceive duality. Located halfway between water and fire on the *sheng* cycle, wood, like the *chongqi*, must fuse these apparent opposites into one. In the primordial five elements, the three return forever back to a chaotic unity. However, in later heaven, habitual conditioning has destroyed the primal unity of the five elements and the mind seeks explanations and reasons for all it perceives. *Yin* and *yang*, water and fire, separate as we embody the vision of duality in the world. This separation is ultimately reflected in compromised integrity of the heart/kidney axis and a tearing apart of the *yuanqi*. Cut off from these sources of intuition the mind now governs alone. It is the wood element that governs the quality of our vision and empowers our balanced perception of both duality and unity in life.

The Nature of Wood

Bamboo offers a perfect model of healthy growth in nature. It derives its strengths from its emptiness, rootedness, and flexibility. When a wind blows, bamboo bends in exact proportion to the strength of the wind blowing it. Its rootedness allows it to yield without falling over, and its emptiness represents nonattachment in the moment to its goal of rapid directional growth. Hence it is "empty" in the sense of not trying to fight the direction it is being momentarily taken. We may resist and become frustrated when faced with obstacles while pursuing a goal. To emulate the virtue of bamboo would be to remain calm and unattached to momentary deviations from our course while maintaining a steady view of the big picture. As the wind subsides, bamboo springs up to immediately reassert its purpose and pursue its path. Exhibiting the virtue of benevolence, bamboo carries no grudge toward the wind that has temporarily waylaid its progress. It continues unencumbered in its journey toward heaven.

In assessing the quality of a patient's wood element, it is useful to draw on imagery of the many ways that wood itself is present in nature. For example, does the patient appear like a tall tree that has overshadowed the growth of all other life around it? Is he like an evergreen continually striving to grow so the soil surrounding him becomes acidic and nothing else can thrive in his presence? Or is he like a banyan tree, always sending out another branch sideways and never progressing very far toward his goal? Perhaps he appears like a piece of brittle wood deprived of water. Although tall, his lack of flexibility may cause him to snap in a strong wind while other more supple trees bend to accommodate heaven's will.

The Nature of Wind

The environmental condition associated with the wood element is wind. In nature, wind moves in an unpredictable fashion, making it difficult to navigate through the world. When external events are rapidly changing, the facility of the liver and gallbladder to make decisions and implement plans is critical if we are to remain oriented.

If the integrated functions of liver and gallbladder are compromised by our habitual reaction to anger, then an internal state of wind may be engendered. Internal wind may be indicated by any symptom that exhibits chaotic and unpredictable movements. For instance, convulsions, muscle twitches and spasms, headaches, or pains that change location rapidly may signal the presence of wind. Emotionally, wind may manifest as anger that blows up like a storm whenever we must alter our plans in order to accommodate present circumstance. With vision so obscured by anger, we may be unable to contact the fixed reference point provided by the liver's plan. In such a scenario, dizziness may present as a symptom indicating our inability to navigate when life changes so rapidly and unpredictably. Indecisiveness and poor planning may make it difficult for us to chart a course as we appear to be blown through life "like a leaf in the wind."

The Spirit of Wood

The character *hun* is composed of the character *yun* (云) on the left, signifying clouds, and *gui* (鬼) on the right, representing a spirit with the head on top and legs on bottom. The *hun* is composed of the three

Daoist treasures, the *jing*, *qi*, and *shen*. The *jing*, associated with the kidneys, is the storehouse for all of life's varied manifestations. The *shen* of the heart is that creative spark which must illuminate potential to make it manifest. Situated between water and fire, the liver regulates the smooth flow of *qi* between these two microcosmic poles of water and fire that represent the duality of heaven and earth. This relationship is depicted in Figure 10.3. In fact, the *jing*, *qi*, and *shen* are the innate influences that empower the implementation of the plan stored in our seed of potential granted us at the moment of conception. The *hun* is the evolutionary spirit that is raised in virtue as we strive toward manifesting the highest which heaven has placed within. Upon death the *hun* exits through the extremity of the liver meridian at acupuncture point Governor Vessel-20 located on the vertex of the head, and ascends to the Big Dipper. Here it reports to the spirits that preside over destiny on the degree to which each of us has cultivated virtue during our lifetime.

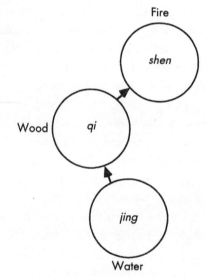

Figure 10.3
HUN: *JING, QI,* AND *SHEN*

The wood element is located between water and fire along the *sheng* cycle. A function of the wood element is to regulate the smooth flow of *qi* between fire and water just as the *chongqi* must harmonize the dual poles of heaven and earth. Physiologically, the liver and gallbladder that regulate *qi* are located in the middle heater, and the *jing* stored in the kidneys and the *shen* stored in the heart are located in the lower and upper heater, respectively. Dysfunction of the wood officials may lead to *qi* stagnation in the middle heater so the interpenetration of water and fire is constrained. It is the liver's virtue of benevolence *(ren)* that allows *shen* and *jing* to interact in an unconstrained manner.

The Rhythm of Wood

The rhythm of wood is qualitatively different from each of the other four elements in that it is continuous with no beat. The wood element ensures that life never proceeds in a circle but always in an upward evolutionary spiral. Hence the rhythm of wood is a continuous streaming that never falters, joining each moment to the next in the endless progression of all things toward heaven.

The circles found in a cross section of a tree are composed of channels known as phloem and xylem. These channels ensure that the tips of the outermost branches and the deepest root are joined in a way that promotes healthy growth. It is this connection that allows the growing branch to be always connected to the deepest root when discerning its direction. Similarly, the function of the wood element is to empower, through the virtue of benevolence, the interpenetration of the deepest aspects of self *(jing)* with the outermost radiation of our branches *(shen)*.

Illumination

To see the small is called illumination (ming).
To abide by the soft is called strength.
Use the bright light (guang),
But return to the dim light.
— DAO DE JING[55]

It is our vision of "things" that creates the phenomenal universe. The two eyes are emblematic of the fall from the unity of the one, where all things are implicit within each other, to the two, where distinctions arise between the good and the bad and, ultimately, between the self and the *dao*. The balanced functioning of discrimination and judgment are important tools for making our way in the world. The sage is able to use these faculties without being deluded that personal discriminations and judgments constitute ultimate reality. We must be able to use the faculties of the mind, such as discernment, to know the world as it manifests in the bright light of day. However, we should not be deluded by our judgments and forget it is the unity which all things return to at night that is ultimately real. When the *Dao De Jing* tells us in Chapter 41 that the "[i]lluminating *dao* appears dark," it is referring to the inward gaze of the sage, who always returns to the vision afforded by the dim light represented by the moon in the character *ming*.

The character *ming*, meaning illumination, has two halves. The left half is the sun (日) and represents outer illumination: the vision that brings "things" into the world. It is the vision of creation that proceeds from the opening of the senses which allows us to perceive the phenomenal world. The right half of the character represents the moon (月): the quality of light at night that "blends all things into one." This inner illumination is the vision that results from shutting off the senses, allowing a look into the depth of things. For Zhuangzi, it is the man of "far-reaching vision" who is able to roll the ten thousand things back into one, "illuminating all in the light of heaven."[56]

The character *ming* may serve as an icon for the functional relationship between the liver and gallbladder, which are the *yin* and *yang* officials that comprise the wood element. In a state of functional balance, these officials empower the integrated vision of our inner and outer world. Internally the liver (moon/*yin*) empowers the vision of *dao* contained in our primordial endowment. The gallbladder (sun/*yang*) must bring the internal vision of the liver into the world as well as convey clearly the reality outside our self back into our depths. It is in this balanced alignment of inner and outer vision that the sage finds clarity.

A Discussion on the Nature of Virtue

One's everlasting virtue being full,
One again returns to the uncarved wood.
— DAO DE JING[57]

According to the Daoist view, the Confucian concept of virtue is artificial because it imposes an external moral standard for proper behavior that is dictated by society. Hence the Daoists consider the virtue *ren* to be the outward manifestation of what they call *de* (virtue). This is evidenced in Chapter 38 of the *Dao De Jing*, which states, "When *de* is lost there is *ren*." Laozi elaborates how the Confucian concept of virtue arises as we humans lose touch with the natural virtues *(de)* that emerge spontaneously when we are in touch with original nature. The *Dao De Jing* emphasizes this in Chapter 5, stating,

"Heaven and earth are not benevolent. . . . The sage is not benevolent."
Daoist commentator Wangbi explains that the sage rules by his own
internal virtue *(de)*, which is based on the spontaneity and nonattachment of the *dao*. Through inaction, he lets the outcome of all things rest
with heaven and earth and finds no use for the overt humane action that
is *ren*.[58] Zhuangzi also belittles the Confucian concept of virtue when he
says, "The way I see it, the rules of benevolence and righteousness and
the paths of right and wrong are all hopelessly snarled and jumbled.
How could I know anything about such discriminations?"[59]

The Daoist concept of virtue denoted by the character *de* may be
considered the unity from which the specific aspects of virtue named
by the Confucians emerge. Therefore Zhuangzi tells us, "When virtue
(de) embraces all things, we have benevolence."[60]

Virtue and Transformation: Belligerence into Benevolence

How is it that the liver corresponds to benevolence?
The liver is the essence of [the element] wood, and
benevolence likes to be actively productive. The East is
[the quarter of wood and of the actively productive]
yang, and is where all first things are born. Therefore,
the liver resembles wood, being green in color and
[shaped as if] having branches and leaves.
  – BAI HU DONG[61]

The character *ren* consists of the *man* radical on the left (亻) and the
character for the number two *(er:* 二 *)* on the right. Its etymology is generally interpreted to indicate the benevolence and reciprocity that
exists between each person and his or her neighbor.[62] However, the
number two itself represents the reciprocal relationship between heav-
en and earth, and the character *ren* could be taken to depict a person
standing upright between these two poles of the cosmos. In this context, *ren* would indicate the upright *(zhen)* behavior, which leads us to
fulfill destiny by perfectly blending the qualities of heaven and earth.
In relationship to the wood element I define the virtue of benevolence
as that which empowers the unconstrained evolutionary journey of all
things from earth toward heaven. Benevolence is the virtue that
emerges when the sage embraces his elevated perspective without being
arrogant, using his all-embracing vision to promote the evolution of
humanity through the elevation of their own perspective.

Some of the ways in which benevolence may harmonize the life issues of this constitutional type are given in Figure 9.3. As we move away from the virtue of benevolence toward life themes of either belligerence or timidity, anger manifests as either an excess or deficient emotion. Excessive anger manifesting as belligerence presents as the tendency to assert plans and decisions over any other considerations. Lack of anger manifesting as timidity presents as an inability to assert their inner direction even when their own life depends on it.

Relative excesses and deficiencies often occur simultaneously, and the practitioner is likely to encounter the presence of both unbalanced displays in different arenas of a patient's life. Hence patients may manifest both the remarkable presence and absence of anger in different realms of life as they habitually react to issues such as judgment and justice. The excess presence of judgment may manifest as an inability to consider anyone else's point of view in their family as they force their vision of "what is right" on spouse and children. Simultaneously, patients may evidence a complete inability to stand up for themselves in the workplace, appearing quite meek to their supervisors. Compromising themselves thus at work they project their lack of self-esteem on others by judging everything and everyone.

The *yin* and *yang* officials paired in the wood element are the liver and gallbladder, respectively. In its *yin* aspect, as associated with the liver official, benevolence emerges as we gain a vision of the plan stored in our depths. Able to see the big picture of how external circumstance complements our own inner plan, the benevolent sage moves through life in an unconstrained manner, holding nothing against anyone and no self-judgments. In its *yang* aspect, as expressed through the gallbladder official, benevolence manifests in the unconstrained implementation of our inner plan and in reading external signs appropriately so the events of life are well used in furthering our own endeavors. In describing the course of the sage through life, Zhuangzi states, "They forget liver and gall, cast aside ears and eyes, turning and revolving, ending and beginning again, unaware of where they start or finish. Idly they roam beyond the dust and dirt; they wander free and easy in the service of inaction. Why should they fret and fuss about the ceremonies of the vulgar world and make a display for the ears and eyes of the common herd?"[63]

As treatment progresses, the practitioner expects the patient's tendencies toward both belligerence and timidity to diminish along with a reduction in the behaviors and illnesses associated with anger. Over time, the virtue of benevolence is expected to become increasingly present. The dynamics of destiny and transformation as they emerge in the wood constitution are evidenced in the case studies presented later.

The Nature of Anger

The man of benevolence is tranquil.
– CONFUCIUS[64]

The emotion associated with the wood element is anger *(nu:*怒*)*. Another bipartite term for anger, *shengqi* (生氣), may be interpreted to mean literally "the *qi* that accompanies the growth of plants." Whenever growth is blocked, anger arises as a call to vision regarding the nature of the obstacle lying in the chosen path of wood constitutional types. The *qi* that supports the manifestation of anger also supports creativity, which emerges in the naturally balanced expression of the wood element in directing growth. Growth may be blocked either by an external circumstance or by their own inability to either contact or express some aspect of inner being that is called for in the moment. Anger in excess may, like the wind, confuse their vision, frustrating them from overcoming life's obstacles. Similarly, the inability to become angry appropriately may cause stagnation in life as resentment builds internally. Lost in habitual functioning, the ignorant lose touch with the creative aspects of anger that further life. Suppression of their natural expression of anger simultaneously suppresses their capacity for directional, creative growth. However, once they have moved past any momentary obstruction, it is imperative that they let go of their anger. Otherwise, they proceed through life belligerently projecting past anger on current circumstances. In this scenario healthy growth becomes constrained and life stagnates as they focus habitually on every perceived obstruction. It is interesting to note that the Chinese character *kun* (困), which means "constraint," depicts a tree growing inside of a box.

Resolution

The virtue of benevolence entails the blending of all duality back into a harmonious whole. Hence resolution of conflict is the result when the habitual emotions of belligerence and timidity are transformed into benevolence. Resolution involves the forgiveness of self and others, releasing all judgments about right and wrong and accepting the past actions of self and others as representing the very best that was able to be accomplished at the time. Resolution thus manifests as letting go of conceptions about how things should have been, should be, or ought to be in the future.[65] Resolution of past conflict therefore empowers unconstrained growth in the present moment.

The Life Thesis of Wood

It is the nature of life that the cutting edge of our growth is always blocked. This resistance empowers the process of natural selection by helping assure that the strongest survive. When a seed is planted, the sprout must first poke through the shell of the seed and then navigate its way through the resistance of the dirt to the surface. It may encounter rocks or other obstacles that it must grow around. After finally beginning to grow, it may need to seek out sunlight in the shadow of other, taller, plants. That resistance accompanies growth is a natural part of life. However, those of the wood constitution interpret this resistance as indicating a fundamental truth about both the nature of life and self. Externally their unconscious reaction to anger is projected on life, which they believe is unjust. Internally, they direct anger toward themselves and interpret any resistance to their plans as constituting a personal failure that results in insecurity based on poor self-esteem.

The key life themes for those of the wood constitution involve the integration of planning and decision making in a graceful manner and in a way presided over by the virtue of benevolence. If habitual reaction to the presence of anger in self or others obscures their access to this virtue, then their life theme is distorted into a thesis which compromises their balanced relationship to growth in every aspect of being. In this case themes typified by arrogance or humility are established that represent distortions of the virtue of benevolence.

The archetypal life theme for wood constitutional types that reflects excess may be stated as, "My vision is so accurate that my plans and decisions must be asserted continually, regardless of the consequences to anything or anyone that gets in their way, including myself." The theme that reflects deficiency may be stated as, "Every time I try to grow in any given direction, life cuts me down."

Irony: Truth Without Compassion Is Tyranny

The irony at the heart of the wood element is that *there is something more important in life than being right.*

Habitual reaction to the emotion anger drives the liver and gall-bladder officials to either over- or underutilize creativity in directing the process of growth. If wood constitutional types are overly determined to assert their direction, then arrogance may be displayed as they rigidly pursue their chosen course. Any impediment to their initiative is habitually interpreted as signifying that life is unjust. With the initiation of each new direction, satisfaction is felt for only a short while before their reaction to anger reasserts itself. Driven by rage to push increasingly hard against each new perceived block in life, their experience of growth is ultimately unfulfilling.

In contrast, if they are resigned to the notion that life's impediments are unmovable, then no new direction or progress may ever be asserted. Every new direction taken results in collapse the moment any resistance is encountered. Only through realization of the virtue of benevolence toward self and others can those of the wood constitution attain a state of tranquility in the process of evolution.

Testing Emotions: Perspective

People of the wood constitutional type habitually respond to the presence of the emotion anger. By offering perspective and noting the quality of the patient's reaction, the practitioner may assess the qualitative function of the patient's wood element. Offering perspective means providing a new and broader context for patients that empowers them to view their situation in life differently. When wood is in a functional state of balance, then perspective from the practitioner should help resolve anger that the patient harbors toward self or others stemming from past events. However, a hallmark of the wood constitution is that habitual reaction to the presence of anger is the unconscious motivating force behind the habitual behavior. Therefore, when offering the patient perspective, the practitioner may find the patient's anger is quelled only briefly, if at all. Perspective provided by the practitioner comes externally, and only with the vision afforded by the virtue of benevolence can those of the wood constitution find resolution of the internalized conflicts which keep them from being fulfilled.

A defining characteristic of the wood constitution is that once

perspective is offered, it will be either continually elicited or rejected by the patient throughout the interview. Belligerent patients
habitually reject any external perspective because they are convinced
their interpretation of events is perfectly right in conforming to reality.
Any external structure offered by the practitioner is habitually turned
by their minds into a prison which constrains their ability to grow
instead of a stairway that might promote evolution. For to be wrong
about the interpretation of any event subconsciously implies they could
be wrong about their interpretation of whatever event initiated their
separation from true self. To consider this possibility would mean the
collapse of their life thesis, leaving them in the presence of their original
pain. The entire functional basis of their ignorance and habitual anger
is perpetuated solely to avoid ever directly encountering this pain.

However, patients may also respond to any perspective offered by
the practitioner by attempting to rely on it in a dysfunctional way.
Their poor self-esteem makes them lose faith in their own ability to
make plans and decisions. In this scenario patients assume the practitioner's interpretation of events is correct and continually fail to look
inward in an attempt to assert their own inner truth.

The practitioner may also offer perspective by providing opportunities to engage patients' functions of planning and decision making. A
simple way to do this is to pay attention to the facility with which
patients are able to make appointments and show up for them on time.
I have found that merely opening my appointment book, showing it to
a patient, and asking him or her to pick a time for treatment can bring
up an entire continuum of dysfunctional behavior involving the wood
element. On the one hand, patients may insist there is only one possible time slot in a given month with no flexibility fifteen minutes either
way. On the other hand, patients may be willing to come at any time
and then call to change their appointment several times during the
month or to ask when their appointment is, because they have forgotten. Finally, it is important to note if a patient shows up on time
because punctuality is the end product of successful planning and decision making. Patients who show up half an hour early for every
appointment may do so because they do not trust their own faculty of
planning to get them anywhere on time. Patients who are chronically
late, miss appointments altogether, or perpetually arrive on the wrong
day are also indicating a functional imbalance in the wood element.

When offering perspective, the practitioner must note the momentary changes in the patient's color, sound, odor, and emotion. The
finding that these signs intensify and the patient becomes green, shouting

or lack-of-shout, rancid, and expresses either excessive or deficient anger is enough to confirm that the patient is wood constitutionally.

The Suggestive Process in Treatment

Imbalance of the wood element is typified by the patient's inappropriate relationship to the issues of decision making and planning. Initially in treatment the practitioner must either provide all perspective or yield to that provided by the patient. When offering suggestions to those of the wood constitution, it is important to place any therapeutic goals in the future. In this way patients are afforded enough perspective that they are able to adequately visualize their goal. Speaking in the language of the wood element is the best way to motivate people by aligning them with their own inner vision. For example, in motivating a patient whose constitution is wood to quit smoking, the practitioner must offer the suggestion in one of two ways. If the patient is excessively attached to personal decisions and plans, the practitioner might say, "I would like you to set a date that you will be able to quit by and plan how many treatments you think it will take to reach that goal." Alternatively, the practitioner may initially need to direct the course of treatment. In this case, setting smaller, more easily accomplished goals, which build in magnitude, can be effective. The practitioner might say, "First let's work on reducing the amount you smoke to one pack a day. When you have accomplished that, we can look ahead to the next step."

As healing progresses, patients' ability to plan and make decisions will proceed in a more functional manner. As this occurs, they will evidence less habitual need to either determine the course of treatment or receive continual direction from the practitioner.

The Wood Officials

The liver holds our internal plan, and the gallbladder's function is to channel the events of life in toward the liver accurately and to implement the liver's plan in the world. We must hold the vision of how heaven's plan, manifesting as the events in our life, complements the internal plan that heaven has stored within. Only by aligning heaven's plan externally and internally may we evolve in a less constrained way. Next I elaborate how the various virtues associated with the wood element express themselves through the liver and gallbladder officials.

The Liver Official

The liver holds the office of general of the armed forces.
Assessment of circumstances and conception of plans stem
from it.
— NEI JING SU WEN[66]

In storing the *hun* spirit, the liver is in contact with the *jing*, *qi*, and *shen*. These are the primordial influences that govern the ascension of the human spirit. The function of the liver is to provide a perspective broad enough so evolution can occur in an unconstrained manner. Hence the liver official empowers the vision of our life from the deepest root as symbolized by *jing* to our outermost branch as symbolized by *shen*. In order to communicate with each other, the *shen*, which is stored in the upper heater, and the *jing*, which is stored in the lower heater, must pass through the middle burner where the liver resides.

The virtue of benevolence empowers the liver to promote the interaction of *jing* and *shen* in a way that is unconstrained. On the one hand, the liver provides the emperor (heart) with a vision of the depths *(jing)*, which is a basis of the emperor's facilities of insight and intuition. On the other hand, the liver must tap the potential of *jing* and implement its internal organization in the world in the same way a tree must send down roots to tap reserves of water, manifesting them on the surface as new growth.

The Art of War

To lift an autumn leaf is no sign of great strength;
to see the sun and moon is no sign of sharp sight;
to hear the noise of thunder is no sign of a quick ear.
What the ancients called a clever fighter is one who not only wins,
but excels in winning with ease.

— SUNZI[67]

The liver as general in our inner kingdom is charged with the initiation of plans and strategies. An examination of Sunzi's (Sun Tzu) advice to generals in his military treatise "The Art of War" (*Yingyi Sunzi Bingfa*) yields several principles that relate to the highest function of the liver official. Sunzi states that the enlightened general must simultaneously hold a vision of his true nature as well as the nature of what he contends with in life. He is clear that ultimately this vision rests with a knowledge of heaven and earth. Thus he advises, "If you know the enemy and know yourself, your victory will not stand in doubt; if you know heaven and know earth; you make your victory complete."[68] The liver situated halfway between water and fire on the *sheng* cycle must maintain contact between our *jing* and *shen* which mirror internally our connection to the dual poles of heaven and earth. It is the interpenetration of our *jing* and *shen* afforded by the benevolent action of the liver that empowers the self-knowledge to which Sunzi alludes.

When the liver and heart are in the proper relationship, the heart is the sovereign who possesses insight and intuition. The liver as general must convey our internal plan accurately to the heart as well as inform the sovereign accurately of external circumstances in life as conveyed by the reconnaissance of the gallbladder. The general must also implement the orders of the sovereign in the world by initiating movements consistent with the heart's purpose by commanding the *qi*. However, our capacity of discernment must always temper our intuition and must not waver if the intuitive capacity of the heart falters. Therefore, Sunzi states, "In war, the general receives his command from the sovereign, but there are commands of the sovereign that must not be obeyed."[69]

In accurately assessing the merits of any given situation we must be unconstrained by past experiences. Hence Sunzi warns, "Do not repeat the tactics that have gained you one victory, but let your methods be regulated by the infinite variety of circumstance."[70] The vision of the liver constitution becomes compromised because of a tendency to habitually project our reactions to past perception of injustice on present situations. Quick to anger, we ignore consulting our inner plan and merely lash out in a vain attempt to defend our position. Therefore Sunzi warns that a hasty temper which can be provoked by insults is one of the great faults that may compromise a general's abilities to command. He tells us, "The victorious strategist seeks battle after his plans indicate that victory is possible under them, whereas he who is destined to defeat first fights without skillful planning."[71]

Ultimately, Sunzi knows that cultivation of virtue is more important than merely always being right in life. He alludes to the highest that the virtue of benevolence has to offer a general in performance of his duties when he states, "To fight and conquer in all your battles is not supreme excellence; supreme excellence consists in breaking the enemy's resistance without fighting."[72]

Archetypal Image

Differing qualities of liver function may be illustrated with the following analogy about how a person handles obstacles in life. Imagine a man walking down a road who comes eventually to a brick wall blocking his progress. Much can be told about the quality of this traveler's liver function by how he handles his predicament. The appropriate response of the liver is to assess the situation by standing back and gaining perspective. If the virtues associated with the liver are empowered, he may find an easy course around the wall. Appropriately, he gains all available information about the situation, such as (1) the hardness of the wall, (2) whether or not he is able to make his way over it, around it, under it, or to knock it down, or (3) determining if he is able to reach his destination using another, more fruitful path. He then reassesses his plan and implements a decisive course of action based on the unique merits of the situation.

Like a mighty river that flows around all obstacles, eventually turning mountains into valleys, and finally reaching the sea, the healthy liver empowers the flow of *qi* with the virtue of flexibility so the traveler may always reach his ultimate goal. The *Dao De Jing* alludes to this quality of *dao* when it tells us "to be crooked, is to be straightened."[73] Being flexible in pursuing its path, the *dao* always reaches its objective.[74]

If the liver is unhealthy and responding inappropriately, the scenario may play itself out in several ways. One such way is for the traveler to continually throw himself against the wall in an attempt to knock it down. Here he is exhibiting a deep inner rage aimed at some past injustice that the wall presently represents. This individual perpetually knocks his head against this and all other walls encountered in his life's journey. This scenario represents liver excess, which is to say that, at least for a while, the traveler possesses enough internal strength to fight against the situation blocking his progress.

Liver *qi* and *yang* deficiency is another expression of the liver's unbalanced functioning. In this instance, our traveler comes up to the wall, looks at the seemingly impenetrable barrier, and proclaims, "This is where my journey ends." This person's life thesis may be stated in this way: "No matter how hard I try, life always blocks my plans, so what's the use of trying?" He continually gathers evidence that life is trying to block his self-expression and chosen direction. Rather than using challenges in life as opportunities for growth, instead he resigns himself to inevitable failure.

The net result of both situations, excess and deficient, is stagnation as the individual remains stuck in front of the wall that confronts him. The real nature of this blockage is the wall erected by the liver, which blinded by reaction to its own anger in turn blinds the heart *shen* from perceiving our deep plan stored in the depths of *jing*. Over time, the external conflicts that confound us in life become embodied as physical pathology. Liver *qi* stagnation presents as inner walls that impede the smooth flow of *qi* internally. Symptoms predicated on such stagnation include menstrual cramps, uterine fibroids, tightness in the sternum and center of the chest, constriction of the throat, and pressure in the head. All these symptoms may indicate a person is unable to proceed gracefully through transitions.

Individuals who rage against the injustice symbolized by the wall develop symptoms of heat as they overwork, trying to defeat the obstacle that confronts them. This heat may manifest as hypertension, headache, visual problems, and arthritis as the traveler's joints become twisted like a knotted tree from raging against every perceived obstacle encountered.

Lastly, travelers who suffer from liver *qi* and/or *yang* deficiency exhibit despair and hopelessness as all life's goals are considered unreachable. Constant weak sighing presents as a way of dissipating whatever inner steam is left to fuel their growth. With their life purpose so hindered, resignation and depression come to typify their experience in life.

Self-Esteem: The Vision of Self

Self-esteem emerges from the vision of those principles that spring from our essential nature which root us to the foundation of life itself. This is the vision afforded by the liver when it is in contact with the innate influence of *jing* and *shen*. In pruning a plant, we may cut unessential branches so growth may be channeled more fruitfully. However, the roots that anchor the plant into its ground of being must not be compromised. When actions are taken that compromise basic principles in life, self-esteem slowly erodes. Compromise becomes gradually easier until we may no longer possess a vision of our true nature. This imbalance is often evidenced in individuals who act belligerently as though any compromise is a personal affront. In contrast, having made mistakes in the past, timid individuals may no longer trust their internal vision and continually acquiesce to others when challenged in life. Hence a life issue for liver constitutional types is to learn to discern which aspects of self may be compromised (the branches) and which aspects are fundamental principles (roots) that must be adhered to.

Irony: Good Planning Entails Flexibility

The irony at the heart of the liver constitution's life is that *at any given moment, our liver can access only half of life's plan.* The other half of every plan lies in heaven externally. Having discerned the internal plan, those of the liver constitution may habitually stick to it in the face of changing external circumstances that require flexibility and compromise. Rather than look within for the answer as demanded by each new twist and turn of fate, the mind of the liver constitution becomes habitually focused on a vision of how things ought to be, based on a past assessment. Trying to force their personal vision on the world, liver constitutional types become belligerent and inflexible. Ultimately growth becomes unfulfilling as life seems to thwart plans at every turn. Only by embracing the virtue of benevolence and joining heaven's plan within with heaven's plan without can liver types find peace in the process of growth.

Gallbladder

> *The gallbladder is responsible for what is just and exact.*
> *Determination and decision stem from it.*
> — NEI JING SU WEN [75]

In the scenario of the traveler just discussed, the gallbladder official expresses itself somewhat differently than the liver. In balance, the well-functioning gallbladder empowers the ability to be decisive when it comes to choosing between alternatives. The healthy gallbladder is able to integrate the inner knowing of the heart as it is expressed in the liver's plan with its own faculty of data analysis and decision making. The force propelling our growth springs internally from the liver, and the gallbladder's job is to actualize this impulse, decisively birthing it into the world. Sunzi describes the functional balance of the liver and gallbladder metaphorically when he says, "The quality of decision is like the well-timed swoop of a falcon which enables it to strike and destroy its victim. Therefore the good fighter will be terrible in his onset, and prompt in his decision. Power (the impulse for growth generated by the liver) may be likened to the bending of a crossbow; decision, to the releasing of the trigger."[76]

Out of balance, the tendency of the gallbladder constitution is to lose perspective and to make decisions based on reason alone, ignoring the plan of the liver, the heart's insight, and the kidney's wisdom. This dynamic is expressed by the image of the traveler going right up to the wall and scrutinizing every aspect of it so closely that all perspective is lost. Here the individual becomes obsessed with the details of the situation. This is like standing an inch from a pointillist painting and, while staring at a specific dot, proclaiming there is no picture. In contrast, if those of the gallbladder constitution are overly sure of the scope of their vision, they may fail to attend to details as they arrogantly pursue their lofty aspirations. The net result of either scenario is that decisions are not made properly and healthy growth toward personal goals is compromised.

Another tendency of the gallbladder is to impulsively send out a new branch laterally each time its direction meets any resistance at all. Rather than survey the situation, the gallbladder constitution may continually change directions and goals in a seemingly random manner. In this case, direction in life is completely dictated by momentary reaction to external circumstances.

Archetypal Image

> *Those who discriminate fail to see.*
> – ZHUANGZI[77]

The hallmark of each constitutional type is that individuals under stress habitually resort to the function associated with their constitution in a dysfunctional manner which undermines the fulfillment of their life's purpose. Hence gallbladder constitutional types invariably resort to excessive decision making or are indecisive when confronted with obstacles in life. The way in which vision, decisiveness, and timidity are functionally related in the gallbladder constitution is well demonstrated by the natural dynamics seen in certain animals when confronted with life-saving decisions.

In the face of an oncoming car, for example, both the deer and rabbit fall prey to their own indecisiveness. The deer, unsure of whether to move to the left or right, becomes frozen in the headlights and is run over. A rabbit in the same situation runs in a zigzag pattern from left to right and back to left. Of course, its fate is the same as the deer, for it too has failed to get out of harm's way. Timidity is associated here with indecisiveness in each scenario, and the result is the same. The external expression is different, however, as the deer becomes frozen and the rabbit moves in any direction quickly but in a way ungrounded in a plan and equally devoid of perspective.

Emulating the functional dynamic of either animal, gallbladder constitutional types build a life thesis that life is not fair and they do not get what they deserve. Continually "run over" in life, they fail to accept their responsibility for appropriate action and instead project their frustration and resentment for failure on others, onto life, and ultimately onto the will of heaven, which is characterized as being unjust.

One-Sidedness

> When all under heaven know beauty as beauty, there is
> then ugliness; when all know the good as good, there is
> then the not good.
> – DAO DE JING[78]

Gallbladder constitutional types generally see the world in terms of clear-cut relationships like good or bad, or right or wrong. Eventually, this one-sided perspective becomes embodied in a way that manifests as symptoms which tend to appear unilaterally. These may include one-sided flank pain, headaches, or sciatica. Such individuals may evidence a restricted range of motion in the neck that limits perspective in accordance with their one-sided view of life. Conversely, range of motion may be restricted bilaterally, reflecting the fact they are only able to look straight ahead toward their goal to the exclusion of all else. The polarities reflected in the character *ming* (明: "illumination"), as an icon for the function of the gallbladder, are indicative of the tendency of people with this constitutional type, when out of balance, to see things in only one light. Hence Zhuangzi states, "What one calls right the other calls wrong; what one calls wrong the other calls right. But if we want to right their wrongs and wrong their rights, then the best thing to use is clarity."[79]

Irony: There Is No Such Thing as Human Justice

The liver tends toward a failure of internal vision that manifests as poor self-esteem. The gallbladder tends toward a failure of external vision so the key events of a lifetime are interpreted in terms of issues of justice. Those of the gallbladder constitution are not free to pick their fights but are habitually drawn into the fray every time they perceive an injustice in the world. However, with each new "victory" they feel at peace for only a brief while before their habitual drive toward justice compels them to take on a new larger battle. In actuality, the irony for those of the gallbladder constitution is *there is no such thing as human justice.*

Whenever a dispute is settled, some degree of damage is always left.

For example, if someone you love is killed in the commission of a crime, human justice can only incarcerate the party responsible. It cannot bring your loved one back to life or restore that aspect of yourself which may have been lost in the process. Only heaven administers ultimate justice, so eventually people each reap what they sow.[80] Resolution for the wood constitutional type often lies in the virtue of forgiveness, which manifests as grace. It is only by the grace of forgiving one's self first, and then others, that habitual rage may subside. Our *shen* may once again have access to our *jing* in a way that empowers the vision of true self. Only when the pain of injustice does not obscure original nature has justice truly been administered. Hence the *Dao De Jing* advises us to "repay injury with the restoration of original nature *(de)*."[81]

Wood: Case Studies

Example of the Liver Constitutional Type

JACKIE: DESERVING OF SELF-ESTEEM

Complaints: Depression, lack of energy.

Background: Jackie for several years had been in a relationship to which she was quite committed. Her mate, however, had engaged in several affairs during this time, which had hurt her quite deeply. Yet she chose to remain in the relationship out of what she described as a sense of "commitment." After about six sessions, Jackie announced she had separated from her mate and was going to take some time to gain a perspective on her own needs relative to relationships in general. On one occasion, however, she expressed anger that her ex-mate did not seem to be doing significant emotional work in "processing" their relationship in the same way she was. She felt he owed her this, and she was quite angry.

Analysis: Jackie's inability to leave her relationship was based on her own lack of self-esteem. This lack of esteem contributed to her inability to trust that if she refused to compromise on the issue of her partner's affairs and left him, she would be able to find another suitable mate. Given the kindness of her nature and her general attractiveness, this belief seemed to stem from a great lack of inner vision about her own nature.

This case is an example of how individuals may interpret their life experience according to the dictates of their constitutional type. A theme that occurs repeatedly for Jackie is anger over not being held in the proper regard by the men in her life. She believes she deserves better treatment, yet is unable to hold herself with the same esteem that she seeks from others. By staying in this relationship, she continued to compromise her fundamental principles. Pulse diagnosis suggested Jackie's depression was predicated in part on liver *qi* and blood deficiency.

Treatment: Initially, I helped Jackie make the distinction between the concept of her being deserving of a man's fidelity and care and the notion she was "owed" that. I pointed out that each human's contract is with heaven and no other. Ultimately, her partner owed heaven the fulfillment of his own destiny, but he owed her nothing. It was her decision to be with him, and the pain she was feeling was the consequence of having compromised her fundamental principles. In fact, the pain had nothing to do with him. In truth, she deserved to be held in high esteem by others only to the extent that she stood up for the principles she discovered in her own depths.

My initial treatments of Jackie focused on draining pathological *qi* ("aggressive energy"), which had to be done several times. For Jackie, this treatment helped clear the functional basis on which her resentment was predicated. An archetypal combination of acupuncture points used in treating Jackie might be Liver-1 ("great esteem"), Liver-13 ("chapter gate"), and Heart Protector-9 ("rushing into the middle"). The wood points on the liver meridian (Liver-1) and the heart protector meridian (Heart Protector-9) are needled together. Hence the virtue of the liver's vision is empowered within the function of the heart protector official. The point "chapter gate" was added to help her turn a new page in life and move on from being stuck in a dysfunctional relationship.

Example of the Gallbladder Constitutional Type

JOHN: LOOKING BACK WITH JUDGMENT

Complaint: Polyneuropathy attendant to diabetes.

Background: John was one of my very first patients. In his early sixties, he came to me for severe leg pain resulting from a polyneuropathy that his physicians attributed to his diabetes. After the first several treatments, John began to recount to me his experiences as a belly gunner on bombing missions during the Second World War. In the same sentence, he would pass judgment on those he had killed while simultaneously breaking into tears at the very thought. His life was a dichotomy of running from his regrets and judgments against himself for his past actions, and projecting his judgments outward onto others in the form of prejudicial comments. John had smoked as many as ten cigars daily since his army years.

Analysis: John's leg pain made a clear path down the gallbladder meridian. This symptom may be viewed as an embodiment of John's inability to reconcile his vision of life and the judgments he holds against both himself and others. I viewed his incessant smoking as an attempt to sedate both his grief and anger regarding the events in his past.

Treatment: John's first acupuncture treatment included a draining of aggressive *qi* followed by the acupuncture points Liver-3 ("happy calm") and Gallbladder-37 ("bright and clear"). After this initial session, John evidenced a nearly complete remission of his polyneuropathy symptoms. This seemed miraculous to me. As a neurobiologist, I could think of no mechanism that could produce immediate and long-lasting relief of the pain that accompanies nerve degeneration. Several sessions later I treated the exit/entry combination of Liver-14 ("gate of hope") and Lung-1 ("central treasury"). John returned the following week to say, "I don't know what you did, but I have given up smoking." From that session onward, John felt no desire to smoke. During the next year and a half John remained pain free yet continued to cry during his sessions about his regrets for having "murdered" people during the war.

In one particular session, I treated John with acupuncture points Gallbladder-41 ("just before crying") and GB-12 ("eye window"). This combination of points helps release frustration and judgment against oneself and others for past events. Within two days of this treatment, John's pain returned in his leg. Evidencing rather poor judgment, he had been out shoveling snow in his tennis shoes and, not feeling the cold because of his diabetes, he was stricken with frostbite. Soon afterward his symptoms returned, and he was diagnosed with lung cancer that spread quickly and aggressively throughout his body.

I believe the initial treatment session had given John access to his last store of pure primordial *qi*. It was this reserve of *qi* that was responsible for the immediate cessation of his symptoms. In striving to assert itself, this *qi* forced into consciousness past events that John had managed to suppress since the war. Ultimately, however, he could find no resolution to the inner judgments and anger that plagued him. John died early that spring just as the first blossoms appeared on the trees.

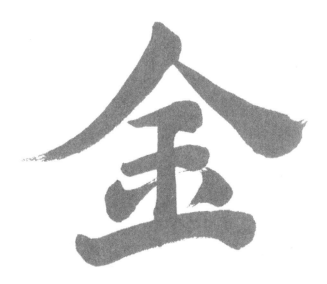

Though the grease burns out of the torch,
the fire passes on,
and no one knows where it ends.

– Zhuangzi[82]

METAL—THE RETURN

The fourth stage of *dao* represents the return from the height of self-awareness back to the origin. This is signified by either the return of self back to *dao,* which occurs at the death of the body, or the return of *dao* back to the self, which occurs as we transcend the material world and begin to manifest destiny. This transition is mediated by the metal element as the yearly cycle moves from the bright light of summer into winter's darkness. Here we return to seed; if we have fulfilled our destiny, this return occurs at a higher, more evolved functional level for having been "stirred" through another round of existence. The officials of the metal element are the lungs and large intestine, which provide a circuit for the accumulation and discharge of all things in the microcosm. Here we examine the metal element as it is embodied within human beings.

The Nature of Metal

The character for metal, *jin* (金), depicts a mine shaft covered by a roof containing two nuggets of gold. Gold is the metal of most value and therefore identified as possessing the qualities that comprise the essence of the metal element. In nature, metal occurs as minerals that give the earth, plants, and all life upon it inner value and structure. Metal manifests as the crystalline lattice of a diamond, that imparts to it both hardness and strength. If a diamond is overly rigid, however, it may crack when being cut and in a single moment be rendered worthless. Therefore suppleness is an important quality for metal to possess. Metal's virtue is that it may be recast or remolded many times. Like water, metal may be induced to take any form, yet, unlike water, metal will hold that form on its own. Metal is used to make weapons, and its ability to be honed to a fine edge enables it to cut to the core of things. Metal is brilliant and in shining may inspire all who gaze upon it.

The metal element is often the most difficult for students of Chinese medicine to understand in relation to the human being. Physically, metal occurs within as the minerals that nourish and give strength to the structure of our bones and tissue. In Chinese internal alchemy, the metal cinnabar represents transformation because it is the only material the ancient Chinese possessed that is stable as both a solid and liquid at room temperature. In its solid form, mercuric sulfide represents mundane consciousness, only able to perceive the fixed nature of material reality. In its liquid form, mercury represents the flow of flexible consciousness that promotes the generation of water from metal along the *sheng* cycle as each new round of evolution is initiated. Cinnabar also figured prominently in external alchemy's attempt to turn lead (mundane consciousness) into gold (illuminated awareness).

In assessing the quality of a patient's metal element, it is useful to draw on imagery of the many ways that metal itself is present in nature. For example, are patients cold and piercing with their view of reality remaining fixed and unyielding? Are they like brittle metal, tarnished and cracking, with no sense of self-worth? Or are they radiant like a diamond, inspiring others with their brilliance and intrinsic value?

The Nature of Dryness

A function of the lungs is to allow water which rises in the body to condense and to then descend in the same way that heaven contains clouds which create rain. Healthy moisture in the lungs and large intestine forms the interface between our internal and external world. Moisture helps the lungs and large intestine draw quality into our being and discharge what has been metabolized and no longer serves. The direction associated with the metal element is the West, which in both China and the United States is where the deserts are found. Hence dryness is the environmental condition that affects the metal element. On a physical level, dryness may manifest in the lungs in association with respiratory ailments and in the large intestine as constipation. On a psychospiritual level, dryness may embody a sense of loss and feelings of having been "burnt" by heaven, which has taken away what one has valued.

The Spirit of Metal: Po

魄

The character *po* consists of the character *bai* (白) on the left, meaning white, and *gui* on the right, signifying earthbound spirits. White is the color of metal, and the *po* is the *shen* associated with the lungs. Whereas the character for *hun* includes on the left the image of clouds that exist in heaven and signifies the ascension of spirit, the *po* includes the image of the color white, the color of bones that lie buried within the earth. Upon death the *po* descends through the anus and returns to earth.

For every action in life there is an equal and opposite reaction. Whereas the ascension of the *hun* is related to the process whereby the spirit evolves through the manifestation of the physical body, the *po* is related to the process whereby the body is created out of the radiation of spirit *(shen)*.[83] The *po* consists of the seven emotions (fear, anxiety, anger, joy, sorrow, worry, and grief) which are the primal urges that facilitate the grasping of life.[84] As an earthbound spirit, I think of the *po* as relating to gravity, a force that draws things in toward the center of our being and holds them there. The function of the *po* is to contact what is of essential worth, receive it into (lungs), and retain it within (large intestine) while returning the *yin* mundane influences back to the earth from whence they came.

The *hun* empowers us to raise the potential stored in the earthly influence of *jing* up back toward heaven through the fulfillment of destiny during our life. The *po* turns the nourishing *yang* (sunlight) of later heaven, which is contained in air and captured by all that grows, into the body. Upon death the *po* becomes fertilizer, returning to earth in a way that empowers new growth.

The Fall

It is the spontaneous generative force of life that fuels the ascension of *qi* from water up to fire along the *sheng* cycle as the seasons change from the winter to the summer solstice. Externally, this process may be viewed as an ascension of being, as the ten thousand things manifest in the world. However, on an internal level this rise may symbolize the fall from original nature as we move away from the *dao*, which is the true source of self as symbolized by the water element and winter.

The season associated with the metal element is termed the *fall* in English. On an external level, it is a fall from the height of life back into the void and barrenness of winter. On an inner level, however, this may be seen not as a fall, but a return to origin in a more highly evolved state. This return is often depicted as an evolution in Daoist mythology as the sage, who, in gaining immortality, ascends to heaven on the back of a dragon or crane (see Figure 10.4).

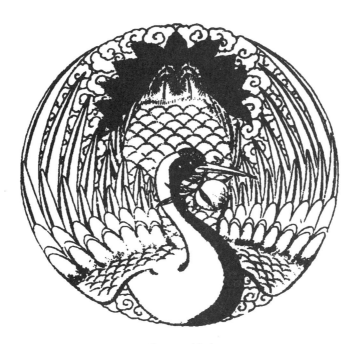

Figure 10.4
ASCENT TO IMMORTALITY[85]

The crane and peach are both symbols of longevity. Here the crane symbolizes the spirit of the dead being conveyed to heaven.

Virtue and Transformation: Loss and Grief into Righteousness

> *How is it that the lungs correspond to righteousness?*
> *The lungs are the essence of [the element] metal, and*
> *righteousness makes decisions. The West is also*
> *[the quarter of] metal, where all things,*
> *having reached maturity, are destroyed.*
> *– BAI HU DONG[86]*

Yi (義), the character for righteousness, is a composite of the character indicating the self (我), placed underneath the character for king (羊).[87] In this sense, *yi* may be thought of as the subjugation of the self to what ultimately lies above, which is the will of heaven. Righteousness may be considered to correspond to divine justice. It is in being at peace with the notion that heaven gives and takes according to its own divine plan that loss and grief *(you:*憂*)* may be healed. For this is the divine balance governed by the breath of *dao,* which is embodied as the metal element.

As we move away from the virtue of righteousness toward a life theme of loss, grief arises as the unbalanced emotion. As we move away toward a life theme of gain, longing (grief directed toward the future) arises as the unbalanced emotion. Metal constitution types may manifest either the remarkable presence or absence of grief or longing as they habitually react to loss or gain as themes in life. Habitual reaction to these emotions may manifest as an inability to let go of what has lost value in life. This dysfunction may be embodied as the symptom of constipation or asthma as they find it difficult to fully exhale. Conversely, they may manifest an inability to hold on to what is of value. This dysfunction may be embodied as diarrhea or asthma, resulting from an inability of the large intestine to retain value or the lungs to fully grasp the *qi*. In contrast, longing as a disordered emotion may unconsciously motivate them to strive for material possessions of increasing worth or to covet what they value, identifying their own source of self-worth with their possessions.

Dong Chongshu tells us that the standard for righteousness lies in rectifying the self, not in rectifying others.[88] As a habitual reaction to our grief we may become obsessed with connecting to purity in life. Convinced their own path is of the highest value, metal types tend toward zealotry, pontification, and the willingness to cut off relations with anyone or anything considered to sully their chosen path.[89] This dynamic is typified by a lack of grief and an emotional coldness that allows them to cut off feelings of attachment to anything or anyone who is not valued.

As treatment progresses, the practitioner expects the emotions of grief and longing to diminish, along with a reduction in the behaviors and illnesses associated with these emotions. Correspondingly, the virtue of righteousness is expected to become increasingly present. The dynamics of destiny and transformation are evidenced in the case studies presented later.

The Rhythm of Metal

The breath of *dao,* as described in Chapters 4 and 5 in the *Dao De Jing,* is a "whirling vortex," a great inhaling and exhaling that gives rise to all creation while receiving it back in the next moment. Upon exhaling *(yang),* the *dao* moves away from itself, imbuing the ten thousand things with their own natures. Inhaling *(yin)* in the next moment, it receives back all to which it has given birth. Chapter 4 of the *Dao De Jing,* which corresponds in number to the metal element as the fourth stage of *dao*,[90] describes the breath of *dao*:

> Dao *is a whirling emptiness* (chong),
> *Yet in use is inexhaustible.*
> *Fathomless* (yuan),
> *It seems to be the ancestor* (zong) *of ten thousand things.*
> — *DAO DE JING*[91]

Chen interprets this chapter as describing the *dao* as "dynamic self-diffusive creativity," pouring out and receiving back all beings.[92] *Dao*, as the origin of all origins, is termed "the ancestor of ten thousand beings." The character *zong* (宗) for ancestor is the same character used for *zongqi* (宗氣), the ancestral *qi* of the lungs in the chest.[93] The *zongqi* is what empowers rhythmic movement in every aspect of our being. It is the breath of *dao* that powers our own breath as we mirror the basic functioning of the universe. The idea that breathing is a basic process of *dao* is supported in the *Dao De Jing*, Chapter 5:

> *Between heaven and earth, how like a bellows it is!*
> *Empty and yet inexhaustible,*
> *Moving and yet it pours out ever more.*[94]

The movement of *dao* is like a great whirlpool, rising and falling like a bellows, giving birth to all things at its periphery and receiving them back at its center.

The Life Thesis of Metal

The key life themes for metal constitution types involve contacting and retaining what is of value in life in a way presided over by the virtue of righteousness. If habitual reaction to grief or longing obscures their connection to heaven and the virtue of righteousness, then their life theme is distorted into a thesis that compromises their balanced relationship to value in every aspect of being.

The archetypal life theme for metal constitutional types that reflects excess may be stated as, "That which I value is of such great worth that it must be coveted regardless of the consequences to anyone or anything including myself." The theme that reflects deficiency may be stated as, "Nothing of value can be truly attained or held on to in life."

Irony: Rust Never Sleeps

The irony that lies thematically at the heart of the metal constitution is that *what is of the most essential worth is least substantial.* Habitual reaction to the emotions of grief and longing drive the lung and large intestine officials to inappropriately hold on to or let go of what is valued in life. We can live for twenty or more days without food (earth/physical nourishment), but we die within minutes if cut off from air (heaven/spiritual nourishment). Yet air is invisible and far less substantial than earth. Those who are spiritually separated from heaven fail to value spiritual connection to the essence of things and focus instead on material possessions that may be acquired in life. However, the acquisition of each new material possession is fulfilling for only a short while before its value is soiled by some fatal flaw. For in time, all material things lose their luster. Ultimately, only our spiritual connection to heaven can sustain us, as the material form of what we have valued slips away.

An internal abyss lies at the center of all things that connects them to the primordial *dao.* The nature of this abyss is that no amount of material gain can ever fill it. For metal constitutional types, this void may be experienced as isolation, lack of self-worth, loneliness, and grief. Feeling cut off from the *qi* of heaven, they may become uninspired and depressed. Driven by feelings of emptiness, individuals may seek to fill their internal void by acquiring material possessions and worldly success. Hence the *Yijing,* in hexagram 58 (*Tui,* "the joyous," which corresponds to the lungs), tells us, "True joy must spring from within. But if one is empty within and wholly given over to the world, idle pleasures come streaming in from without."[95]

A major therapeutic principle in treating people who are metal constitutionally is to help them experience the "emptiness" inside as the essence of life that is most subtle and valuable and to understand that joy dependent on external circumstances is transitory. Confucius states, "The superior man understands righteousness *(yi:*義*);* the inferior man understands profit *(li:*利*)."*[96] For Confucius, profit seeking and the virtue of righteousness are opposites. Righteousness may be viewed as the virtue that springs from connecting to the transcendent value of things without attachment to their material form.

The Nature of Self-Worth

Self-esteem, as governed by the wood element, emerges from the vision of who we are in our depths. Self-worth, as governed by metal, is the virtue of valuing what we find there. Self-worth is based on the essential quality instilled by heaven at conception and what we are able to acquire and retain in life. However it is not enough to merely possess quality internally; we must also be able to connect to and appreciate what is of value, a facility presided over by the balanced functioning of the lung and large intestine officials.

Our inherent quality is instilled by heaven at conception and, on earth, is transmitted through the father's *jing*. This *jing* is transmitted by the father at conception via the mother's "metal gate" through which the fetus enters being out of the void. In life, the father remains the embodiment of heaven in transmitting the virtue of self-worth to the infant, whereas the mother is the embodiment of earthly nourishment. Ideally, the mother's connection to her child provides unconditional nourishment. However, the father's connection is predicated on appreciating the child for manifesting the potential he, as an emissary of heaven, has placed within at conception.

Often individuals' ability to appreciate what is of value in self and others reflects the nature of their relationship with their father throughout life. Interestingly, I have found that often asthma in young children reflects a longing for the father, who is either emotionally or physically unavailable because of death, divorce, or work.

Image: Poignancy

A predominant feeling of metal constitutional types manifests as a sense of poignancy emerging from the dynamic between appreciating the beauty of life and simultaneously mourning its loss. This dynamic is evident in the fall as the leaves on the trees turn beautiful colors in their process of dying. Turning bright yellow, red, orange, and purple, the dying leaves display the essential beauty that lies within. In the moment metal constitution types stand transfixed by the tree's beauty, the wind stirs and one brown leaf falls slowly to its final rest upon the earth. Simultaneously spectators are filled with appreciation of the tree's beauty and sorrow at the knowledge that as soon as tomorrow, the tree will be barren.

Habitually reacting to feelings of loss leads metal constitution types to one of two dysfunctional behaviors. In its excess display, metal types may try in vain to hold on to the physical manifestations of life. Here their grief drives them to obsessively guard anything valued in life. In this regard I recall a patient who refused to drive a car he had spent years restoring for fear it might be scratched and therefore ruined. In contrast, convinced that value is elusive in life, we may not be able to bring ourselves to even look at the momentary beauty of the tree for fear of the inevitable pain of loss that is sure to follow. In this case our life becomes barren as a desert for the failure to acquire and retain the essential quality that life has to offer.

Testing Emotions: Acknowledgment

Metal constitutional types habitually respond to the presence of the emotions grief and longing by losing connection to value in life. By offering acknowledgment and noting the quality of the patient's reaction, the practitioner may assess the qualitative function of the patient's metal element. By offering acknowledgment, the practitioner is actively valuing some aspect of the patient's essential worth. When metal is in a functional state of balance, acknowledgment from the practitioner should help allay the grief and longing displayed by the patient. However, a characteristic of metal constitutions is that reaction to grief is the unconscious force motivating their habitual behavior. Therefore, when offering acknowledgment to patients, the practitioner may find their grieving and longing subside only temporarily, if at all. Once acknowledgment is offered, it will either be continually elicited or rejected by patients throughout the interview. For example, patients with a poor sense of self-worth may be unable to take a compliment in the spirit it is offered. Or patients may be rather narcissistic and continually provide examples of how they shine the brightest of all. Acknowledgment from the practitioner comes externally. Only the internal virtue of righteousness can restore the connection to heaven and rectify one's habitual relationship to the disordered emotions associated with loss.

When offering acknowledgment, the practitioner must note changes in the patient's color, sound, odor, and emotion. The finding that these signs intensify and the patient becomes white, weeping, rotten, and expresses either grief or longing confirms the metal constitutional type.

The Suggestive Process in Treatment

Metal constitutional types are unconsciously motivated by their reaction to experiences of loss. The practitioner must pay particular attention to instituting a relative balance of gain and loss when making a suggestion to metal constitution patients. Hence metal types are most easily empowered to let go of something after taking in something new or, conversely, to receive something new after letting go of something old. For example, in motivating metal types to stop eating candy the practitioner might suggest replacing it with raisins. Motivating metal types to accept their own self-worth, the practitioner may suggest they let go of a relationship that has lost its worth as a token of their new emphasis on finding value in life.

Using the language of the metal element to motivate this constitutional type to quit smoking, the practitioner might say, "I'm sure the fresh air in your lungs will be inspiring. I can see that stopping smoking is really in line with your commitment to quality. It will feel great to be clean again inside."

The Metal Officials

The *yin* and *yang* officials paired in the metal element are the lungs and large intestine, respectively. The lungs and large intestine form a functional yoke whereby the lungs bring quality into our life while keeping impurity outside, and the large intestine lets go of impurity while keeping what is precious within. Together, the lungs and large intestine empower us to be in touch with the essential spirit of things and to let go of their superficial material form.

In a sense, the normal relationship between the *yin* and *yang* officials is somewhat altered when considering the large intestine and lungs. Generally the *yang* official is the interface to the outer world and the *yin* official provides connection to the deeper aspects of self contained in the *jing*. On first glance, however, this relationship is reversed in metal where the lungs bring essence into our life and thus interface with the outer world and the large intestine looks within to eliminate any impurities that it finds. Upon closer consideration, however, it is apparent the lungs are an interface between early heaven within in the form of inherited essence and later heaven without in the form of acquired essence.[97] The large intestine, in contrast, contacts mundanity within (in the form of feces) which represents the acquired habituating influences gleaned from earth and returns these back to earth whence they came. Therefore, the lungs, in the upper burner, preside largely over our connection to heaven, and the large intestine, in the lower burner, predominantly governs our connection to the earth. Next I elaborate on how various aspects of being associated with the metal element express themselves through the metal officials.

The Lung Official

The lungs hold the office of minister and chancellor. The regulation of the life-giving network stems from it.
— NEI JING SU WEN[98]

The character *xiang* (相), translated as minister, also means "reciprocity" and signifies the close functional relationship of the heart and the lungs, which are the only officials residing in the upper burner. The upper burner corresponds to heaven with the heart representing the sun and the lungs representing the upper arc of heaven as the canopy that covers the earth. The heart is relatively *yang* compared to the lungs and governs the blood, which is *yin*. The lungs, relatively *yin*, govern the *qi*, which is *yang* compared to blood. Synchronization between the rhythm of the heart and lungs plays a crucial role in empowering the quality of an individual's presence and connection in life. The rhythm of the heart empowers us to be consciously present in each moment, tying the flow of our life into the instantaneous pulsation of *dao*. The rhythm of fire is a repeated cycling of on, then off, then on again, signifying the *dao's* rise and fall from nonbeing to being, and back to nonbeing again for eternity. The rhythm of the lungs empowers a broader connection to the breath of *dao* in the act of creation and dissolution of being.

Blood is a substance unique to living beings. The heart instills *shen* into our blood so our own consciousness circulates to every aspect of who we are. The heart *shen* also radiates our awareness so we may connect with the world outside. The lungs with each inhalation draw in air and, in so doing, assimilate that aspect of *qi* trapped by air as sunlight (heavenly *yang*) and reject what has no value in promoting life. The lungs thus construct a barrier between our inner and outer world in a way that defines what is self and not-self. The protective boundary established by the heart is an expansive force and its outer limit, as conveyed by the triple heater official, represents the outermost level that our consciousness can extend. The boundary established by the lungs is a contractive force that represents the outermost limit of where we are able to draw quality into our life. I think of this limit as the edge of the force of people's "gravitational pull," which defines where they end and the outer world begins.

The lungs are said to be the sensitive official because they are most vulnerable to the attack of external pathogens that invade the body like wind/cold or wind/heat. The lungs govern the *weiqi,* which defines our outermost boundary, and prevents all that does not conform to true self from penetrating inward toward our core. Habitually reacting to the presence of grief, the function of the boundary empowered by the lungs may become compromised. If this boundary becomes too dry, then assimilation into self is hindered because moisture serves as the interface that allows the lungs to draw things internally. If the lungs hold on to water and fail to help it descend, then phlegm in the lungs may also obscure our connection to essence in life.

Later heaven radiates as sunlight toward humanity in an attempt to nourish the seed placed within by early heaven at conception. Sunlight that lies at the heart of all things is the source of nourishing *yang* extracted from air with the first breath and with all assimilated that is healthful during life. The lungs must identify sources of *qi* that contain this essential quality in life while filtering out what is purely mundane. It is the lungs' connection to quality and essence that enable them to empower the virtue of inspiration. As quality is drawn into our lives with each inhalation, the lungs must surrender with each exhalation what is of no value.

If we lose in life what we have valued, then grief is the resulting emotion. In health, the lungs empower us to stay connected to the essence of value even after the material form of a thing has disappeared. For example, after mourning the death of a loved one, the healthy lung official empowers connection to the spirit of the person who has passed even though the material body is gone. However, lung constitutional types may interpret loss by fixating on the material aspect of what has vanished. In this way they fail to grasp the essence of what has empowered their life and become habitually lost in grief, limiting their appreciation of each present moment.

Reacting to past loss, the lungs may eventually fail to contact essence in life due to anticipation of its inevitable loss. In this scenario lung constitutional types come to feel empty inside, losing touch with the essential aspects of self that empower self-worth. Uninspired, and uninspiring, individuals pass through life as though followed by a cloud that obscures their connection to the sun and heaven. This cloud of grief may become embodied as phlegm in the lungs, a chronic cough representing the lungs' rejection of heavenly *qi,* and constant clear sinus dripping symbolizing the embodiment of grief as internal tears.

The lungs, as the arbiters of divine justice, empower the virtues of exactness and balance in the transaction of value in life. Hence in China autumn was the time that merchants in the marketplace attended to calibrating the scale's weights and measures.[99] In health, the lungs empower the virtues of a good merchant. This manifests as balance and precision in our relationship to acquisition and loss in a way that is governed by the virtue of righteousness. A successful merchant understands the true value of each possession, as well as the price paid for holding on to it too long. To the degree that lung constitutional types react to grief in life, the virtue of righteousness may be distorted into the habitual behaviors of either coveting or rejecting material possessions.

Image: Clouds of Grief

Grief in those of the lung constitution tends to occur as a quiet weeping tone in the voice and the presence of pervasive sorrow directed toward either the past or the future. It is as though what a person values is continually receding through a thin veil of fog. Patients may give many names to what they seek, identifying money, love, or some material possession as the object of desire. However, the source of their quest is always reconnection to heaven and spirit as it manifests in all of life.

Grief directed toward the past manifests as a sense that value has slipped through their fingers and, even in the moment of trying to grasp it, it recedes slowly into the past, ever eluding capture. Grief directed toward the future manifests as longing. It is as though they are pursuing something through fog only to find that as they approach what is valued, it disappears ahead of them through the clouds, again eluding their grasp.

Large Intestine Official

> *The large intestine is responsible for transit. The residue*
> *from the transformation stems from it.*
> *– NEI JING SU WEN*[100]

The lungs, located in the upper heater, are the internal representation of heaven above and therefore contain the most rarefied and essential *qi.* The large intestine, located in the lower heater, corresponds to earth and governs the elimination of mundane *qi,* which has lost its value. However, as the large intestine eliminates what no longer serves, it must also absorb minerals that are of value into the body. In nature, the earth absorbs the heavenly *yang (shen),* which radiates down as sunlight and then condenses within the earth to form minerals and gemstones. Hence minerals in nature represent the condensation within the earth of heaven's spiritual light, which is evidenced in their radiant brilliance and intrinsic worth. Minerals, as condensed *yang,* represent the most essential rarified *qi* as it exists materially on earth, compared with air that represents the *qi* of heaven, which is significantly less substantial.

Just as the rhythm of the lungs draws heaven in toward our being, the peristaltic action of the large intestine draws all waste from the upper regions of the body, which represent heaven within, down toward the lower heater where it is eliminated and returned to earth. Similarly to the lungs, the large intestine constructs a barrier between self and not-self by sorting out which acquired influences need to be retained and which need to be let go.

Whereas the lungs must receive heavenly *qi* and exhale all that does not conform to true self in the next moment, the large intestine empowers the longer term process of ensuring purity within by eliminating all mundane influences acquired during life. Confucius alludes to this function when he states, "A good merchant hides his treasures as if his store was empty and a gentleman with full virtue *(de)* appears like a stupid man. Get rid of your proud air and many desires, your overbearing manners and excessive ambitions. None of these are good for you."[101] Failing to respond in a balanced way to loss in life, the large intestine constitution reacts to the presence of grief and longing. The habitual nature of such reactions distorts the virtue of righteousness into dysfunctional behaviors that result in either the inappropriate letting go of value or holding on to what no longer serves. These dysfunctions may be embodied as diarrhea, a process whereby minerals are lost from the body, or constipation, a process whereby waste is inappropriately retained. The result of either behavior is a pervading sense of inner worthlessness as personal value either slips away or is completely obscured by life's mundane influences. This dynamic may be evidenced by a general grossness of behavior including poor grooming habits and a general lack of cleanliness.

Failure to contact essence within and the accretion of mundanity are often expressed as pessimism, cynicism, and general negativity in all domains of life. In this scenario the large intestine loses functional contact with the lungs' connection to heaven within and without. The dysfunctional large intestine fails in its task of maintaining a state of internal purity and projects its failing on the external world. Large intestine constitutions may imagine themselves the arbiters of divine justice, coldly proceeding through life endeavoring to purge all influences that do not conform to their mind's image of spiritual purity. This is the dynamic present in all religious crusades where the leaders, separated in their own hearts from heaven, mistake all that does not conform to their belief as constituting impurity. In this scenario the mind has distorted the appreciation of whatever value lies within as signifying that we alone are closest to heaven. In a less dramatic display this state may manifest in excessive pride and a holier-than-thou attitude.

Image: Closing the Iron Door

Habitual reaction to the presence of grief and longing may cause large intestine constitutions to lose touch with the true nature of value in life. The minds of the large intestine constitution come to interpret life's events as proving the thesis that they are not appropriately valued by others. Conversely, feelings of not being valued are often paired with the self-assurance that, in fact, this represents a failing in others who lack the facility to appreciate their elevated worth. The resulting feeling of being cut off and separate from other human beings in life is predicated on their own rejection of heaven, which is perceived as having taken away what was valued.

Failing to feel valued by others, large intestine constitutions easily find fault with others in life. In this scenario, lack of connection to quality within leads to the inability to find value in others. Focusing instead on the negative, the minds of the large intestine constitutions become overly critical. Once any flaw is found, the nature of the entire relationship is experienced as being soiled, as the habituated mind is unable to let go of the negative and connect to the positive. The ensuing tendency is to sever the relationship as if closing an impenetrable iron door that is rusted shut. In an attempt to avoid the pain of loss associated with perceptions of not having been valued, the mind has severed connection with what was valued, resulting in feelings of separateness, loneliness, and poor self-worth.

Metal: Case Studies

Example of the Lung Constitutional Type

SANDY: A LESSON IN SELF-WORTH

Complaints: Inability to have a rewarding relationship, smoking cessation.

Background: Sandy is a very attractive woman who could easily be a high-fashion model. She maintains an immaculate appearance and wears only the finest clothes and jewelry. Every hair seems to be in place. A rigid perfectionist, Sandy finds very little room for flexibility around the ideals and behaviors that she values. Her main issue in life has been to find a man with whom to have a meaningful relationship.

Sandy has a history of choosing men for relationships and then using them to test her self-worth. She often becomes involved with men without first determining whether they are attracted to her merely for her looks. She habitually overlooks her partner's glaring faults, such as previous abuse of a spouse, believing he should value her enough to change his ways. When in a relationship, Sandy holds so tightly to her partner that he feels suffocated. If he withdraws on even the subtlest of psychic levels, she experiences it as rejection. However, she makes herself unavailable for a relationship by finding a fatal flaw in each lover and then distancing herself from him.

Although Sandy has no overt history of sexual abuse, she characterizes her relationship with her father while she was growing up as having poor boundaries. On several occasions, he told her, "With your looks and my money, we are going places." One day during a treatment session while discussing her father, she stated, "I don't need him, I'll show him I can succeed with my *own* looks and money."

Sandy had started smoking when she was 16 during her parents' divorce and had tried to quit several times unsuccessfully.

Analysis: Like a diamond—shiny and pretty on the outside but ultimately both cold and hard—Sandy subjects every lover to her discriminating perfectionism in an effort to estimate their value. She continually looks for proof that she is not valued by setting challenges that her lovers must meet. Every time a test is passed, however, she raises the ante until eventually all must fail. She then interprets the failure of the relationship as indicating she is not valued, and her deep unspoken fear of worthlessness is then confirmed. Ironically, Sandy simultaneously overlooks glaring faults in her partners to which her own sense of self-worth, if it were functioning properly, should alert her.

Her statement that her success is based on her own looks and money may be taken as a reaction to her feeling that her father did not value her appropriately. It also suggests that she herself fails to value what is her essential worth and focuses instead on her own "looks and money." Both of these attributes are superficial and transitory aspects of one's true worth. Her smoking may be seen as a habitual behavior predicated on her grief resulting from her separation from her father.

Treatment: Sandy did not feel ready to address her smoking at the beginning of the treatments. In order to help her stop smoking, I helped her pair letting go of this habit with a renewed commitment to her own self-worth and value. I helped Sandy experience her smoking as a screen cutting her off from others and limiting the quality of her intimate contacts. In this way, the act of stopping smoking became a logical extension of her own desire to have a fulfilling relationship.

When the issue of her father arose in treatment, I pointed out her habitual drive to substantiate her value and avoid feelings of emptiness and worthlessness. I suggested she was failing both to value her father for having loved her in the only way he was able and to value her own essential worth that lay beyond her "good looks" and financial success. In this session, I treated acupuncture points Large Intestine-1 ("merchant *yang*") and Lung-8 ("lightening"). Both are horary points associated with their respective officials and thus are particularly effective at empowering the embodiment of balanced metal. These were paired with the "window of heaven" on the lung meridian (Lung-3, "celestial storehouse"), a point empowering the experience of self-worth. After this treatment, Sandy reported feeling she had let go of a substantial portion of her issues with her father and felt that perhaps she had the basis for a new kind of relationship with him. Concurrently, she reported she had quit smoking on her own and she has not returned to smoking since that time.

As treatment continued, I helped Sandy focus attention on the ways her own sense of deficient self-worth prevented her from attaining the closeness she desired in relationships. I pointed out her pattern of either overlooking glaring flaws in her partners or discarding seemingly good relationships because of relatively minor flaws. After gaining awareness of her patterns and resolving her issues with her father, Sandy finally found a long-term relationship that endured for several years.

Example of the Large Intestine Constitutional Type

LINDA: CLOUDS OF GRIEF OBSCURE THE HEART'S FIRE

Complaints: Glaucoma, ankylosing spondylitis, chronic constipation.

Background: Linda is a 44-year-old woman who initially came into treatment for some relatively serious complaints. My first impression was of a woman with an all-pervasive grief hanging over her like a cloud. Linda was slowly becoming blind as a result of glaucoma. In fact, her internal vision was turned entirely onto her past as she grieved for lost friends and lovers, and for her health, which was slowly slipping away.

A telling symbol of Linda's deep grief was a silver "dog tag" with the name of a soldier who had died in the Vietnam War. She had worn it for twenty-one years. Although she had never known the man, she wore this necklace as a token of the era and the pain she felt about the war.

Linda was treating her chronic constipation by giving herself daily enemas at the recommendation of her holistic physician. In our initial session, she informed me that I was her "knight in shining armor," who would rescue her from her illnesses.

Analysis: Linda's glaucoma may be considered an embodiment of her grief, which covers her eyes like a veil of mourning. I considered her ankylosing spondylitis, a disease resulting from the calcification of the upper thoracic vertebrae (an area associated with the lungs and the location of the lung *shu* points on the bladder meridian), to also be the embodiment of her grief. Calcification of this region associated with the lungs is an inappropriate concentration of metal (minerals in the form of calcium) in the upper part of the body. In this regard, it is important to note that a key function of the large intestine is to abstract minerals from the stool. Her chronic constipation may be seen as the embodiment of her inability to let go, manifesting in the lower half of her body.

Linda's constant use of enemas actually undermined the large intestine's ability to function normally. Because the enema in effect does the work for the large intestine, that organ becomes further disempowered from adequately performing its function. One strength of Chinese medicine is that it does not impose on the organ functions but rather gently supports them in improved functioning by creating a better balance from within.

Linda's statement designating me as her "knight in shining armor" is highly evocative of imagery associated with the metal element, and I took it as one sign of her metal constitutional type.

Treatment: In the course of treatment, Linda's slowly released her grief about past events and people as she gained awareness of how it limited her capacity to experience a wide range of other emotions in the present. She eventually removed her dog-tag necklace as a potent symbol of her willingness to let go of the past, but this act came too late to have a significant effect on her physical condition. She had already progressed past the point of being able to make substantial improvements with treatment.

A point selection that captures Linda's functional dynamic might include Large Intestine-4 and -18, paired with Lung-7. Large Intestine-4 and -18 both empower the letting go of that which no longer serves us in life. These points helped enable Linda to let go of her old grief as symbolized by her tarnished metal dog tag. Lung-7, as the *luo* point on the lung meridian, joins the lung's function of receptivity to quality with the large intestine's capacity for eliminating impurities in life. In this way Linda was empowered to bring new quality into her life, which helped to balance the loss of what she had let go of.

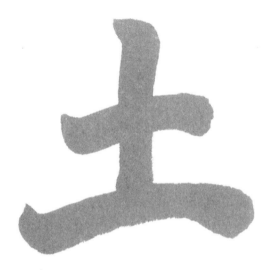

I alone am different from others.
For I treasure feeding on the mother.
– LAOZI[102]

EARTH—THE AXIS

The earth element corresponds to the number five in the enumeration of creation. The number five in Chinese (五) signifies the primal *yin* and *yang*, giving birth to the five elements (十) between heaven and earth (二).[103] Earth, as center, provides the fulcrum around which the other four transformations take place. The earth element governs our connection to the earth in a way that empowers utilizing and integrating all sources of available nourishment in life so the potential of the inherited constitution may be actualized. Hence the source points on the *yin* meridians are all earth points that pull each official back to its center, helping it derive nourishment from connection to our inherited and acquired influences.[104]

The earth element helps establish an appropriate boundary regarding the nourishing of self and others in life as mediated by a balanced response to feelings of need. The quality of this balance is predicated in part on the nature of our relationship to our mother as it guides the course of our development from conception to adulthood. From conception through birth, the fetus is connected to its mother through the umbilical cord whose place of attachment defines the physical center of the human body. Through this connection the fetus is nourished continually and unconditionally. The quality and nature of this connection is that the fetus is feeding directly from the primordial *dao* as embodied by its earthly mother. The severance of this connection and the ensuing inhalation of the first breath signify the infant has left the womb of *dao* and is now being nourished by the acquired *qi* of later heaven. With the cutting of the umbilicus the mother puts the child to her breast and reestablishes the connection of the infant to the primordial *dao*.

Eventually the infant, toddler, or child is weaned from breast-feeding and its mother becomes the earthly symbol of connection to the universally available source of nourishment that is *dao*. Each successive stage of development between our first breath and leaving home as an adult entails a distancing from the mother as provider of connection to nourishment. As time passes, an increased responsibility is placed on each of us to appropriately meet our own needs in life by connecting to *dao* as it is present both within our self and without in the world. It is the quality of our connection to mother early in life that sets the stage for our balanced relationship to the issues of need and nourishment in every aspect of being. Earth constitutional types are destined a priori to attach special significance to this relationship in life because they are prone to interpreting life in terms of the fulfillment of needs.

It is in centering ourselves that we gain stability and avoid being swept along by the whirlpool of fate. Through the act of centering and aligning our self with the primal axis of *dao,* we may become masters of our own destiny. For it is only in connection to the center which never varies that our movement through life may occur in a stable fashion. Centering may be accomplished by meditation and, in the *Yijing,* the hexagram for meditation is *ken,* "keeping still": "Keeping his back still so that he no longer feels his body/He goes into his courtyard and does not see his people."[105] *Ken* is the trigram for mountain doubled and is strongly representative of the stability of earth.

Symptomatically, people who are earth constitutionally may suffer from a lack of center, or from an excessive centeredness, on every level of being. Symptoms such as prolapsed uterus, diarrhea, or poor balance may all evidence a lack of physical centeredness. On an emotional level, uncenteredness may show up as excessive thought manifesting as worry. To the other extreme, accumulations of excess weight, stagnation of food in the digestive system, fibroid tumors, or selfishness may be considered signs of excessive centeredness.

The Nature of Earth

The quality of the earth's roundness is often reflected in the physical features of the earth constitutional type. Conversely, a person who is undernourished may appear overly thin. The earth as center processes all that comes to it in a way that nourishes life from conception to death. Hence the earth absorbs sunlight, rain, the decay of old growth, and the seed of new growth, transforming all of these into the abundant life that ideally thrives on it. As earth empowers the physical center of all things, so does the center of the body reflect the quality of the earth element. In Chinese medicine the body's center is comprised of the area just under and including the umbilicus. This region is referred to as the *hara* in Japanese, which reflects a translation of the Chinese characters *qihai* (氣海), or "sea of *qi.*" In internal alchemy this area of the body is called the lower cinnabar field *(diantian:*丹田*),* which corresponds to the function of *mingmen.* Any signs of the center sagging, as occurs with excessive weight or the prolapse of an organ, is a sign of deficient earth.

In late summer (roughly the middle of August until the first frost), the season associated with earth, the fields are filled with nourishment representing the fruits of our labors. In such a state of harmony, the earth maintains a reciprocal relationship with human beings whereby it yields an abundant harvest to those who adequately cultivate and care for it. Out of balance, earth may be dry and cracked as in a barren desert that yields hardly enough nourishment to support all but the simplest life-forms. Earth may be cloying like quicksand that grabs onto and slows the progress of anything or anyone that stumbles into contact with it. Representing years of slow geologic process, earth may manifest as a landslide or earthquake that in one moment displays devastating force and unyielding strength. The quality of the earth element in each individual may be compared to the quality of the different types of earth that exist in nature. Hence, like a desert, earth constitutional types may have little nourishment to support their own functioning, let alone enough to share with others. Like quicksand or mud they may appear needy and cloying, appealing for sympathy to all those who become stuck in a relationship with them. Or they may be altruistic and, having enough for themselves, be happy to share selflessly in a way that allows others to thrive.

The Nature of Dampness

Dampness is the environmental condition present as humidity that injures the balanced functioning of the earth element. Internally, dampness is an accumulation of everything that should have nourished us but has instead been transformed into burden. Dampness represents stagnation that slows the function of an official in all aspects of being. Psychospiritually this may present as lethargy, boredom, slow thought process, obsession, or brooding. On a physical level, dampness may present as phlegm or mucus that tends to accumulate in the organs of the digestive system, notably the spleen, stomach, lung, and large intestine. Sweetness is the flavor associated with the earth element, and the excessive need to either give or receive sympathy is the psychospiritual attribute of dampness.

The Spirit of Earth: Yi

The character *yi* is composed of the radical *yin* (音), which signifies an uttered sound, placed over the character *xin* (心), meaning heart.

Wieger defines *yi* as the intention of those who speak manifested by the sound they utter and, by extension, the meaning conveyed by their words.[106] The character *yi* may also be thought of as composed of three components. Hence the 117th radical *li* (⊥), meaning "to establish," is placed over the character *yue*, meaning "to speak," which depicts a mouth (⊟) with words in it, which in turn is located over the character *xin*, depicting heart. Thus we may describe the character *yi*, meaning intention, as signifying the process of establishing meaning in the world with words that come from the heart.

The *yi* empowers the integration into self of only that which corresponds to the template provided by our inherited constitution. In so doing, the inherited and acquired constitutions are united in a way that produces a fully integrated human being. On a physical level this means allowing the digestive system to abstract from all sources of acquired *qi* the necessary ingredients for nourishing, building, and maintaining the body. In psychospiritual aspects of being, the *yi* allows us to integrate our life experiences in a nourishing way that produces the virtue of integrity *(xin:*信*)*. This integrity is evidenced by the quality of our intention and the degree to which our words conform to the truth in our heart.

Hence the *yi* preside over the digestive functions of thought that allow the processing and assimilation of our life experiences in a way that is nourishing. Unbalanced function of the *yi* is evidenced by brooding, worry, and obsessive thought patterns. These states are typified by constant thought on emotional material that yields no productive action in the world. Those who think obsessively become stuck in a pattern of thinking for thought's sake alone and are never nourished by the experiences they are processing. This dynamic may be likened to chewing on the same mouthful of food forever without swallowing.

Virtue and Transformation: Selfishness and Selflessness into Integrity and Reciprocity

How is it that the spleen corresponds to good faith [xin]?
The spleen is the essence of [the element] earth. The highest function of earth is to nourish all creatures so as to give them form. It produces creatures without partiality which is the acme of good faith.
– BAI HU DONG[107]

Two virtues are associated with the earth constitutional type: *xin*, which I translate as "integrity," and *shu*, meaning "reciprocity." The character *xin* (信) depicts a man (亻) standing by his words (言). Wieger translates *xin* as "sincerity; the quality that the words of every man should have."[108] He also translates *xin* as meaning faith and truthfulness, which are the effects produced on a person by the words of another.[109] The virtue of integrity emerges from the alignment between our thoughts, actions, and words.

The earth nourishes all to which it gives birth without discerning between the good and bad and so is called "impartial." Hence Chapter 49 of the *Dao De Jing* tells us that the sage trusts *(xin)* both the trustworthy and the nontrustworthy, which it equates with having trust in nature *(de)*. The earth nourishes all of creation, using the virtue exemplary of faith, trust, and loyalty, all of which are translations of the character *xin*. For these are the traits that emerge when the destiny of the earth is fulfilled. Although the earth may nourish humans, this abundance is not unconditional. The reciprocity *(shu:恕)* of nurturance and care between the earth and humans is exemplary of the virtue that emerges when the expression of the earth element is balanced in any relationship (see Figure 9.3). Reciprocity becomes manifest in our relationships as we comprehend the interrelatedness and interdependence of the earth and all beings.

Reciprocity and integrity are those virtues that empower meeting the needs of others and self in a balanced way, which manifests as altruistic behavior. Expecting nothing in return, the altruistic person is able to care appropriately for self and others without attachment to the results. Confucius makes this clear when he tells us, "The superior man is on good terms with [his fellow man] and is not identical, the inferior man is identical but is not on good terms."[110] Elsewhere, he states, "Clever words, an ingratiating demeanor, and excessive respect . . . I am ashamed of them."[111] Confucius clearly felt that we must not be ingratiating but show our true nature. People must act with integrity, in accord with their own feelings and natures, and not by ingratiating themselves with others.

The emotion associated with earth is sympathy *(si:思)*, which is also translated as thought, concern, worry, and obsession. Wieger tells us that the etymology of the character *si* indicates that, "When one is thinking . . . the vital fluid of the heart ascends to the brain."[112] In balance, the earth element's capacity for thought empowers the integration of the inherited and acquired constitutions in a way that promotes integrity. When the earth element is unbalanced, excessive thought manifesting as worry can drive people to cater obsessively to their own needs or to the needs of others. The transformation of self-ishness and ingratiation into integrity and reciprocity is one of the key themes in the life process of earth constitutional types. As they move away from these virtues toward a life theme of selfishness, an excessive need for sympathy arises as an unbalanced emotion. As they move away from these virtues toward a life theme of ingratiation, excessive sympathy arises as it is directed toward the needs of others.

Self-centeredness may lead them to look out for their own needs regardless of the needs of others. Selfishness may actually motivate them to give to others, always hoping to receive back what has been "invested." We may experience this dynamic when a person comes up from behind to rub our shoulders and the overall feeling is that the person rubbing is taking more *qi* than they are giving. Ingratiation means taking care of the needs of others without considering our own needs first. This behavior always leads to the accumulation of resentment, with the net result that relationships which should nourish us eventually become burdens.

As treatment progresses, the practitioner expects the aberrant behaviors of neediness and selfishness to diminish, along with a reduction in ingratiating behavior. Over time, illnesses and symptoms predicated on habitual reaction to the earth constitutional types' need for sympathy should abate, and the virtues of sincerity and reciprocity steadily increase. The dynamics of destiny and transformation as they pertain to the earth constitutional type are exemplified in the case studies presented later.

The Rhythm of Earth

The cycle of the seasons around the earth creates a continuous rhythm that empowers humanity to find stability through all of life's changes. Hence Chen notes that the character *xin* (信), the virtue of earth, is connected in its meaning to the regularity and rhythm of life that inspires confidence in nature and the stability of humanity's place in the world.[113]

The Life Thesis of Earth

The key life themes for the earth constitution involve integrating and distributing what is nourishing in life in a way that is presided over by the virtues of integrity and reciprocity. The habitual need to give or receive sympathy obscures their connection to earth and the manifestation of these virtues. In this case their life theme is distorted into a thesis that compromises their balanced relationship to nourishment in every aspect of being.

A common theme in the life of earth constitutional types is that the aspects of life which should have been nourishing are transformed into burdens. From the outside, their life might appear bountiful in terms of available sources of nourishment, such as money, career, hobbies, and family. However, all these are related to as though they are weights that must be dragged around rather than as sources of nourishment.

The archetypal life theme for earth constitutional types that reflects excess may be stated as, "My need to give and/or receive is so great that it must be manifested regardless of how overbearing it is in affecting the ability of others to be nourished or care for themselves." The theme that reflects deficiency may be stated as, "I am not enough to nourish others and life is not enough to nourish me."

Irony: The Balance of Production and Consumption

The irony at the heart of the earth element is that *their ability to be truly nourished lies in the balance of producing and consuming what is nourishing in life.* Nourishment, like all aspects of being, has both inner and outer attributes. Externally, nourishment is what may be integrated into our being to support our process of evolution and fulfillment of destiny. Earth constitutional types often become habitually fixated on external forms of nourishment and fail to assess whether those sources are consistent with their internal needs. Hence consumption of nourishment may become focused on fulfilling the habituated desires of the mind rather than manifesting inborn potential. The mind, of course, seeks whatever makes the person feel most comfortable in the moment, which rarely is deeply nourishing in the long term. Pursuing nourishment in an external fashion predicated on habitual drive is ultimately unfulfilling. Therefore, individuals become increasingly driven to ingest increasing amounts of both food and experiences at a faster rate in a vain attempt to be satiated. A typical image of this scenario is provided by people who eat their food too rapidly while reading, listening to the news, and talking simultaneously. Here input is received through every sensory orifice, overwhelming their capacity to process and be nourished by what they ingest.

The inner aspect of nourishment lies in being nourished by producing good effects in the world rather than by consuming. When in balance, the earth element is nourished by drawing on the endless resources that lie within the *dao*. Hence the *Dao De Jing* tells us the *dao* is like an ocean that use can never drain.[114] But, out of balance, individuals may continually draw on their own resources by giving to others. These persons seek nourishment by taking care of others and giving up their own internal resources of time and energy. Seeking to make the world right by endlessly catering to the needs of others, they ultimately end up unfulfilled with their resources exhausted. Only through the healthy balance of caring for self and others, empowered by the virtues of integrity and reciprocity, can earth constitution types feel fulfilled in a way that endures.

The Hypochondriac

The tendency of earth constitutional types toward worry can result in excessive concerns regarding the state of their own health. Their minds can turn inward in a self-centered way that magnifies every perceived discomfort into an issue thought to require the immediate attention of a health-care specialist. Hence earth constitutional types may often arrange to see many healers and medical specialists simultaneously. The tendency of such people is to terminate treatment immediately if the practitioner attempts in any way to empower them to make a lifestyle change that they perceive as reducing their level of comfort.

Reciprocity and the Issue of Balance

Reciprocity emerges in the healthy balance between consuming and cultivating nourishment in life. The notion of balance may pose particular difficulty when treating earth constitutional types who are prone to eating disorders that affect the digestive system. Reaction to sympathy prevents those of the earth constitution from appropriately fulfilling their own needs. Hence they are prone to either eating too much or too little, as well as choosing inappropriate sources of nourishment in life. This dynamic may manifest as symptoms as serious as anorexia, bulimia, or merely the craving for excessive amounts of sweets. These addictive behaviors pose a unique therapeutic challenge because the practitioner is unable to separate the patient completely from them.

When endeavoring to end any other habitual behavior, whether it be addiction to heroin or nicotine or merely nail biting, we can stop the behavior completely. However, the need to eat means that patients cannot merely stop the destructive behavior but must actually come to terms with their issues if health is to be restored.

This dynamic is reflected in the physiology of pathological conditions that are characterized by internal dampness. The fragrant smell associated with the earth element emanates most explicitly from stagnation and fermentation of food in the digestive tract. The physical basis of both fragrance and dampness is often proliferation of the organism *Candida albicans,* a normal part of the bowel flora (the organisms that coexist in the lower digestive tract). In health, the virtue of reciprocity emerges in the symbiotic relationship between humans who provide a home for the organism and the organism that helps humans digest their food. Excessive intake of sweets and poor dietary habits create an internal environment in which the Candida bacterium may proliferate and contribute to many of the symptoms of dampness experienced by the earth constitution. These symptoms may include vaginal infections, sugar cravings, sinusitis, ulcers, indigestion, constipation, and diarrhea. Treating Candida is difficult because the therapeutic goal is not to eliminate it entirely but to create an internal condition of health that naturally maintains a healthy balanced relationship between the organism and its host. This balance emerges only when the psychospiritual basis of the behaviors leading to poor eating habits is addressed in a way that leads the individual to embrace the virtues of the earth element.

Image: Momentum versus Inertia

The dysfunctional behaviors that typify the imbalances of the earth element occur on a continuum from complete inertia to unrelenting momentum. Hence the central tendency of earth constitutional types is to remain at rest or to be unstoppable once moving in a given direction. As earth imbalance manifests in deficiency, they may give the impression they are lying in a hammock on a hot and humid summer day. Movements and thought processes are slow and heavy, evidencing the thickness and weight of the late summer heat. This characteristic manifests as lethargy and boredom and often appears in illnesses typified by chronic fatigue. Like a tractor stuck in mud, spinning its wheels and getting nowhere, patients' minds may race with all they need to accomplish while their bodies refuse to budge.

In contrast, the earth element in excess may manifest as sheer momentum, making it difficult to slow down once engaged in an activity. In this case patients may be likened to a bull charging straight ahead, unable to slow down or change course. It is as though they are stuck in the fields relentlessly harvesting, driven by the worry that even a moment's rest will cause them to miss a grain of wheat and thereby lose a potential source of nourishment. This characteristic may manifest as stubbornness in a variety of life situations. The net effect of both the excess and deficient presentation of earth is one of being stuck, either unable to move at all or caught in a direction of movement like a train that cannot be derailed.

Testing Emotions: Sympathy

Earth constitutional types habitually react to the presence of need as it is perceived in self and others. By offering sympathy and noting the quality of the patient's reaction, the practitioner may assess the qualitative function of the patient's earth element. When earth is in a functional state of balance, sympathy offered by the practitioner should help fulfill the need the patient is displaying. However, a defining characteristic of those of the earth constitution is that reaction to sympathy is the unconscious force that motivates their behavior. Therefore, when offering patients sympathy, the practitioner may find their needs are met only momentarily.

Sympathy may be offered explicitly by merely saying, "I am sorry, that must have been difficult," when the patient is expressing emotional pain. Sympathy may also be offered in a less obvious way through physical touch, for example, by touching a knee or hand if they are displaying sorrow or grief. The practitioner may also merely offer a sympathetic glance while offering patients a tissue if they are crying. Regardless of how sympathy is offered, if patients are earth constitutionally it will trigger their habitual reaction of either downplaying the level of their own need or of increasing the degree of their complaining in an attempt to elicit sympathy from the practitioner.

The practitioner may also note the quality of sympathy that patients display toward others. This quality is most readily apparent when patients are providing medical information relative to their families' health history. Noting patients' quality of care for friends and relatives when they are discussing their health offers an opportunity to assess the quality of patients' sympathy.

Sympathy offered by others comes from outside patients whose life lesson involves establishing an appropriate boundary in meeting their needs and the needs of others appropriately. Only by embracing the internal virtues of integrity and reciprocity can earth constitution types ever find fulfillment. In the moment of offering sympathy, the practitioner must note changes in the patient's color, sound, odor, and emotion. The finding that these signs intensify and the patient's face reflects the yellow color, their voice manifests the singing or lack-of-sing tone, their odor becomes fragrant, and they express either excessive or deficient sympathy is enough to confirm the patient is earth constitutionally.

The Suggestive Process in Treatment

Earth constitutional types are unconsciously motivated by reaction to the desire to fulfill the needs of self and others in life. Hence the practitioner's suggestions are most effectively made by implying that following a given course of action will result in feelings of comfort. Using the language of the earth element to motivate this constitutional type to quit smoking, the practitioner might say, "I'm sure you will feel wonderful within days of quitting smoking. Just imagine how good you will feel to really taste food again once you've quit." The practitioner may also imply that the patient will be more effectively caring for others by following whatever suggestion is offered. Thus the practitioner might state, "Stopping smoking will be a great example of your caring for your children. If you find the strength to stop, perhaps your husband will follow your lead."

The Earth Officials

The earth element plays a major role in governing the acquired constitution. Next I elaborate on how the various virtues associated with the earth element express themselves through the earth officials.

The Spleen and Stomach Officials

*The Spleen and Stomach are responsible for the storehouses
and granaries. The five Wei (tastes) stem from them.*
– NEI JING SU WEN[115]

The *yin* and *yang* officials paired in the earth element are the spleen and stomach, respectively. The *Nei Jing* discusses the function of each of the other ten officials as discrete entities with specific charges. In the quote here, however, the function of the stomach and spleen officials are addressed together.[116] These two officials form a functional yoke whose concern is acquiring and distributing all nourishment in life. The stomach is the interface between the internal world of the spleen and all potential sources of nourishment that exist outside of the self. The virtues of earth manifest through the stomach official in the appropriate gathering and processing of all resources that are available in the external world. The spleen official must integrate into self that nourishment acquired by the stomach, which it accomplishes through the production of blood. Through the blood, the spleen distributes the appropriate nutrients to every aspect of self internally in a way that nourishes the healthy function of every *yin* official. The spleen empowers the virtue of integrity by incorporating into the self that part of life which is consistent or *sympathetic* with one's inner being. This is the process whereby later heaven, as it exists in the form of nourishment, is combined with our endowment of early heaven in the internal alchemical process that empowers the fulfillment of destiny.

The separation of heart and mind perpetrated by our reaction to the emotion sympathy effectively prevents the stomach from looking inward to the spleen when assessing the reality of our needs in life. Divorced from this reality, the mind of the stomach constitution seeks poor sources of nourishment in life that are ultimately unfulfilling. The thought process of the stomach constitution becomes obsessive as it either rejects all forms of nourishment or tries in vain to acquire anything and everything that might have nutritive value. The spleen official, failing to receive appropriate sources of nourishment, is unable to empower the blood with the subtle essences needed for maintaining life. The function of every official suffers as internal reserves of *jing* must be drawn on to support the continued function of the individual.

Failing to adequately procure and process nourishment, the boundary between fulfilling personal needs and the needs of others becomes compromised. The breakdown of this boundary manifests as either excessively drawing on other people for nourishment or attempting to be nourished by dysfunctionally taking care of others. In the first instance, individuals may become like a sponge, soaking up sympathy like dampness. Overly sweet, they use ingratiation as a way of manipulating others to take care of them. This dynamic may be betrayed by the person who unconsciously reaches for food off another person's plate as a way of breaching the boundary that healthy earth must establish between self and other.

Unable to meet their own needs, earth types may look for intimate relationships with needy and sick people whom they endeavor to nourish back to health. In this way they seek to care for another with the quality of care they wish *they* had received from their own mother and, ultimately, from earth and life itself. Relationships based on this dysfunctional dynamic are unfulfilling because earth constitutional types become exhausted from catering to the other party. Should they persevere and nourish the other party back to health, they are generally rewarded with the end of the relationship as the other party, having gained independence, no longer needs them. A typical reaction to this scenario is resentment and a feeling of having been "owed better treatment" for the quality of care that was given. Only through the virtues of integrity and reciprocity can earth constitutional types come to care for others and self in a balanced way.

Earth: Case Studies

Example of the Stomach Constitutional Type

PAULETTE: CAUGHT IN THE MIDDLE— INGRATIATION AND RESENTMENT

Complaint: Poor digestion.

Background: Paulette is a 32-year-old massage therapist. She has a history of both anorexia and bulimia, which exhibited itself between the ages of 16 and 24. Although she has not engaged in the extreme behaviors that typify these illnesses in eight years, she does exhibit a wide variety of digestive disorders. These range from bowels that fluctuate between constipation and diarrhea, poor appetite, and general tightness and occasional burning in her esophagus. This latter symptom is accompanied by a feeling of constriction in her throat, which results in constant attempts to clear it. Paulette had her appendix removed at age 14 and her gallbladder removed at 21. Upon initial examination, Paulette's pulses were both deep and extremely thin.

Paulette's parents were divorced when she was 12 years old, and she describes a family situation where she was constantly "caught in the middle trying to take care of them and help them get along." She seems to be in constant conflict with herself regarding anything in life that could be considered as a source of nourishment. Her typical pattern is to deny herself whatever she craves until her emotional pain and internal conflict reach a breaking point. Then she overindulges in the object of her desires until she becomes repelled by it. She typically treads a thin line between food cravings and guilt about overindulgence. The logo on her business card included the phrase, "Health Through Integration."

Analysis: Paulette's eating disorders may be viewed as an embodiment of the conflict in her family situation growing up. Just as the stomach resides in the center of the body and integrates all that we ingest, Paulette was always at the center of her family, mediating between her parents. She absorbed her parents' anger and resentment toward each other as she attempted to help them get along. This may be considered an example of ingratiating behavior harming one's earth element.

Paulette's functional dynamic is one of wood invading earth in a way that leads to feelings of constraint when engaged in any process in life. I have described here a typical etiology of this dynamic that involves being stuck at a young age between warring parents. The virtues of wood are clarity and decisiveness in implementing one's inner evolutionary plan. Hence the power of wood is to be able to hold the vision of a goal during the entire journey. This is in distinction to the nature of earth, which is to empower the process that takes place between the conception of a project and its completion. These two elements, both necessary for healthy growth, often become unbalanced with each other.

Patients may feel constrained by the process they are engaged in, often feeling impatient about reaching their goal. Thus a tension may be created as the earth element is put under the burden of having to process at increasing rates so that wood may attain its goal more quickly. The process of nourishing self may become a burden, which may be evidenced as eating very quickly or irregularly. The earth element is not being nourished, because patients fail to appreciate the importance of adequately nourishing themselves during the journey. Or they may eat excessively in an unconscious attempt to provide "grounding" for their creative instincts, which are proceeding too quickly for their earth element to process and support.

In my experience, a function of the appendix is to absorb anger, resentment, and undigested pain. The fact that Paulette lost her appendix so early in life is a telling sign of the degree of stress she internalized. Generally, I find that once the appendix is removed, the gallbladder takes over its function of absorbing the resentment that comes from ingratiating behavior. Eventually, it too may become ill and need to be removed, as seen in this case. Once the gallbladder is removed, if there is no change in awareness and behavior, resentment moves deeper and serious illness is often the result.

Paulette's anorexia and bulimia may be viewed as her literally not being able to "stomach" anything else. Similarly, the tightness in her throat may be thought of as representing both her unexpressed anger at both her parents and her own inability to stand up for and communicate her own needs. The sour taste Paulette complains of may embody the bitterness and resentment she has had to swallow through her ingratiating behavior.

Paulette's pulses indicate both extreme *qi* deficiency, by virtue of their depth, and blood deficiency by virtue of their thinness. Her eating disorders likely contributed to the depletion of these vital reserves. Further, these disorders have probably undermined the long-term functioning of her digestive system as evidenced by her varied symptomatology.

Paulette's line of work may be considered to reflect her constitutional type and its expression of imbalance. The earth element is said to govern the muscles and flesh, and as a massage therapist, she endeavors to heal others at this level. Further, as a caregiver, she is at peril of absorbing her patients' pain in the same way she did with her parents. Paulette's business logo speaks directly to a central function and virtue of the stomach, which is integration.

Treatment: The initial stages of Paulette's treatment involved helping her become aware of her habitual tendency to take care of others to the point that she grew resentful. I also had her focus on the ways her neediness was transferred onto her eating habits as a tendency to deny herself and then binge. Early in treatment, I prescribed the Chinese herb formula "ginseng nutritive combination" (Renshen Yingyang Tang), which I have found to be one of the most deeply nourishing formulas for extreme depletion of blood and *qi*. An archetypal point combination for Paulette might include Stomach-36 ("leg three miles"), Stomach-9 ("people welcome"), Conception Vessel-12, and Liver-3 ("happy calm"). Stomach-36 as the earth point on an earth meridian is a transmitting point and especially strong in empowering all the virtues of the stomach official. Stomach-36 is paired with Liver-3, the earth point on the liver meridian, and therefore transmits the virtue of groundedness and stability to the liver official. The point "people welcome" is the window of heaven on the stomach meridian and especially strong in empowering the virtue of reciprocity with others as it is mediated by speech.[117] Conception Vessel-12 is a main point that harmonizes the middle burner and thus provides a central focus for the rest of the treatment.

In time, Paulette gained significant control over these patterns and they gradually abated. Concurrently, her digestion improved, as did the tightness and burning in her throat and esophagus. Paulette's relationships also improved as she now found herself better able to express her own needs and set boundaries regarding her expenditure of time and energy on others. Interestingly, after approximately a year of treatment, Paulette decided to leave her massage therapy practice and become a farmer. This allowed her to work directly with the earth in a way she saw was more in line with her intention of receiving and providing nourishment in a balanced way.

Example of the Spleen Constitutional Type

RONA: STUCK SPLEEN—THE ACCUMULATION OF BURDEN

Complaint: Fatigue, depression, chest pain.

Background: Rona, a women in her seventies, possessed intelligence, wealth, and creativity that manifested in her art, which she had exhibited at major galleries. Her painting studio always seemed to be disorganized, and she complained it was impossible to work in such a cluttered environment. After having miscarried during her early twenties, Rona had never had another long-term relationship, choosing instead to live alone in relative isolation.

Rona complained of her solitude, and it seemed as though her primary relationships were with therapists from whom she purchased emotional support. Without fail, she would abandon these therapeutic relationships as each practitioner, in turn, would inevitably challenge her self-destructive behaviors, which included alcoholism. Rona had a deep love for Venice, and although she possessed the means and freedom to travel there, she felt trapped by her responsibilities. She continually engaged in lawsuits and bickering with those she would hire to help free up her "obligations" in life, and she became increasingly mired in her current situation.

Although she lived locally, Rona would continually show up late or miss her appointments. Frequently, she would grow indignant if I could not accommodate her. I had the feeling that every time I went out of my way to take care of her, she would immediately up the ante by trying to prove I did not care for her in some other way.

Analysis: Although she had the means to enjoy life, all of Rona's pleasures were continually transformed into burdens, rather than nourishing her as they might have. Her barrenness, literally and figuratively, mirrored the accretions of clutter and burden that she carried along throughout life. This accumulation may be thought of as representing the manifestation of unprocessed pain from her own past, particularly regarding her miscarriage. Her feelings of being stuck and so unable to travel are another example of the spleen failing to aid in the "transportation and distribution" of acquired influences in life in a way that nourishes.

The pain in Rona's chest may be attributed to an entry/exit block between acupuncture points Spleen-21 and Heart-1.[118] Hence the function of her spleen is unable to nourish and support the heart.

Treatment: In the initial stages of treatment, I prescribed the formula "Prosperous Farmer."[119] The imagery in this formula's name suggests its usefulness for helping the earth element transform life into nourishment. Treatment on the meridians associated with her earth element helped empower Rona to feel more free in her movement through life. Her digestion improved and, after twenty years of thinking about it, she returned to Venice and eventually moved there. A point selection that may be considered to contain the essence of Rona's elemental dynamic is the exit/entry combination of Spleen-21 ("great enveloping") and Heart-1 ("utmost source"), combined with points Spleen-3 ("great white") and Heart-7 ("spirit gate"), both earth points on their respective meridians, to "ground" this powerful combination.

Questions

Each element is associated with certain virtues the expression of which represent the external manifestation of innate potential. When an element becomes unbalanced, excess and deficient behaviors supplant the expression of the associated virtue.

1. Can you think of any virtues I have not listed that you would associate with a given elemental type or official?

2. What are the excess and deficient behaviors that would result if the integrity of the virtue was compromised?

3. What are the likely ways that these behaviors might contribute to illness?

4. What is the nature of the beliefs that would likely motivate the expression of these behaviors?

NOTES

1. Not all the points referenced here are covered in this text. For the inner functions of many of these points, see Jarrett, 1994b, 1995b, and my Web page at http://www.spiritpathpress.com.
2. Mathews, 1931, p. 984.
3. Mathews, 1931, p. 284; Porkert, 1982, p. 110.
4. Chapter 8; my translation
5. Fung Yu-lan, 1983, vol. 2, p. 41.
6. Fung Yu-lan, 1983, vol. 2, p. 39; Dong Chongshu (179–104? B.C.E.).
7. Note that determination of constitution is ultimately verified through effective treatment.
8. My initial introduction to this topic in the context of the five-element system was a lecture given by practitioner Jonathon Klate at the third national conference sponsored by the Traditional Acupuncture Institute, Columbia, Maryland, 1985.
9. See Dumont (1972) for a wonderful book on the suggestive process in therapy.
10. Larre and Rochat, 1987, Chapter 8, p. 76.
11. I paraphrase this story from memory, hoping to convey its essence. I believe it is from a collection of ghost stories by Bu Songling (1640–1715), "Strange Stories from a Chinese Studio" *(Liaozhai Gushi).*
12. Larre and Rochat, 1987, Chapter 8, p. 84.
13. The *taiyang* (great *yang*) meridians (bladder and small intestine) are equated with the nervous system by Leon Hammer in his book *Dragon Rises, Red Bird Flies* (1990), p. xxiv.
14. Sold by Jade Pharmacy, Eugene, Oregon.
15. See the poem by Zhuangzi in reference to acupuncture point Kidney-23 in Chapter 13.
16. In my clinical practice, patients are often amazed that I am able to describe personal characteristics (after only a brief interview or taking their pulse) more accurately than more intimate people in their lives who have known them a long time. This emphasizes the point that all information is available in the moment to the skilled observer.
17. From Confucius's commentary to the *Yijing,* hexagram 30, which corresponds to fire, "the clinging," in Wilhelm, 1967, p. 538. Note that *li,* denoting the hexagram for fire, is a homophone of *li* (propriety), the virtue of the fire element.
18. Fung Yu-lan, 1983, vol. 2, p. 41.
19. Wieger, 1965, p. 239; Wilder and Ingram, 1974, pp. 41, 61.
20. Fingarette, 1972, p. 16.
21. Often, in medical literature, the character *xi* (喜) is used to denote pathological joy, whereas the character *le* denotes the healthy expression of joy.
22. Fung Yu-lan, 1983, vol. 2, p. 41.
23. Larre and Rochat, 1985, p. 23.
24. Cleary, 1986b, pp. 126–127.
25. Note that homophones for the character *xin* have meanings of sad and bitter as well as happy, all words associated with the fire element.
26. In a very real sense, we can only fantasize about past and future events because they do not exist. Reality exists only in the momentary present.

27. Chapter 39; translation mine.
28. Key acupuncture points that address the balance of the *ling* and *shen* are Kidney-23, Kidney-24, and Kidney-25, as discussed in Chapter 13.
29. Fingarette, 1972, p. 4.
30. Ibid.
31. Chapter 17; in Henricks, 1989, p. 220.
32. Watson, 1964a, p. 17.
33. So named because, reportedly, purple mortar was used in its construction. The color purple is associated with the emperor as well as with the heart's blood.
34. In my experience, the influence of the heart is rarely unavailable for healing on a spiritual level. Most often, in severe illness, the dysfunction of the other officials prevents the practitioner from accessing the heart. The only cases I have seen where the heart was absolutely unavailable were "clear" cases of "possession."
35. Larre and Rochat, 1985, p. 69.
36. Hence a main cause of sexual abuse is also a primary result of abuse. This may contribute to understanding why victims of incest show an increased incidence of perpetrating incest.
37. With this definition I avoid judging private practices of others that do no harm to anyone including themselves. We may also define as perversion all "unconscious" sexual activity. Here the term "unconscious" implies the participants are unaware of what motivates their behavior.
38. Wilhelm, 1962, pp. 41–42.
39. Chapter 8; in Larre and Rochat, 1985, p. 23.
40. Larre and Rochat, 1985, p. 82.
41. Another cause of inability to orgasm is dissociation. The term "frigid" is often used derogatorily in reference to women. In my usage a man could evidence the same qualities of frigidity.
42. I use the term "ministers" here to refer to the other eleven "officials" that constitute the organ systems and functions of Chinese medicine.
43. This condition is effectively treated by acupuncture point TW-1, named "rushing the frontier gate."
44. In this regard, I often treat Liver-1 ("great esteem") in combination with either Heart Protector-1 ("heavenly pond") or Heart-9 ("little rushing in").
45. "Flying tiger" is the name of acupuncture point Triple Heater-6, the fire point on the triple warmer meridian. It is useful in helping drain excess heat from the triple warmer, which presents either physically or psychospiritually as initiating excessive contact in life in a way that burns others.
46. I have found that Chinese medicine is unique in its ability to provide access to this "missing" information. It is relatively more difficult to reestablish a balance in the functioning of boundary when the "memory" of abuse is stored in this "primordial language," as opposed to memories stored in a more "concrete" [literal] form. See Jarrett, 1995a, 1995b, 1995c.
47. *Qi*-wild conditions imply a fundamental separation of *yin* and *yang* that creates a picture of chaos throughout one's being. See Hammer, 1990, pp. 336–338; 1993, parts I and II; and Jarrett, 1994a, pp. 29–45.
48. The herbs prescribed were Chinese formulas Yunan Pai Yao ("White Medicine from Yunan Province") and Sheng Mai San ("Generate Pulse Soup"). I have discussed the use of these formulas for this purpose in Jarrett, 1995b, p. 133.
49. I have covered the topic of treating sexual abuse with Chinese medicine at length elsewhere. See Jarrett, 1995a, 1995b, 1995c.
50. Herbs and acupuncture points that "open" the orifices generally have the effect of promoting conscious awareness. See my analysis of the herb formula Niu

Huang Qing Xin Wan at my Web site: http://www.spiritpathpress.com

51. The relationship between these points is discussed in Chapter 13.

52. Sold by Jade Pharmacy, Eugene, Oregon.

53. Interestingly, the term for "far away" is denoted by the character *yuan,* which is a homophone for the character *yuan,* meaning origin or source. Hence to be far away is to return.

54. Watson, 1964a, p. 65.

55. Chapter 52; in Chen, 1989, p. 178.

56. Watson, 1964a, p. 36.

57. Chapter 28; translation mine.

58. See Chen, 1989, pp. 64–67.

59. Watson, 1964a, p. 41.

60. Watson, 1968, p. 171.

61. Fung Yu-lan, 1983, vol. 2, p. 41. Note that I have changed Fung Yu-lan's translation of the character *ren* from love to benevolence.

62. Wieger, 1965, p. 28.

63. Watson, 1964a, p. 83.

64. Legge, 1971, p. 192.

65. Note that the capacity to let go in this way can be empowered by the balanced functioning of the metal element, which regulates the function of the wood element across the *ke* cycle.

66. Larre and Rochat, 1987, p. 34.

67. Chapter 4.2, verse 9.

68. Sunzi, Chapter 10.6, verse 26.

69. Chapter 8, verses 1–3.

70. Chapter 6.6, verse 28.

71. Chapter 4.3, verse 12.

72. Chapter 3, verse 2.

73. *Dao De Jing,* Chapter 22; in Lin, 1977, p. 40.

74. Note that the quality of flexibility is empowered by acupuncture points Liver-8 ("crooked spring") and Gallbladder-43 ("valiant stream"), which are the water points on the liver and gallbladder meridians, respectively.

75. Larre and Rochat, 1987, Chapter 8, p. 43.

76. Chapter 5.3, verses 11–13.

77. Watson, 1964, p. 39.

78. Chapter 2; in Chen, 1989, p. 55.

79. Watson, 1964, p. 34.

80. Resolution of human injustice is often empowered by the metal element, which controls wood across the *ke* cycle. Hence the virtue associated with metal, *yi* ("righteousness"), signifies the peace restored after a conflict (Wieger, 1965, p. 179). It is in letting go (metal) of one's resentment that the virtue of benevolence empowered by the wood element is able to be restored.

81. Chapter 63; in Chen, 1989, p. 200.

82. Watson, 1964, p. 49.

83. An elegant formulation by practitioner Thea Elijah.

84. According to Daoist enumeration, the three *hun* correspond to the unity of heaven, human, and earth and therefore the human spiritual ascent toward heaven. The seven *po* correspond to the return of mundanity back to the earth.

85. Figure 10.4 originally appeared in M. Ridley (1977), *Style, Motif, and Design in Chinese Art* (Poole, U.K.: Blandford Press). My thanks to Blandford Press for their permission to reproduce this figure.

86. Fung Yu-lan, 1983, vol. 2, p. 41.

87. Chen, 1989, p. 147.

88. Ibid, p. 38. Note that fanaticism often denotes an imbalanced metal element.

89. Interestingly, this dynamic is visible today in some Islamic sects, which have developed in desert nations characterized by dryness. The pathology of this zealotry may be characterized as lung heat in the terminology of Chinese medicine.

90. The Chinese character for the number four, si (四), is a homophone with the character si (死) meaning death. Hence the fourth stage of dao may correspond to the death of primordial dao and the fall to the ten thousand things. Or it may correspond to the death of the body and the end of life or of ego, signifying the rebirth of the true self.

91. Chapter 4; in Chen, 1989, p. 61.

92. Chen, 1989, p. 62.

93. The character zong refers to the building from which emanates the influence of the deceased ancestors over their posterity. Wieger, 1965, p. 101.

94. Chen, 1989, p. 64. Metallurgy was a highly developed art in ancient China. The use of the bellows as an image for the "whirling vortex" of chongqi between heaven and earth provides a tie between the lungs as the earthly manifestation of the breath of dao, the zongqi, and the metal element.

95. Wilhelm, 1968, p. 225.

96. Fung Yu-Lan, 1983, vol. 2, p. 28.

97. It is interesting to note that the function of the lungs in receiving the external world as governed by the sensory orifice of the nose is mediated by acupuncture point Large Intestine-20 named "welcome fragrance."

98. Larre and Rochat, 1987, Chapter 8, p. 30.

99. Larre and Rochat, 1989, pp. 12–13.

100. Larre and Rochat, 1989, Chapter 8, p. 67.

101. Chen, 1989, p. 7.

102. Dao De Jing, Chapter 20; in Chen, 1989, p. 102.

103. Wieger, 1965, p. 107. Note that the right section of the character denoting the four directions and center is bent down to avoid confusion with the character wang (王).

104. On the yin meridians, the earth and source points are all the third point, counting proximally. Three is the number of the primordial dao and emphasizes the role of the source points in helping to "feed off the mother."

105. Wilhelm, 1968, p. 652. Acupuncture point Stomach-44 is named "inner courtyard." As the water point on the stomach meridian, it represents the depth of water within earth. The name of this point evokes the image of meditation.

106. Wieger, 1965, p. 187.

107. Fung Yu-Lan, 1983, vol. 2, pp. 41–42.

108. Wieger, 1965, p. 186.

109. Ibid.

110. Legge, 1971, p. 273.

111. Ibid., p. 182.

112. Larre and Rochat, 1995, p. 189.

113. Chen, 1989, pp. 106–107.

114. Chapter 4; in Chen, 1989, p. 60.

115. Chapter 8; in Larre and Rochat, 1985, p. 64.

116. For this reason I have not provided a separate discussion or image for each of the earth officials as I have done with the others.

117. For more on acupuncture point Stomach-9, see Chapter 15.

118. See Jarrett (1994b) for a presentation of the nature of exit and entry blocks.

119. "Prosperous Farmer" is a modified version of "Six Gentlemen Soup" (Liu Jun Zi Tang) written by Ted Kaptchuk and marketed by Jade Pharmacy, Eugene, Oregon.

II

THE
PHYSIOLOGY
OF *QI* AND BLOOD

O UR ENDOWMENT OF *YIN* AND *YANG* REPRESENTS THE
dual poles of heaven and earth as they occur within the individual. *Qi* and blood exist between these two poles as the human being
stands between heaven and earth channeling each to the other. *Yin* and
yang as the poles that define the two cosmic centers are beyond the
level of human conscious awareness. In a sense, they are impersonal
forces that create the basis of movement and structure for all of existence. An individual's blood and *qi*, however, are personal attributes
intimately tied to awareness. Here we examine the physiology of *qi*
and blood as it pertains to the manifestation of virtue and the fulfillment of destiny.

The Nature of Physiology

The Western concept of physiology pertains to the purely physical
workings of the human body. The Chinese concept of physiology is not

a purely physical but rather a functional concept. When I use the word "physiology" pertaining to the practice of Chinese medicine, I refer to the dynamic functioning of every aspect of a human being, both physical (e.g., digestion) and nonphysical (e.g., thought) as they are inherently integrated with each other.

Qi, *Blood, and Virtue*

Although distinctions may be made between *qi* and blood, the functions of each are intimately tied together. Blood is derived from and held in place by *qi*. In turn, the officials that produce and regulate the *qi* are nourished by blood.

One whose virtuous actions arise spontaneously from his or her own embodiment and experience of virtue may be said to exemplify the balanced relationship of blood and *qi*. The differences between *qi* and blood may be summed up in the difference that lies between "being" (blood) and "doing" *(qi)*. Blood as a composite of inherited and acquired influences may be viewed as the present embodying the past. *Qi,* in contrast, may be considered the present creating the future.[1]

Heaven may be thought of as the source of virtue ultimately embodied on earth. The ability to act in a virtuous way and embody the experience of a specific virtue spring from *qi* and blood, respectively. *Qi* enables us to move our body and act in a way that is virtuous; however, this is quite different from embodying and consciously being aware of the virtue inherent in the act. For example, our liver *qi* may empower us to "act" benevolently toward one another, thus exemplifying the external virtue of "just" behavior. It is the blood of the liver that empowers us to "feel" benevolence toward ourselves, thus exemplifying the internal virtue of self-esteem (see Figure 11.1 for a summary of these relationships by organ system. It is blood which houses the *shen* that empowers us to "be" virtuous.

Qi

The concept of *qi* is pervasive in Chinese medical and philosophical thought. Porkert suggests that the term *qi* is nearly equivalent to the English word "energy." He identifies thirty-two distinct types of *qi* that have appeared in Chinese medical literature over the last 2,500 years.[2] These diverse types of *qi* all refer to some unique aspect of the *dao* as it manifests in physiological function.

Qi and Blood: Physiology of Virtue			
Official	**Contribution to Blood**	**Inner Virtue**	**Outer Virtue**
Kidney	Essence/template	Self-assurance	Bravery
Liver	Stores/mobilizes	Self-esteem	Justness
Heart	*Shen*	Self-possession	Compassion
Heart protector	Circulation	Intimacy	Partnership
Spleen	Essence acquired from food	Fulfillment	Altruism
Lung	Essence acquired from air	Self-worth	Acknowledgment

Figure 11.1

QI AND BLOOD: PHYSIOLOGY OF VIRTUE

As with any Chinese character, no single English word serves as a direct translation of *qi*. Kaptchuk has described *qi* as "matter on the verge of becoming energy, or energy at the point of materializing."[3] I like this definition because it posits a functional relationship between energy and matter. However, *qi* is neither energy nor matter on the verge of transitioning one into the other. *Qi* is a larger concept still, for *qi* supports the manifestation of both energy and matter. I understand *qi* as the quality of the *dao* that supports the emergence of any functional relationship at a specific moment in time. Because a relationship is not a thing, the precise nature of *qi* can never be named with a word that denotes a measurable thing. I believe *qi* has no material substance, and that we are at peril when we assert that any thing measurable "is" *qi*. Rather, all "things" that exist materially depend on *qi* for their existence and function and may not be said to be *qi*.

Qi, then, is that aspect of the *dao* which supports the existence of the material plane, yet it will ever elude our attempts to measure or precisely define it. Modern views of *qi* as energy are, I believe, motivated in part by a culturally founded desire to understand a nonmaterial, functional concept as a thing rather than as a relationship. Further, it is my assessment that the habit of translating *qi* as "energy" is the foundation of much imprecise thinking relative to both the teaching and study of modern Chinese medicine. It is not unusual to hear individuals justify their point selections, herbal prescriptions, and other therapeutic suggestions by claiming that their approach captures the "energetics" of the patient. Chinese medicine offers a very highly developed language for describing the functional dynamics which govern the flow of *qi*. A point combination chosen to empower self-esteem and tonify liver *yang* based on the finding of an empty liver pulse and the observation that the patient yields excessively when confronted is trivialized when merely ascribed to the patient's "energetic." Lastly, thinking of *qi* as "energy" is frequently used to validate an array of dubious electronic diagnostic and treatment devices. These range from acupuncture point locators and stimulators to computers that prescribe herbs based on reading a patient's "energy."

The physiological state of *qi* in any part of any being can only be discerned in the quality of the functional relationship between two things or two processes within the being. A diagnosis of deficient spleen *qi,* for example, may be predicated on the observation that a patient's belly is sagging relative to his or her center. The diagnosis is made by noting the relationship of belly to center. The practitioner may corroborate this assessment by also observing the relationship of the belly to the tongue, to the pulse, and to a multitude of emotional and personal expressions as well. The diagnosis of deficient spleen *qi* emerges from these relationships and may be described as a specific functional dynamic emerging from that individual patient at that particular moment.

In sum, everything is *qi* and yet its essential quality is unknowable by the mind. All manifestations of *dao* are based on *qi* and therefore, like the eternal *dao,* the essential nature of *qi* cannot be known.

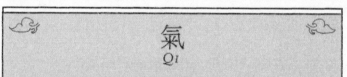

氣

Qi

The top element of the character *qi* is radical 84, denoting "breath."[4] The lower aspect is the character *mi*(米), denoting "rice," the most essential form of sustenance for the Chinese people throughout history. Together, they depict vapor rising from boiling rice.[5] This image evokes the sense of a fine essence emerging from and inherent to each thing that nourishes and sustains life.

Types of Qi

There are two broad categories of *qi*: *qi* granted by heaven at the moment of conception and prior to birth (the *qi* of early heaven, known as *yuanqi,* or *xiantianqi*) and *qi* acquired after birth, beginning with the infant's first breath (the *qi* of later heaven, or *houtianqi*). Two types of acquired *qi* are traditionally recognized: *guqi* (穀氣), derived from food, and *kongqi* (空氣), derived from air. A third source of post-natal, acquired *qi* is also available: the *qi* derived from one's interpretation of experience in life. Positive interpretations of experience enhance our resources, and negative interpretations of experience obscure and dilute the quality of our constitutional resources.

Physiologically, the lungs and stomach receive, via the nose and mouth, the physical aspects of later heaven's *qi* (food and air), but the other sensory orifices too must be considered to receive input that is a potential source of nourishment in later heaven.

Functions of Qi

The quality of a given type of *qi* may be discerned by the quality and directionality of any functional process observable in life. In the body, *qi* has five major functions: (1) movement, (2) protection, (3) transformation, (4) retention, and (5) warming. These functions exist even at primordial cosmological levels. *Chongqi* —that *qi* at the center of all things, harmonizing all dualities and extremes back to unity—fulfills these functions by preserving the integrity of heaven, earth, and *qi*.

Movement

Chongqi is the cosmological generator of all movement. Physiological movement may be differentiated into willed movement (walking) and involuntary movements such as breathing, growth, and the evolutionary thrust of the human spirit.

Protection

The universe during the time of "cosmic incubation"—heaven, earth, and *qi* existing as unity—has been compared to a chicken egg. Just as the eggshell protects the yolk from pernicious outside influences, so too *qi* supports, surrounds, and protects the healthy individual. The protective function of *qi* emanates from *zhenqi*, or "upright *qi*," which emerges when a person stands between heaven and earth and allows these opposing poles to fuse in him or her, unimpeded by the activity of the mind. *Zhenqi* is present when an individual fulfills personal destiny and becomes the source of his or her own inner strength and immunity. Physiologically, when a person fulfills destiny, then his or her reserve of *qi* becomes strong enough to deter any invasive pathogenic factor in life, whether a virus, a traumatic injury, or a painful emotional event. No external impact will be strong enough to knock the person off center in a way that causes ongoing separation from true self.

Another kind of protective *qi* is *weiqi,* which surrounds the body like a shield. The lungs and triple heater preside over its function. Like the triple heater, *weiqi* may be compared to the Great Wall of China: It must deter any harmful influence from penetrating deeply into the patient's being.

Transformation

The character *chong* in *chongqi* denotes in part a soaring movement toward heaven, suggesting a geyser shooting from earth toward the sky. This represents the evolutionary thrust of the *dao* as it manifests in life. The basis of that movement is transformation that occurs in the process of evolution. A visual analogue of this is the helical structure of DNA: The *chongqi* is like a spiral staircase carrying us ever upward along our respective paths. *Qi* is the basis of all transformation in life, as it occurs simultaneously in corresponding aspects of spiritual and material physiology. Making blood from nutrition or turning a disordered emotion like habitual fear into a virtue like wisdom are examples of processes dependent on the strength and integrity of one's *qi.*

Retention

A primary function of *chongqi* is to blend perfectly the poles of heaven and earth, while maintaining a firm center between them. While blending the two primordial poles, *chongqi* also holds them apart to prevent them from collapsing into each other. It is the center created by *chongqi* that allows heaven and earth to simultaneously penetrate each other while maintaining two functionally distinct entities. Physiologically, *qi* may be said to hold organs in place, keep the blood in the vessels, and help people maintain a strong emotional center in the face of life's challenges.

Warming

The cosmological stage where heaven, earth, and *qi* are united into one may be thought of as a time of "cosmic incubation." *Qi* provides the warmth needed for the *dao* as fetus to develop from one cell into life as the ten thousand things. All physiological processes depend on warmth to progress, and *qi* presides over these functional processes.

Imbalances of Qi

Qi is in evidence in the vigorous and balanced functioning of each organ system, official, and associated physiological process in the body. To the degree that a functional relationship is compromised, a functional disorder of *qi* can be found associated with it. *Qi*, when unbalanced, may be described as being deficient, collapsed, rebellious, or stagnant.

- Deficient *qi* is in evidence when any physiological process is proceeding with less than optimal force. Slow digestion, for example, may be a sign of deficient stomach *qi*.

- Collapsed *qi* is a subset of deficient *qi*. It is in evidence when *qi* is so deficient that it cannot hold things in place. For example, a weak center, denoted by the presence of hemorrhoids, may be a sign of collapsed *qi*. The type of exhaustion where a person is unable to stand up for him or herself physically or emotionally, such as in chronic fatigue syndrome, may be another instance of collapsed *qi*.

- Rebellious *qi* moves in the wrong direction from normal physiological flow. For example, balanced lung *qi* must descend. Coughing is air moving forcefully up and out, counter to its normal flow of in and down, therefore indicating rebellious lung *qi*.

- Stagnant *qi* is a relative excess of *qi* that occurs in a specific aspect of functioning and in a specific location in the body. For example, if the liver does not fulfill its function of "spreading" the *qi*, then distension may be felt around the area of acupuncture point Liver-14. The psychospiritual correlate of stagnant *qi* is meeting a situation in life so challenging that the movement of one's *qi* cannot flow smoothly around it. Physically and psychically, the internal stress generated as the body tries to move the block is expressed as excess heat, pressure, distension, stuckness, and frustration.

Blood

Blood is the soft, receptive part of self that fills us "from the inside up to our skin" as contrasted with *qi*, which takes us past our borders out "into" the world.[6] Each of the *yin* officials both empowers, and is empowered by, the functioning of blood in a unique way. From the viewpoint of the inner tradition, blood may be defined as that aspect of self that allows us to experience the embodiment of virtue.

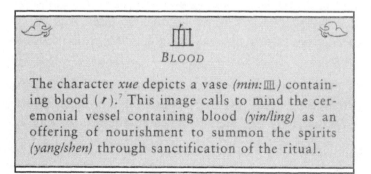

BLOOD

The character *xue* depicts a vase *(min: 血)* containing blood (ﾉ).[7] This image calls to mind the ceremonial vessel containing blood *(yin/ling)* as an offering of nourishment to summon the spirits *(yang/shen)* through sanctification of the ritual.

The Creation of Blood[8]

Blood is co-identified with the self, which, in health, emerges from the integration of the highest aspects of inherited and acquired resources. The kidney essence is said to produce "marrow," which includes the spinal cord, brain, and bone marrow. In modern texts, the bone marrow is said to manufacture blood.[9] Functionally the kidney's contribution to the production of blood consists of the essential aspect of self imparted by heaven at conception in the form of *yuanqi* and *jing*. The kidney also contributes *yin* in the form of fluids. The essence imparted by the kidney serves as an internal template which ensures that only those aspects of acquired *qi* congruent with true self become embodied as blood. The kidney essence rises to the middle burner to combine with *qi* acquired from alimentation and forms the *guqi*, which is the purest *qi* acquired from food that corresponds to true self. Kidney essence also rises to the upper burner to combine with the "clear" *qi* acquired from respiration.

The *qi* of the spleen then serves to transport the refined essence that is *guqi* up to the lungs, where it meets and combines with the *qi* acquired from respiration. Together these three, the *jing, guqi,* and heavenly *qi* acquired from the breath, combine to form *yingqi*, or nutritive *qi*. The nutritive *qi* then passes through the heart, which imbues it with heart *shen,* thus turning it into blood. The heart invests blood with *shen* in the same way that the emperor invests a decree with his authority by affixing his red seal upon it. The presence of *shen* empowers the blood to be a vehicle for one's awareness to penetrate to every aspect of one's self.

Disharmonies of Blood

There are three major disharmonies involving the blood: blood deficiency, blood heat, and blood stasis. The ways in which they manifest are qualitatively different, depending on the organs that are either causing the disharmony or affected by it.

Blood Deficiency

Blood is a fluid and is therefore considered a *yin* substance. If there is significant *yin* deficiency, there may be blood deficiency as well. The Western concept of blood deficiency (i.e., anemia) has more to do with the hemoglobin content of the blood, whereas the Chinese concept has more to do with the serum content of the blood. It is quite possible that an individual could be considered by a practitioner of Chinese medicine to have blood deficiency although a Western medical assay might not evidence anemia. Ultimately, Chinese medicine is concerned with the quality and function of blood, and a patient's blood may be considered to be deficient if one or more of the functions of blood are not being fulfilled adequately. The physical symptoms and signs associated with blood deficiency are a pale tongue, scanty menses, dry skin, and a pulse somewhat yielding and thinner than normal. If the blood fails to nourish any official, then the *shen* of that official will not be nourished and the person may appear ill at ease and thus not comfortable "inside."

Blood Heat

The concept of blood heat is associated with the presence of either excess or deficient heat in the blood. The symptoms and signs associated with blood heat may include headaches, tinnitus, visual disturbances, skin conditions, readiness to anger, increased blood pressure, elevated cholesterol, and hardening of the arteries. The presence of heat in the blood is suggested by the finding that the pulse expands as one's finger pressure diminishes from the organ to blood depth of the pulse. Various causes of heat in the blood include exposure to toxic chemicals, poor digestion, too rich diet, and overactivity of the *shen* associated with *yin* deficiency.

Blood Stasis

The natural flow of blood may become impeded for several reasons, including either physical or emotional trauma, or because the quantity or quality of blood has become compromised due to impairment of the function of one or more organs associated with the blood. The physical symptoms and signs associated with blood stasis are sharp stabbing pain that is fixed in location, purple lips, a tongue that is generally purple or has a purple spot on it, purple engorged veins under the tongue, and a choppy pulse.[9] Emotionally, blood stasis may present as lost memory of painful events, difficulty with intimacy, and feelings of having been betrayed, which may manifest as a fixed stabbing pain in any aspect of a patient's being, reflecting the compromised function of the heart protector official.[10]

Congealed blood refers to a condition of blood stasis where the blood has actually hardened to form a mass. Such a condition is evident in symptoms ranging from blood clots to certain kinds of tumors. The presence of congealed blood generally indicates that some trauma has occurred which is too painful to assimilate.

Functions of Qi *and Blood by Organ System*

Kidney

Kidney *qi* empowers the use of will in the world in a way that may be described as brave. Here bravery may be defined as the outer manifestation of the wisdom that allows us to take proper action in the face of our own fear. Kidney blood enables us to embody the virtue of self-assurance, which may be thought of as our wisdom embodied as faith in the presence of the unknown. Since blood is a fluid, it depends ultimately on the integrity of our endowment of kidney *yin* for its vitality and presence. The kidney is said to rule the bones and the marrow stored in the bones, which emanate from the vitality of one's *jing* and is thought to help create the blood. Hence any deficiency of kidney *jing* is likely to be reflected in the quality or quantity of the blood.

Liver

The liver is said to regulate the smooth flow of *qi*. Because *qi* moves the blood, any failure of the liver *qi* to move the blood may result in blood stasis. The *qi* of the liver may empower someone to act in a way that is benevolent toward others, thus bringing one's embodiment of the virtue into the world in a way that may be described as being "just." In this sense, justness may be thought of as the outer manifestation of benevolence displayed as an equanimity toward all human beings. The liver is said to correspond to vision and to nourish the eyes.

Hence the blood of the liver may be said to nourish one's deep view of self that corresponds to self-esteem. The presence of self-esteem indicates that the virtue of benevolence is being manifested toward one's self.

Just as liver blood may nourish the tendons so that we are flexible, so too does it nourish our capacity for emotional flexibility. When blood becomes either excessive or deficient due to compromised liver function, then we may exhibit the tendency to be increasingly irritated by life's minor details as we become increasingly attached to our vision regarding how things "ought" to be.

Heart

Heart *qi* empowers us to act with propriety toward others. Think of propriety as the effortless display of compassion that an enlightened monarch feels toward his or her subjects. For it is the heart's compassion that empowers the sovereign to fulfill the role of both knowing and utilizing each official's special attributes. Heart blood empowers us to embody the virtue of propriety toward our self. Those who embody this virtue may be said to be "self-possessed" in that they have insight into and truly govern themselves.

The heart rules the blood; the constancy of its beat reflects its commitment to fulfilling its role as sovereign ruler. The virtue of commitment emanates from a heart in which the heart's *qi* and blood are maintained in a healthy, balanced relationship. Any irregularity in the pulse may reflect a weakening of the heart's *qi* and/or blood and its ensuing struggle to maintain control. Signs of deficient heart blood may include instability of the pulse with movement, lack of joy, and a general failing of the heart to be nourished. All these signs may correspond to the heart failing to imbue the blood with *shen* that is synonymous with insight and awareness.

Heart Protector

The heart may be thought of as a pump that circulates the blood throughout one's being. Think of the heart protector as comprising the actual vessels and veins through which the blood flows, as well as its quality of movement in flowing. Hence, in part, the heart protector may be conceived as the vasculature that in essence "protects" the blood as it circulates.

The *qi* of the heart protector may empower us to act in a way that reflects connection in relationship. The blood of the heart protector is that part of self which empowers us to experience intimacy and embody it as warmth and openness. The highest will of the heart protector is to empower intimacy from a position of strength.

Both physical and emotional trauma may result in a "shock" to the circulatory system, which is governed by the heart protector. For example, consider physical injury in which overstepping a physical boundary results in a direct assault to the body. The body's response to this impact includes *qi* stagnation and blood stasis with a corresponding hardening of the area of impact and associated black and blue bruising. The hardening that occurs when clots (congealed blood) form may be viewed as a protective mechanism which results in a physical "separation from self" in response to injury. Similarly, congealed blood patterns may be generated due to psychic assaults such as sexual and emotional abuse that impact on the heart protector.

The heart protector's ability to heal after the trauma of abuse may manifest as the virtue of courage. One of the greatest gifts a healthy adult possesses is the capacity, from a position of strength, to make a conscious choice to be intimate with another.

Spleen

The spleen rules that aspect of blood known as *ying,* which provides nourishment to every aspect of the patient's being. The character *ying* (營) is composed of the character for fire (火火) doubled over the character *gong* (宮), meaning "palace." The character *ying* denotes an encampment of soldiers around a fire over which they cook their food. A homophone of this character is *ying* (盈), which signifies "the abundance that comes to one when, by one's efforts, one arrived to fill with provisions one's vessels."[11] A function of the spleen is to abstract nourishment from food and distribute it throughout our being. This is accomplished by contributing to the production of the functionally nutritive aspect of blood known as the *ying.* If the spleen does not make its contribution to blood of nourishing essence, then an individual may appear needy. If one's earth element (stomach and spleen) is weak, then digestion may be incomplete, leading to excess heat in the blood. Emotionally this excess heat may present as an insatiable appetite for all things.

The virtues associated with the spleen are reciprocity and integrity *(xin).* Our *qi* may empower us to manifest the virtues of the earth element toward others by acting in a way that may be described as altruistic. Altruism may be defined here as the act of selflessly and dependably giving to others so that they may be fulfilled. The blood of the spleen grants the capacity to embody the virtue of integrity within one's self. The formation of blood is the very basis of integrity as the individual incorporates outside sources of nourishment into self. One who is in touch with his or her deepest source of nourishment may be described as being fulfilled in the sense of the character *ying* (盈) just described.

Lungs

The *qi* of the lungs may empower an individual to acknowledge the essential quality in self or others. This type of appreciation is evident in the valuation of another's essential worth, as might be evidenced in a gracious bow denoting respect. The healthy function of blood as it nourishes the lungs may empower one to embody the virtue of self-worth. Here self-worth may be thought of as constituting the appreciation of one's own essence.

If the lungs fail to imbue the blood with the essence gleaned from respiration, then the quality of the blood will suffer. The category of lung-blood deficiency is not typically found in Chinese medicine. Nevertheless, the findings discussed here play a role in my own clinical practice.[12] Diagnostic signs suggesting lung blood deficiency may include a thin right distal pulse or special lung pulse, and feelings of worthlessness.

Summary

No concept in Chinese medicine is purely physical in nature. Modern texts often focus on the physical symptoms predicated on imbalances of *qi* and blood. The language of Chinese medicine is deeply rooted in concepts that pertain to the nature of human awareness and spirit. The physiology of *qi* and blood as it empowers virtue informs both the selection of acupuncture points and prescription of herbs for their ability to promote the healthy presence and balanced functioning of these resources. My interpretations of *qi* and blood in terms of their roles in promoting the manifestation of virtue represent only an initial inquiry into the language of Chinese physiology as it reflects its deepest spirit.

Questions

No concept in the inner tradition of Chinese medicine is purely physical in nature.

　　1. What words in your tradition of practice refer to purely physical aspects of a human being?

2. Can you think of a way to expand your understanding of such terms to include nonphysical aspects of such structures?

3. Are there any aspects of being that are purely physical?

NOTES

1. Note from lecture by Ted Kaptchuk.
2. Porkert, 1982, pp. 168–173.
3. Kaptchuk, 1983, p. 35.
4. Wieger, 1965, p. 241.
5. Ibid.
6. From lecture by Ted Kaptchuk, 1989.
7. Wieger, 1965, p. 322.
8. The generation of blood described here represents my own thinking on the matter, having assimilated many authors' writings on the subject, and my own reflection and clinical experience. It is important to remember that terms such as blood, *jing, yuanqi, guqi, shen,* lungs, and spleen are primarily functional concepts in Chinese medicine. It may be true in a functional sense that the acquired essence from digestion rises to the chest to combine with that essence gleaned from respiration to form *ying.* However, this process is not a localized phenomena in the way that Western physiological processes are thought to be.
9. *Essentials of Chinese Acupuncture,* 1980, p. 26.
10. See Jarrett, 1995a, 1995b, and 1995c.
11. Weiger, 1965, p. 62. I consider this definition to capture the essence of the highest function of the nutritive aspect of blood, also pronounced *"ying."*
12. Note that the herb E Jiao both nourishes blood and enters the lung meridian. This herb is highly effective for dealing with issues of loss and self-worth.

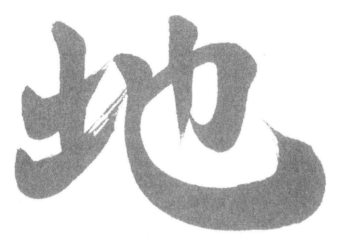

12

HEALTH, ILLNESS, AND HEALING IN THE INNER TRADITION

W E HAVE THE OPPORTUNITY TO ACKNOWLEDGE THE essential nature of life based on our connection to the *dao* or to create meanings that distort events and conform instead to our own belief process. Health is embodied to the degree that we accurately perceive life, and illness is embodied to the degree that our interpretations deviate from reality. If we accept the premise that attitudes, thoughts, and interpretations play a significant role in influencing health, then it becomes of primary importance to intervene therapeutically at the level of the patient's belief system. The habituated mind speaks to patients in their native language and it is with words that patients create their reality. The practitioner must choose words that directly support the therapeutic intention of all other actions taken during treatment. This chapter examines the nature of health and illness in the inner tradition and the role of the practitioner as both sage and healer in the restoration of original nature.

Spontaneity and Habit; Health and Illness

To act without understanding and to do so habitually with-
out examination, pursuing the proper path all the life with-
out knowing its nature—this is the way of the multitudes.
            – MENCIUS [1]

Laozi characterized the movement of *dao* as an eternal "self-becoming" *(ziran:*自然*)*.[2] The expression *ziran* indicates that, at every
moment, the *dao* spontaneously becomes itself, forever cleaving from
and reverting to its original nature. The *dao's* virtue of *ziran,* or natural spontaneity, is the foundation of the Daoist ideal of health. I
interpret the concept of *ziran* to be the model of health espoused by the
Dao De Jing. Spontaneity is the ability to respond to life based on our
commitments, rather than habitually reacting to circumstances and
avoiding our responsibility to fulfill destiny. The virtue of *ziran*
empowers us to respond to each new situation encountered based on
its unique merits in a way that is uncolored by past experience. The
heart is nourished by spontaneity and presence in the moment, whereas the mind always seeks to avoid momentary presence, thereby
thwarting spontaneous action. In contradistinction to the notion of
spontaneity, which is empowered by the primordial influence of early
heaven, is the notion of habitual unconscious functioning. This occurs
due to the conditioning influences acquired during later heaven.

Liu Yiming tells us that at the moment of the first breath, the "generations of history" enter the newborn through its sensory orifices. The
characters that Cleary has translated as "generations of history" are
lunhui. The character *lun* (輪) indicates the revolutions of a wheel as it
spins. Similarly, the character *hui* (迴) means "to revolve." Taken
together, the couplet signifies the transmigration of the soul as it
revolves from lifetime to lifetime.

When Liu tells us that the sage endeavors to "avoid compulsive routine," the characters translated as compulsive routine are again *lunhui.*
Hence compulsive habituated behavior is depicted with characters that
indicate a wheel spinning in circles. The price we pay for such unconscious behavior is being forced to partake in an endless cycle of birth,
death, and rebirth. Liu suggests that obsession is the seed of repeated
birth and death.[3] Ignorant people (*ren bu zhi,* literally, "those who do
not know") are swept along in the whirlpool of fate, always victims of
forces they do not comprehend.[4] They just "go along," following the
endless process of birth and death. A character illustrating this idea is

shun (順), meaning "going along," "docile," "compliant," or "to be in accordance with." *Shun* depicts a person with his head aligned with the direction that water is flowing in a stream, representing, in this case, a person being swept through life by the whirlpool of fate.[5] Liu used the character *ni* (逆) to indicate the action of the sage, who "reverses" the habituating process of later heaven by returning to original nature.[6] Referring to ignorant people Liu states, "What such people do not realize is that reversal means going back to the origin of life. It is like someone who has left home and gone far away returning home."[7]

Liu also uses the term *xiqi* (習氣) to refer to the conditioned *qi* on which habits are predicated. The first character in this couplet refers to "the rapid, frequent motion of the wings in flying." This motion is symbolic of habitual thought and the repetitive action to which it leads. In Buddhism, the term refers to the tendency of an habitual thought or delusion to continually resurface even after one has largely overcome the habit.[8] These characters are also used to refer to the Buddhist concept of *vasana*, which means to "becloud" in the sense that ignorance may obscure the mind.[9] Humphreys tells us that the ignorance of *vasana* is caused by habitual *qi* conditioned by our past actions.[10] The phrase *vasana* literally means the fragrance of a plant which expels noxious influences, thus obscuring our senses in the same way that ignorance may cloud our mind.[11] Interestingly, in Chinese herbal medicine, the aromatic properties of fragrant herbs are believed to cut through accumulations of phlegm and dampness that obscure the sensory orifices and thus perpetuate ignorance and delusion.

Another term for habit is *gu* (痼), meaning "chronic," or "a deeply rooted illness or habit."[12] Thus we may understand that the spontaneity which emerges when we are in touch with *dao* as the motivating force in our life is synonymous with health. Illness is a state of unconscious habitual reaction to life based on our past actions and interpretations of experience.

Engaging the Mind

You have heard of the knowledge that knows, but you have never heard of the knowledge that does not know. Look into that closed room, the empty chamber where brightness is born!
— ZHUANGZI[13]

The Daoist texts assert the role of human thought in initiating and perpetuating separation from true self. This separation is conceived of as constituting the functional basis of illness. The practitioner of the inner tradition endeavors to use language to engage the patient's mind in a way that contributes to healing by helping to break habituated thought patterns. The precedent for this approach in Daoist healing was set by Zhuangzi, who repeatedly used language as a device for shocking the mind of the reader into awareness of original nature. The practitioner's intention in engaging the mind of the patient must cohere with the intention of the acupuncture and herbal prescriptions administered to engage the patient's *qi*.

In Zen Buddhism the concept of *ziran* refers to the spontaneous emergence of enlightenment that occurs when one perceives the true nature of original mind.[14] Emphasis is placed on gaining a perspective on how one's mind operates to obscure one's innate capacity for clarity. The mind of the Zen practitioner is compared to a mirror that must be free of dust (mundane influences) in order to perfectly reflect the true nature of self and life. Zen teachings emphasize that the ignorant must attempt to meet a "good and learned friend" who may scatter delusions and falsehoods and illuminate the free and easy character of original nature.[15] The practitioner of the inner tradition must aspire to be such a friend in guiding each patient's path of healing. Hence Zen master Yixuan tells us that he possesses no tricks to help people reach clarity but merely cures disease and sets people free.[16] Here Yixuan is equating the shackles of separative thought with illness.

The precise use of speech affords the practitioner several advantages in treatment. The first is to be able to use language in a way that reinforces all other therapeutic messages administered. Second, suggestions may be offered in a subtle way that naturally speaks to the patient in the "language" of their constitutional type. Third, language itself may be used as a method to accelerate the dawning of open awareness as in the example of the Zen koan described later. Fourth, the patient's degree of habituation and progress in treatment may be continually assessed through the process of testing emotions. Lastly, language may be used to establish the context for an acupuncture treatment prior to needling and initiate movement of the *qi,* which may enhance the efficacy of the entire session.

I consider the use of language to mobilize the patient's *qi* and promote healing to be perhaps the most highly refined skill that a practitioner may possess. Language is an interface where one engages the patient's mind, yet the primary force initiating healing resides in the place such language arises, the internal alignment of the practitioner's own *shen* and *jing*. The power *(ling)* of transformation that emanates from this alignment may reinforce the alignment of the patient's own heart and kidney axis and thus initiate the return to true self.

Here I present several techniques I have found complementary to my use of acupuncture and herbs in helping guide people to the restoration of original nature. It is imperative to be aware that with these, as with every therapeutic technique, timing is everything. I might engage the patient in these types of conversations during the first session or after several years of continual work. The patient's readiness to receive any given therapeutic suggestion is always of primary importance.

Habits and Perspective

When coaching patients on how to gain awareness of their habits, I often liken the dilemma of unconscious behavior to that of drowning in a river. Imagine a man who continually finds himself the mediator between hostile parties. At home his children fight, at work he is stuck between his boss and the people he supervises, and his best friend is getting divorced and looks to him to mediate with his soon to be ex-wife. The patient complains of burning pains in the epigastric area and a sour taste in his mouth, both of which worsen with stress.[17]

Initially, the patient is engaged in habitual behavior in the same way that one who is drowning might thrash around uselessly in the water. He is just going along through life and then, all of a sudden, finds himself in another situation as mediator. His habit to engage in this dynamic is so unconsciously motivated that he does not realize such a situation is developing until it is too late. He only discovers that he is stuck once the burning in his stomach alerts him to the stress he is under.

Upon recognizing his situation, a better course of action would be to determine which way the river is flowing and to align himself with the flow of the water. Rather than being unconsciously engaged in the situation, he may learn to become aware of it in its initial stages and then respond appropriately to extricate himself before he becomes ill.

In time, he can imagine he is on the shore, watching himself align his head with the current while aware of the threat at hand. With further practice he may take another step back and see himself at the shore watching himself align his head with the current. Eventually, sufficient distance between true self and events may be created so he is able to disengage from habitual reaction to any given situation and instead take appropriate action based on his commitments. Rather than unconsciously jumping into the river of discord every time a conflict arises, he learns to recognize his impulse to do so and then step back from the shore and evaluate what action he is committed to. We must cultivate the ability, given any immediate stress, to find that place inside which is eternally unmoved and unaffected. For it is in this place that we are aligned with *dao* and empowered by original nature.

Feeding the Dog

Another useful image is to liken the habituated *qi* which drives the patient's behavior to a dog that keeps coming to the back porch begging for food. If the patient does not continually feed the dog, it will eventually stop coming to visit. Habits are fueled in large part by belief systems and are reinforced when we continually respond to the presence of a belief with a specific behavior. For example, a young woman who believes she is overweight and unattractive may engage in the habitual behavior of bulimia. Her behavior of purging is paired with her erroneous self-image. Every time she has the thought "I am unattractive," the impulse to engage in the behavior is stimulated. The therapeutic task at hand is to disengage the belief from the behavior by empowering the patient to understand that the belief does not reflect reality.

Every time the patient uses her will to avoid the behavior, the habitual *qi* loses its force of association with the belief. Like the dog that is not fed, eventually the belief itself will be less likely to appear. I would point out to the patient that if she had a friend who told her what she is telling herself, she would choose not to spend any time with that person. For example, if her friend continually told her, "You're unattractive, and purging is the only answer. You'll never be able to break this habit," she would end the friendship immediately. However, when her own mind tells her this very same thing, she empowers its presence by feeding it with her belief as if the thoughts reflected reality.

The belief itself is purely a mental construct created by the patient, and it is important that she comes to perceive it as such. I would inform her that in such situations she should simply "thank her mind for sharing" and pay no further attention to such negative thought patterns. By becoming aware of the thoughts, beliefs, and attitudes that drive her behavior, she is provided with a perspective which empowers the freedom to act spontaneously in a way that reflects virtue rather than merely unconscious habituated responses.

My comment to "thank her mind for sharing" is a lighthearted way of pointing out that she has a source of knowing and acting that is different from that aspect of her mind which continually gives her disempowering messages. Often it is appropriate to be lighthearted in treatment and there are times when a different approach is called for. It is imperative that with every communication the practitioner reinforces the patient to create meaning in life in a way that adds to, rather than detracts from, vitality.

The Koan

One of the primary tools of Zen utilized to awaken accurate perception of reality is the koan (*gongan* in Chinese). Literally the term "koan" signifies an official document yielding the sense of an important decision and the final discernment of truth and falsehood.[18] To this end Zen masters made use of language to defeat the habituated mind of the disciple and help return spontaneous mental functioning. This technique may trace its origin to similar linguistic devices used by Zhuangzi. An example of a Zen koan is the statement, "If you meet the Buddha on the road, kill him!"

An example of the therapeutic use of this type of technique was provided in the case study in Chapter 9. The patient in this example had been unconsciously motivated since his childhood by the pain felt when his father had left home. His entire life thesis and ego identification was built on his evidence that nothing of value could be retained in life. Sensing that the patient had reached the turning point in his path of healing I informed him that his father had not left him and that, in fact, he had left his father. The patient was not able to interpret what I had said in terms of any previous life experience. He was, in essence, brought fully present into the moment. The silence that emerged in this instant signaled the collapse of the habituated mind and the reassertion of the primordial *qi* as a guiding influence in this patient's life.

I consider this type of technique to be perhaps the single most powerful use of language as it occurs in my practice. It is only administered as the patient approaches the turning point in treatment and when I am certain that the full force of the primordial influences are moving to reassert themselves in the patient's life. Prior to this moment there has been a much more subtle use of language continually to both support and assess the patient's progress in healing.

The Nature of Cure and Healing

After ten years of the study of [medical] books
[one believes] that there is no incurable disease.
After ten more years of study of [medical] books
[one is certain] that there is no curable disease.
– HUAI YUAN[19]

Generally, when people think of the word "cure," they take it to imply that a specific condition is treated to the point it no longer exists. In truth this is rarely, if ever, the case. The manifestation of any given symptom indicates by its presence an a priori constitutional weakness that allowed it to be expressed. In other words, the patient had either a genetic and/or karmic predisposition that allowed this symptom to become manifest. The inner tradition focuses on constitutional issues which comprise that aspect of self that can never fundamentally be changed because it comprises one's inborn nature. Medicine can help compensate for our constitutional weaknesses but cannot ultimately change what has been present from conception. Hence the inner tradition does not focus on achieving a cure as an end point of treatment. Rather, the focus is placed on guiding the patient through the process of healing. A condition is considered to be healed when it no longer limits a patient's self-expression or hinders quality of life.

Even after substantial improvement, all symptoms, like habits, have a tendency to return. After all, the constitutional basis that allowed them to manifest in the first place is still present, and all people tend to fall back into their old patterns of behavior. When a patient initially comes for treatment, he or she may be suffering from migraine headaches four days a week. The condition may be so debilitating that the patient is virtually unable to function. After a successful course of treatment, the patient may have only one or two migraine headaches a year. The patient whose quality of life is now greatly improved may tell friends that the headaches have been cured. It is clear, however, that the patient still has the same inner disposition that created the headaches in the first place.

Ultimately, symptoms are warning signs of deeper imbalance. Patients must learn to recognize their symptoms in their early stages before they become fully manifest. They may then learn to make the appropriate internal shifts necessary to avoid becoming ill. As people heal, they must be encouraged to think of their symptoms as signs that some internal matter needs attending to. By taking responsibility for maintaining their own health, patients are less dependent on the healer and should need treatment with decreasing frequency.

The Three Levels: Body, Mind, and Spirit

Using the language of classical Chinese medicine it is impossible to talk of the separation implied by the English words *body, mind,* and *spirit.* Hence the character *xin* refers to the physical, emotional, and spiritual heart. The Chinese language uses one term, *xin,* that has a multitude of meanings implicit within it. On the other hand, the English language uses three terms, *body, mind,* and *spirit,* to address what is implicitly thought to represent a unified whole, namely, the human being. Think of each of the five elements as comprised of spiritual, emotional, and physical realms of being. For example, the spiritual aspect of the wood element corresponds to the *hun* and its ability to be in contact with *jing* in a way that informs one of his or her life plan. The mental aspect of wood involves the decision-making faculties of the gallbladder which transmit the potential of that plan into the world. The physical aspects of wood are comprised by the actual organs of the liver and gallbladder, as well as all material aspects of being associated with these officials such as the tendons, ligaments, eyes, and the course of the liver and gallbladder meridians.

The functional basis of disharmony may emanate primarily from the physical, emotional, or the deeper realms of spiritual being. For example, a lack of benevolence and the presence of belligerence indicate dysfunction in the spiritual and emotional realms of the wood element. It is quite possible, however, that at the time of the assessment the patient exhibits no physical symptomatology in the wood element. A patient diagnosed with hepatitis C, a severe physical illness of the liver, however, may be perfectly healthy in the spiritual and emotional domains of liver function. Hence the patient may be tranquilly benevolent and possess healthy self-esteem. Identifying the level of being that perpetuates dysfunction in each patient is a primary task for the practitioner of the inner tradition.

Of the three depths, the spirit possesses the capacity to move most quickly. In just one moment, the spirit may heal in a way that binds one again to true self and one's life purpose. Healing in this way is signaled by increased experience of the virtues associated with one's constitutional type. Hence a person who is wood constitutionally will be better able to experience the virtue of benevolence as it exists at his or her core. Increased contact with one's source of virtue corresponds to a restitution of the basis of one's capacity for intuition.

The mind's capacity to heal is somewhat slower than the spirit's. Although profound insight may occur in a moment, the tendency of the mind is to continually fall back into habituated patterns of thought and belief. Only commitment to manifesting innate virtues paired with conscious vigilance can prevent the mind from seizing control and motivating one's attitudes and actions. Healing of the mind is signaled by an increase of behaviors that reflect one's constitutional virtues. While the spirit may know virtue, it is the mind that governs the movement of *qi* and wills actions that are consistent with fulfilling destiny.

Of the three depths, the body takes the longest to heal. Once a functional imbalance has manifested physically, it is relatively more concrete and harder to influence through treatment. Spirit is that which allows us to be in contact with virtue, and mind is that which allows our actions to reflect virtue. After original nature is lost and one is separated from the source of virtue, it takes many years of dysfunctional thought and behavior for illness to become embodied. Although spirit and mind may move toward healing relatively quickly, it will again take years for correct thought and action to be once again embodied as physical health.

This last assertion may contradict what some believe to be true about acupuncture. After all, many people experience long-lasting relief from chronic pain with just a few acupuncture treatments. One such example is John discussed in Chapter 10, whose pain associated with eight years of polyneuropathy disappeared after only one session. However, immediate relief of this nature is predicated in large part on movement of spirit and mind and often does not reflect a true physical healing at all. Despite his decrease of pain and renewed positive outlook, any objective measure such as a test of nerve conduction velocity would have revealed that my patient still had polyneuropathy. Imbalances of spirit and mind take years to become embodied as physical illness. Rectification of the spirit and mind may lead a person to feel better long before the physical embodiment of dysfunction is actually healed. It is therefore imperative to guide people to live in a healthier way so that true healing is promoted and the tendency to recreate one's illness is mitigated.

This preceding discussion illustrates an important premise in the inner tradition: Therapeutic measures administered with the intention of promoting healing will be received by the deepest aspects of self that perpetuate dysfunction. Of course, the focus of constitutional diagnosis is to direct healing toward the deepest aspects of the patient's being. One's constitutional dynamics are the basis for all expressions of true self in life. In directing treatment to this depth, the practitioner lays a foundation for subsequent healing by attending primarily to the most essential aspects of being. These principles are also present physiologically. Functional imbalances often begin with excessive physical and/or emotional work and then proceed to *qi,* blood, *yin, yang,* and ultimately *jing* deficiency. Deficiency of *jing* signifies the physiological depth of an imbalance. If a patient is *jing* deficient one must tonify this root of the imbalance to promote substantial healing.

If the symptoms of dysfunction are suppressed, illness will be driven deeper into the level of being that perpetuates imbalance and subsequently increase dysfunction in the other levels of being. If an imbalance of spirit is treated in a way that suppresses its expression, then the root of the imbalance will continue to perpetuate dysfunction as the patient becomes increasingly distanced from original nature. Eventually what began as a spirit-level dysfunction may become embodied as physical illness. For example, a patient who has been physically abused and subsequently experiences rage and depression may be given antidepressants as a long-term intervention. These drugs do not address the root cause of the problem, however, that may be located in the spiritual depth of the liver official. In time, the spiritual dysfunction that has been unattended to will undermine the functioning of the mind and body, ultimately leading to physical illness.

In contrast, illness may begin in the physical realm with the invasion of an external wind/cold pathogen. In this case antibiotics may be administered that eliminate the bacterial source of the infection but do nothing to eliminate the wind/cold. Excess heat generated as the body attempts to move the stagnation of cold will, over time, consume fluids. Depletion of fluids, in turn, will predictably lead to the more serious state of lung *yin* deficiency. By the time the *yin* of the lungs is injured, the imbalance is likely to have entered the spirit and emotional realms and the patient may evidence grief, longing, and difficulty receiving quality in life. Note that the suppression of symptoms is not limited to the inappropriate use of Western medical interventions. Treatment in any modality that eliminates pain but does not educate the patient has the potential to perpetuate ignorance and drive illness deeper.

The Path of Healing

At the moment original nature is lost, a separation occurs between the heart and mind that compromises the functional integrity of the heart/kidney axis. Original nature as a guiding force in life is obscured to the degree that *shen* is unable to access *jing*. During healing, as the connections between heart and mind, and *shen* and *jing* are rectified, psychospiritual issues that have been sublimated will begin to move toward the surface and into consciousness. The force of original nature being restored will, like a flood, erode the foundation on which ignorance is built. As the edifice of imagined self that is predicated on habituated *qi* begins to crumble, the potential exists for physical and emotional states that occurred in proximity to the loss of original nature to be reactivated.

Constantine Hering (1800–1880), a founder of homeopathy in America, formulated a framework that describes the general process of healing when patients are treated holistically. The "law of cure" states that symptoms disappear from within to without, in the reverse order in which they occurred, and from top to bottom.

Though the "law" of cure originates from a tradition of practice outside of Chinese medicine, I find that it is generally accurate in predicting the overall course of a patient's path of healing when they are treated in the inner tradition. To designate these principles as "law" in the same way that the laws of physics are considered to govern the motion of physical bodies is to state the case too strongly. In fact, I find the third principle to be wholly irrelevant to my experience in clinical practice. However, the first two principles do influence my assessment of every patient's progress toward health.

Of particular importance is the relationship between the turning point, as conceived in the *Yijing*, and the healing crisis as conceived of in homeopathy. Both the turning point and healing crisis signify that the patient has reached a crucial juncture where the restoration of original nature is imminent and symptoms may be temporarily exacerbated. By following a patient's progress according to these tenets, the practitioner may be alerted in advance to the arrival of the turning point and be better prepared to guide the patient during this most critical time.

From Within to Without

At the depth of each human being is the central reality of primordial *dao*. This exists physiologically as the *jing* and the *yuanqi*. The most external aspect of self is the *weiqi*, the defensive *qi* that surrounds each person. This *qi* protects us from invasive pathogenic influences, whether they be environmental pathogens such as a virus or the negative attitudes of another person. Between the core of self and our outermost projection of defensive *qi* are many successive levels of being that exist on a continuum from internal to external.

Each of the elements contains a *yin* organ that is relatively internal functionally and a *yang* organ that is relatively external. Each element also is paired with an external structure in the body. For example, in the metal element the lungs represent the inner aspect of function and the large intestine represents the outer aspect. Both these organs are relatively internal compared with the skin, which is associated with the functioning of the metal element.

We can illustrate the course of illness and cure according to these principles with the example of a young girl who had developed eczema. This skin condition initially manifested for her as a red irritation appearing in the crooks of her elbows in the area of acupuncture point Lung-5. Upon seeing her scratching, her parents took her to a physician who prescribed cortisone cream to apply to the area of the rash. The cream worked quickly and, as long as she applied it regularly, the symptoms of the rash were alleviated. This treatment, however, merely suppressed the expression of the symptom that is the outer expression of internal heat in the girl's lungs. With administration of the steroid cream, the heat is unable to exit through the skin and thus builds in her lungs to the point that she eventually develops asthma. The symptoms have progressed from the relatively external manifestation of a skin rash to the relatively internal manifestation of asthma. It is expected with treatment in a holistically based tradition of Chinese medicine that, as the asthma improves, the progression of the symptoms will reverse and start to move more externally. The reappearance of the skin rash signifies that healing, rather than suppression, has occurred.

There is another way to think about how symptoms move along the continuum of internal to external during healing. This continuum proceeds from the nonphysically manifest inner levels of spirit, through the intermediary stage of the mind, to the physically manifest and relatively outer level of the body. Spiritual and emotional imbalances may begin to manifest more physically in a given official as they resolve. For example, a man whose central imbalance manifests in the spiritual realm of the lung official may exhibit depression predicated on his unconscious feelings of having been betrayed by God because of the death of a loved one. As he heals, he may experience a severe flu characterized by the expectoration of a great amount of phlegm from his lungs that corresponds to the physical embodiment of his spiritual grief.

Symptoms Leave in Reverse Order

In the earlier example, a patient reexperienced her skin condition as her asthma improved. This illustrates the principle that symptoms tend to reappear in the reverse order to their first appearance. It is critical at this juncture that the expression of the skin condition not again be suppressed with medications. Rather, life has provided another opportunity to heal the initial issue by treating the underlying heat in the lungs on which it is predicated. Only by conducting a thorough intake that covers the patient's health history can the practitioner know if the appearance of a given symptom signals the worsening or improvement of a functional imbalance.

The emergence into the realm of conscious awareness of issues that unconsciously motivate a person's habitual behavior is another example of pathology moving from inside (the unconscious realm) to outside (awareness) during healing. A general principle is that when habituated behaviors begin to subside, a person is often confronted with precisely the same life issue that initiated the habitual behavior to begin with. For example, a teenager may begin to drink alcohol excessively as a way of coping with sexual abuse. Twenty years later the patient may seek treatment to help maintain sobriety. As the momentum toward health builds, and drinking subsides, the issues surrounding sexual abuse are likely to reemerge into consciousness. While confronting these issues, symptoms that occurred in proximity to the abuse such as heart palpitations, anxiety attacks, and nightmares may reappear, signaling a law of cure reaction and the patient's proximity to the turning point.

Symptoms Leave from Above to Below

The law of cure predicts that as a functional imbalance heals, the general progression of symptoms is from the center of the body out to the extremities and from the top of the body downward. For example, a man may suffer from pain localized in his lower back and traveling into the buttocks. As the functional basis of this symptom is balanced, the pain may subside in the back but follow the course of the bladder meridian (which corresponds to the course of the sciatic nerve) down his leg. With initial improvement the pain may move to the back of his knee and then eventually just be felt along the outer edge of his foot until it eventually leaves completely.

I have never found this aspect of the law of cure to occur at a frequency any greater than would be predicted by chance alone. In my experience, sciatic pain is just as likely to become localized in the lower back as healing occurs as it is to move toward the periphery. I therefore disregard this tenet in assessing a patient's progress.

A Mechanism Explaining the Progression of Healing

The notion of functional imbalances moving from inside to outside and in reverse order of occurrence is supported in Chinese medicine in part by the function of divergent meridians.[20] Each of the twelve main meridians is associated with a divergent meridian that runs in tandem with the central channel. The divergent meridians connect each organ to its associated sensory orifice and also serve as channels for the "curious organs" that include the brain. I think of the divergent meridians as playing a significant role in maintaining the functional integrity of each official. A primary function of the divergent meridians is to keep external pathogens, or life events that are too threatening to consciously assimilate, from penetrating to a functional depth which could injure a primary organ. For example, wind/cold/damp that has entered the liver meridian could be diverted away from the liver and into the hip joint. Similarly, rage from physical abuse could be diverted away from the liver by that official's divergent meridian.

The "window of heaven" points, located on the neck between the mind (brain) and the heart, are considered to be some of the strongest points for treating the spirit. In fact, several of these points are the upper confluent points of the divergent meridians. Part of the efficacy of "window" points in treating the spirit may be attributed to their function of allowing sublimated emotional material to resurface at a time in life when a person is no longer in proximity to a threatening event. With the perspective afforded by time, and the influence of heaven empowered by the window point, one may be better able to comprehend heaven's intention in sending us a previous difficulty. In this way one may let go of interpretations of traumatic events that have prolonged one's pain and the dysfunctional state on which it is based. Hence window points possess the dual purpose of bringing up sublimated emotional material that has been repressed and of facilitating our learning from challenging events in life.

Although the divergent meridians and window points may explicitly pertain to releasing latent pathogens and emotional states, it is my belief that all acupuncture points work in this way. That is to say, each point holds the potential to put a patient in immediate contact with some pure aspect of being as it exists untouched by life's traumas. Reconnection to a lost virtue has the potential to cause any *qi* that does not correspond to true self to begin exiting toward the surface of the patient's being. When pathogenic *qi* begins to depart, the patient may experience a healing crisis. In part, the pathogenic *qi* corresponds to the functional basis of those interpretations of events that perpetuate habitual nature and identification with the created self.

The Healing Crisis

As treatment progresses and the patient approaches the turning point, a dynamic tension occurs between the primordial influences struggling to reassert themselves and the habituated influences struggling to maintain the patient's image of created self. As the primordial influences win this battle and flood through the patient's being, the accretions of mundanity acquired over a lifetime are swept away. As this old stagnant *qi* leaves through the same substrate (the patient's body and being) that it initially entered, old symptoms may return and current symptoms may be exacerbated.[21] There are some principles that may allow the practitioner to discern if an aggravation of a symptom constitutes the worsening of a condition or a movement toward healing.

If an aggravation of symptoms represents healing, then it will never be experienced by the patient as worse than the worst it has ever been. For example, if a patient has an asthma attack that represents a healing crisis, it may be as bad as, but never worse than, any previous attack. True healing crises never last longer than 48 hours before the symptoms begin to subside. In every case of a healing crisis, once the aggravation does subside, patients are expected to feel substantially better than they felt before the crisis occurred.

In my practice I have seen that patients tend to experience a healing crisis at the first-, second-, and/or third-year anniversary date marking the beginning of treatment. Often the patient, having felt gradual and substantial improvement, will arrive for a session and announce that symptoms have returned and he or she is "back to square one." Patients describe their situation as if they have come full circle and made no progress. In reality, however, life never proceeds in a circle but always in an upward spiral. As patients have approached the anniversary date, they move toward releasing a deeper level of habituated *qi* on which their symptoms and imbalances are based. While they are dealing thematically in life with the same issue, there is less force of the habitual *qi* driving the manifestation of the symptom, and patients have more tools that empower them to deal with the issue at hand. In fact, they have not come full circle, but are at an elevated position in an upward spiral that affords a better perspective, although the view is similar. In such situations I have found that just treating the source points on the constitutional meridians will often be sufficient to help move them past this critical juncture.[22] Invariably, the patient returns to the next session and informs me that the symptoms abated within two days and he or she has had a renewed sense of vitality since.

Destiny and How Chinese Medicine Works

Who we are at any given moment in life is an expression of the momentary interaction among three variables: our inherited constitution (early heaven), our acquired constitution (later heaven), and our beliefs and attitudes regarding our inherited constitution and life experience. Heaven wills for each of us an inborn nature that roughly corresponds to the modern notion of genetic endowment. This endowment is granted at the moment of conception and falls under the influence of early heaven. Forming our potential for manifestation in life, the contribution of early heaven may be said to correspond to *yin*. Whatever seed heaven plants within us in life is unalterable from the moment of conception to the moment of death. We are given certain innate capacities that set the limit, in every aspect of being, on what can be accomplished in life given the most advantageous environment, coupled with the most arduous self-cultivation.

Heaven, having planted this seed within, then sends life experiences from without in order to cultivate the seed of inborn potential. All situations that come to us in life belong to later heaven and constitute our environment. These active impulses *(shenming)* from heaven correspond to *yang*. The situations that arrive from heaven fall into three categories: (1) all that we have received in the past, (2) all that we receive in the present, and (3) all that we will receive in the future.

Only that sent us by heaven from the infinite sea of possibility that is the future is possibly alterable. Like our genetic endowment, that environment received in the past and that sent by heaven in the present moment are unalterable. The past is gone forever, existing only as memory, and actions cannot affect it. We cannot change the moment, for, as we act, that moment is now gone and a new moment is here. Humans are trapped forever in the moment, and it is "what is" in the moment that the habituated mind seeks to escape. In essence, we can only be aware of what is (i.e., our feelings) in each moment and consciously choose not to react simply out of routine habit in the next moment. In this way, we become a vessel through which the *dao* may flow and spontaneously express itself. By practicing being present in the moment, we are able to influence future circumstances even though present and past circumstances remain unalterable.

Hence what is unalterable—our inborn constitution and previous life experience—and what occurs in the moment is the aspect of life that human will *(zhi)* cannot change. It is this "fixed" aspect of life that may be defined as the will of heaven. The will of heaven constitutes "what is" or, in other words, ultimate reality. By acknowledging and nourishing what heaven has placed within, and accepting all situations in life as opportunities for self-cultivation, the sage manifests destiny. In this way, the individual may, like the *chongqi*, perfectly blend all qualities of *yin* (early heaven) and *yang* (later heaven). Therefore, the appropriate use of the mind is as a tool for self-discovery and as the commander of the *qi*, which allows us to take actions in the world consistent with the intention in our heart.

We have said that the "true self" constitutes that which heaven has placed in our heart of hearts at conception. Everything else about a given individual corresponds to the third domain discussed here, which is our interpretation of life. This is the self we believe our self to be, which is created out of the meaning we have attached to life and its events. This is the habitual self, conditioned by the accretions of mundane consciousness and acquired influences. Here, the individual's mind takes control and acts independently of the truth within the heart.[23] Eventually, due to our inability to distinguish between the true and the created self, our reality comes to be predicated solely on belief and interpretation.[24] This is what the philosophers of ancient China refer to as being deluded or "asleep."

We can run but we can never hide from the will of heaven. The moment we close an avenue of self-expression, heaven begins sending us life events to reestablish the spontaneous flow of *dao* that has been constrained or cut off. Internally, symptomatology is generated according to the dictates of that person's constitutional type. Hence, in the inner tradition, symptoms are seen as warnings that, at a deeper level, some aspect of self has been lost. Externally, heaven will send us life situations that, if heeded, will exemplify the lesson we need to learn which is the consequence of lost self-expression. Heaven will continually call forth that aspect of lost self-expression as the only possible solution to the challenges it sends. By looking at the momentary picture of "what is" in a patient's life, the practitioner may gain immediate access to how the patient is generating his or her reality. Hence the nature of our symptoms and life situation at any given moment is always pointing to a deeper truth which is the aspect of self that has been lost.

If our constitutional type never changes from the moment of conception to the moment of death, how is it that traditional Chinese medicine may effect a "cure"? Although the theme of a life is unchanging, the plot of a life, as it occurs around the theme, may certainly be altered. By harmonizing those aspects of excess and deficiency that at their core imply the separation of *yin* and *yang* and the disordered functioning of the five elements, we may restore the patient to balance. After having bridged the gap back to the lost self, patients are now free to take actions in the world consistent with the truth they find in their own hearts. As they become sages and perfect channels for the flow of *dao*, heaven ceases to create havoc in their lives. Internally the warning signs of imbalance that manifest as illness slowly subside, and externally life becomes less "interesting."[25]

Treatment with the inner tradition actually removes the functional basis that drives the separation from true self. It is not that life does not put obstacles in the way of the sage, but rather that the sage is able to see all obstacles as the will of heaven. Instead of causing pain and generating illness over life's ups and downs, the sage goes along with what has been allotted and each moment returns to original nature.

The Sage as Healer

He recovers the transgressions of many.
In assisting the self-becoming of all beings, he dares not act.
– DAO DE JING[26]

The *Dao De Jing* tells us that "*De* is treasured not by decree *(ming)*, but by spontaneity."[27] Destiny is fulfilled by patterning ourselves on the spontaneous movement of the *dao* and being "self-so" *(ziran)*. In the alchemical texts, the process of returning to original nature is likened to being pregnant. Through cultivating his spiritual embryo, the adept gives birth to himself in his own process of "self-becoming." It is the sage who, in guiding the adept through this process, acts as the midwife in this delivery. "The sage in the world," says the *Dao De Jing,* "mixes *(hun)* the minds *(xin)* of all,"[28] helping to return the conditioned mind *(xin)* of humans to the primal state *(hun)*, which is the heart of *dao.*

The sage may be considered the standard of wisdom aimed for in each practitioner's quest to become a healer. In teaching the return to original nature, the *Dao De Jing* asks us to pattern ourselves on the sage. The term for sage, *shengren* (聖人), means literally "wise man"— he who "listened to and understood the advice given [by the sage] and thus becomes wise."[29] The Chinese character *ting* ("listen":聽) means to have our heart rectified by listening to the words of the sage. It is through listening to the sage within his or her own heart that the practitioner may be transformed into a healer capable of rectifying the heart of another.

Next we examine some of the themes present in this text as they bear on the practitioner as sage and the sage as healer.

Excess and Deficiency: Harmonizing the Flood

The myth of Gun and Yu may serve as metaphor for several fundamental principles of Chinese medicine. Gun built dams to suppress the floods that were symbolic of humankind's fall out of harmony with nature. For attempting to block the expression of this imbalance, Gun lost his mandate from the Yellow Emperor and was destroyed. By suppressing any symptom, we guarantee that it, like the *dao*, will eventually express itself, eventually breaking down all obstacles placed in its path if necessary. Yu, rather than suppressing the floods, tunneled through the mountains to allow the overflowing rivers to find their own way to the sea. Only by opening the passageways and assisting the patient to channel life's flow of *qi* can treatment be successful. The way of heaven is found when a flow and balance is achieved: "What has surplus is reduced, what is deficient is supplemented."[30]

This same notion is expressed nicely by Zhang Cong Zheng in the *Rumen Shiqin* (c. 1228): "[Physicians who] consider a supplementing [therapy] for persons who have been affected by evil [influence] accumulations [already] are followers of Gun who drowned in the great flood [because he applied the wrong method to drain it]."[31]

It was Yu's power of intention in visualizing the spirits on top of Mount Mao that allowed him to summon and transform them into one body, an assembly *(hui)* of all under heaven. His intimate knowledge of the river and mountain spirits (*maili*:脈理,veins of the earth) enabled him to draw the waters off, out the southeastern "door of the earth," and into the abyss of the sea.[32] What Yu did for ancient China in controlling the floods and uniting the kingdom, the practitioner of the inner tradition of Chinese medicine also does for each patient. By learning intimately the nature of the spirits living in the internal structures of the patient's being, and by channeling off the excess and supplementing the deficiencies, traditional treatment is able to maintain and restore harmony to the patient's inner kingdom just as Yu established harmony by unifying ancient China.

Healing and Ritual

Do not place a needle into a patient until
you have already performed a treatment.
– BOB DUGGAN[33]

Wilhelm suggests in his elaboration of the first *Yijing* hexagram (*jian,* "heaven") that the sage operates in the human world through creative action and "through his power awakens and develops [people's] higher nature."[34] The sage's "power" *(ling)* to awaken the highest in others is derived from internal alignment with heaven and acceptance of destiny. When we are in the presence of individuals who are exactly where they ought to be, doing exactly what they ought to be doing, it is a transforming experience. The sage, in perfect alignment between heaven and earth, is able to create the context in which spiritual transformation may occur in those receptive to the sage's presence.

Taking the sage to represent the healer, the concept of *ling* holds special import for those engaged in the practice of Chinese medicine. Just as we cannot force heaven to rain by performing a rain dance, practitioners of the inner tradition cannot make things happen in their patients. Rather, they create the appropriate context for change through each nuance of interaction with the patient. The practitioner's own internal alignment, called forth in performing the ritual of treatment, creates a context for healing even before the needles are inserted or the herbs are prescribed. Ideally, the patient's transformation is initiated by the very presence of the practitioner. This approach deemphasizes the technical aspects of acupuncture or herbalism and places the responsibility for successful treatment directly on the spiritual development and cultivation of virtue by the practitioner.

Summary

The uncarved wood disperses to become vessels,
to be used by the sage as officials.
Therefore a great institution does not mutilate.
— DAO DE JING [35]

When the ministers stick to their posts, the hundred
officials have their regular duties, and the ruler
employs each according to their particular ability.
— HAN FEIZI [36]

Just as the sage's responsibility is to recognize the unique function and purpose of each official, so too it is the healer's charge to perceive and empower each patient's life purpose. The healer has no agenda other than to bring the *dao* uniquely into the world through the patient, and therefore "does not mutilate" by imposing his or her will on the patient. In describing the way of the sage we are told that "He works, but does not contend."[37] Emperor Yu, in diverting the waters to the sea, did so "as if he were acting without any special effort (for he followed the natural tendencies)."[38] So too must the healer follow the natural tendencies of *dao* as they strive to assert themselves in ordering each patient's life. The *Dao De Jing* emphasizes this principle:

Therefore the sage says:
I do not act,
Hence the people transform by themselves;
I love tranquility,
Hence the people are normal by themselves;
I have no business,
Hence the people grow rich by themselves;
I have no desire,
Hence the people are like the uncarved wood by themselves."[39]

The therapeutic goal of the inner tradition is to assist patients in "transforming by themselves." It is as though the patient is on a journey and the practitioner, noticing the patient's own inner direction, travels around each corner just ahead, clearing the path of obstacles. The patient is only aware of effortlessly proceeding on his or her journey and not of being acted upon by the sage's will. In the cultivation of original nature it is necessary to approach our heart and the heart of the patient as if we were trying to entice a deer to eat out of our hand. Hence we must sit still and merely extend our hand, allowing the deer to draw closer with each encounter. The boundary must be set entirely by the deer, whose nature is to be timid and shy. Eventually, with trust established through the stillness of the practitioner's own heart, contact may be made with the truth that lies guarded in the patient's heart.

Mencius too asserts the importance of recognizing each patient's inborn strengths and weaknesses. He states, "The sages never required the same ability from all creatures or made them all do the same thing. Names should stop when they have expressed reality, concepts of right and wrong should be founded on what is suitable. This is what it means to have command of reason and good fortune to support you."[40] The healer as sage assesses each patient in terms of what is appropriate individually as a unique expression of his or her own being. The sole purpose for choosing to treat any condition is to remove the obstacles that prevent patients from bringing themselves more fully into the world.

Zhuangzi advises, "Do not try to develop what is natural to man; develop what is natural to heaven. He who develops heaven benefits life; he who develops man injures life. Do not reject what is of heaven, do not neglect what is of man, and the people will be close to the attainment of truth."[41] What is natural to heaven is the virtue inherent in each patient's inborn constitution. What is natural to humans are the unconscious habits born of socialization. The healer must help each patient cultivate the awareness of heaven's influences and original nature by treating the constitutional basis of any disease. Suppression of symptoms perpetuates ignorance of true self and thus cultivates "what is natural to man."

Any action we take in life has one of two consequences: We perpetuate ignorance or we dispel ignorance. Regardless of the relative seriousness of a patient's symptoms, the commitment of the practitioner in the inner tradition must be to educate the patient about the basis of the illness and to aid in the restoration of original nature. Patients ultimately must be empowered to be the agents of transformation in their own healing process. In so doing, the patient may be restored to the eternal virtue of the *dao*'s *ziran,* or self-becoming.

The wisdom of preventing illness before injury can occur is addressed in the *Dao De Jing,* Chapter 64:

> *What is at equilibrium is easy to maintain;*
> *What has not emerged is easy to plan;*

What is fragile is easy to dissolve;
What is minute is easy to disperse.
Act when there is yet nothing to do.
Govern when there is yet no disorder (luan).[42]

Similar ideas are echoed by the physician Xu Zhunfu (1556), who described the sages' approach to preventive medicine: "The sages treated those who were not yet sick; they did not treat the sick. . . . This treatment consisted of paying great attention to the illness from the very beginning and in applying protective measures when it was still very weak! . . . Then it will never happen that one has to treat it after it has already become manifest."[43] However, once affairs have proceeded too far and illness has become embodied, the *Dao De Jing* is quite clear that true healing involves returning to one's original nature.

In reconciling a great injury,
There is sure to have some injury left.
How can this be good?
Therefore the sage holds the left tally,
He does not blame others.[44]

When a person suffers a great injury there will never be a satisfactory resolution in terms of human justice. As long as we persist in distinguishing between right and wrong, there will be scars and lingering damage. No human resolution can make up the loss created by injury. The only real healing comes from rolling the two of right and wrong back into the one of primordial *dao* in which all opposites are harmonized. Along these lines, the *Dao De Jing* advises us not to seek justice but rather to "repay injury with *de* [virtue]."[45] We may only be considered to be healed when the damaging events of life no longer limit self-expression and the manifestation of life's purpose.

Ultimately, the sage, in healing others, is healed. In order to treat any aspect of being in another person, the practitioner must be able to access that state within, and he or she in turn is rewarded. Through the path of selfless service to others, the sage cultivates virtue. The *Dao De Jing* thus asserts:

The sage does not hoard.
Having worked for his fellow beings,
The more he possesses.
Having donated himself to his fellow beings,
The more abundant he becomes.[46]

Questions

1. What is the difference between a practitioner and a healer?

2. What is the difference between the nature of healing and the concept of cure?

3. To what degree does the practice of healing spring from your life's purpose?

4. To what degree are the virtues you express in the treatment room integrated into your everyday life?

NOTES

1. Legge, 1970, p. 451.
2. *Dao De Jing,* Chapter 25; in Chen, 1989, p. 117.
3. Cleary, 1986a, p. 115.
4. Contrasted with those who are ignorant are those who possess "consciousness of reality" *(daoxin:*道心*)*. The characters translated by Cleary may literally be translated as "path of the heart." Ibid., p. 5.
5. Wieger, 1965, p. 327. The character *shun,* like many Chinese characters, can have diametrically opposed meanings depending on the context of its usage. When applied to those who are ignorant, the character infers that we proceed through life docilely, swept along by fate. In a different context, however, the character *shun* is used to tell us that to survive we must "adapt" to the laws of *yin* and *yang.* Unschuld, 1988, p. 11.
6. Some modern authors translate *ni* as "countercurrent," indicating *qi* that is flowing in a direction opposite to normal physiological process. In this usage *ni* is used to denote an undesirable process resulting in symptomatology. In Liu's usage, *ni* denotes a desirable spiritual return to original nature against the habituating currents of life. In Chinese Buddhism, *ni liu* (逆流) means to set one's course against the stream of transmigration and enter the path of nirvana. See Soothill and Hosous, 1995, p. 340. In Chapter 6 I presented Liu's seven stages of losing original nature. He also elaborates seven stages of returning original nature and nine stages for obtaining sagehood. These last nine stages involve reversing one's relationship to the five elements so that the order of the elements in the *sheng* cycle is reversed. Hence the cycle moves from water, to metal, to earth, to fire, to wood. See Cleary, 1986a, pp. 87–104. Jeffrey Yuen terms this an "involutionary" sequence of the elements, as opposed to the normal sequence, which is an "evolutionary" cycle.
7. Cleary, 1986a, p. 56. Here Liu alludes to the writing of Han Feizi.
8. Soothill, 1937, p. 3.
9. Ibid., p. 467.
10. Humphreys, 1984, p. 210.
11. See Soothill, 1937, p. 467.
12. Mathews, 1931, p. 513.

13. Watson, 1964a, p. 54.
14. Chan, 1963, pp. 443–444.
15. Ibid., pp. 438–439.
16. Ibid., p. 447.
17. This is a pattern of wood invading earth (see the case study of Paulette in Chapter 10). Often people with this pattern absorb the anger of the parties they are mediating. They embody the functional dynamic of being stuck between warring factions as their wood element (liver and gallbladder) on their right side attacks their earth element (spleen and stomach) on their left side. The burning in the epigastric area halfway between wood and earth is the embodiment of the anger being absorbed.
18. Chan, 1963, p. 429.
19. In Unschuld, 1979, p. 104. Huai Yuan (c. C.E. 1808) was a physician.
20. The following discussion of divergent meridians is based on my interpretation of a lecture by Jeffrey Yuen as well as my own clinical experience.
21. For an appraisal of the healing crisis and the law of cure in accordance with the holographic theory of Chinese medicine, see Jarrett, 1985.
22. Each meridian has a source *(yuan:*原*)* point that unites the meridian with the primordial influences which support its functioning. In the order of *qi* circulation these are Heart-7, Small Intestine-4, Bladder-64, Kidney-3, Heart Protector-7, Triple Heater-4, Gallbladder-40, Liver-3, Lung-9, Large Intestine-4, Stomach-42, and Spleen-3. Source points are "grounding" in nature and generally considered to be among the most gentle points for influencing the function of each official.
23. The mind makes a good slave but a cruel master.
24. This underscores the therapeutic importance of suggestion and intervening at the level of the patient's belief system.
25. Remember the Chinese curse: "May you live in interesting times!"
26. Chapter 64; translation mine.
27. Chapter 51; in Chen, 1989, p. 175.
28. Chapter 49; in Chen, 1989, p. 170.
29. Wieger, 1965, p. 211.
30. Chapter 77; in Chen, 1989, p. 223.
31. *Jumen shih Ch'in*, Chapter 2; in Unschuld, 1988, p. 216.
32. Lagerwey, 1987, p. 11.
33. President and founder of the Traditional Acupuncture Institute in Columbia, Maryland.
34. Wilhelm, 1968, p. 3.
35. Chapter 28; in Chen, 1988, p. 124.
36. Watson, 1964b, p. 17.
37. Chapter 81; in Chen, 1989, p. 231.
38. Mencius, Chapter 4b, verse 26; in Chan, 1973, p. 76.
39. Chapter 57; in Chen, 1989, p. 190.
40. Watson, 1964, p. 116.
41. Watson, 1964a, p. 120.
42. Chen, 1989, p. 203.
43. Unschuld, 1988, p. 32.
44. Chapter 79; in ibid., p. 226.
45. Chapter 63; in Chen, 1989, p. 200.
46. Chapter 81; in Chen, 1989, p. 231.

13

THE
INNER NATURE
OF ACUPUNCTURE
POINTS[1]

To truly appreciate the function of acupuncture points, it is helpful to understand how the ancient Chinese thought about their world. Their conception of the universe is well reflected in the early Chinese mythology presented earlier in this text. When we understand this mythology (literally, spirit talk, *shenhua:*神話), the spirits of the points come alive and talk to us. Just as Emperor Yu traveled throughout China and became familiar with the spirits of the deep structures, so too must the acupuncturist know intimately the nature of the spirit present in each acupuncture point.

The meridians *(mai:*脈*)* running through the body are the internal rivers of the microcosm, each acupuncture point along a meridian representing and harmonizing a specific aspect of being in the individual's inner kingdom. The acupuncture meridians and points reflect the way in which the Chinese saw the macrocosm of the universe as it is mapped onto the microcosm of the body. This map guides the skilled practitioner to balance the functional relationships that maintain the integrity of the human being.

Just as the *Yijing* is a tool to guide our intuition to an understanding of the *dao's* implicit movement in the world, so, too, a knowledge of the imagery of the points may give us access to the ways in which the *dao* strives to express itself through each individual and the ways in which that effort is blocked, resulting in imbalance and ill health. It is often the practitioner's knowledge of the symbolism of each point that spells the difference between treating patients superficially and reaching them at their depth.

The unique property of acupuncture points is their ability, with stimulation, to restore our memory of original nature. Each point has the capacity to evoke some aspect of functioning that has been lost, buried under the accretions of life's habituating influence. The general characteristics of each of the five elements—water, wood, fire, earth, and metal—are elaborated in the discrete functions of the twelve "officials." The function of each official is further elaborated in its associated acupuncture points. For example, the general qualities of the wood element are elaborated into their *yin* and *yang* aspects as the liver and gallbladder officials, respectively. A function associated with the liver official is "planning." Thus the fourteen acupuncture points on the meridian of the liver official each address some discrete aspect of the function of planning.

The practitioner's developed knowledge of the individual points then guides her to identify and minister to subtle aspects of being that the patient is failing to access. For example, on the liver meridian, acupuncture point Liver-14, named "gate of hope," may allow the practitioner to empower that quality of being called hope within the patient. Hope can help to ease internally generated constraints on our plans as we project them into the future. Liver-14, by empowering the balanced expression of "hope," may help harmonize unbalanced emotional extremes on a continuum ranging from despair to blind optimism. We could devote a lifetime to writing volumes on Liver-14 and the nature of hope as it presents in humanity. In fact, this job would be endless because the human understanding of the aspect of being we call "hope" continually evolves. Hence the nature of any acupuncture point function evolves as the human understanding of being evolves. The nature of acupuncture points is limitless and cannot be defined as narrowly as they have been in most modern texts.

The images contained in the point names do not define point functions, but serve as foci for discussion about particular aspects of being harmonized by the point.[2] For example, discussing destiny *(ming)* in the context of the point Governor-4, *mingmen*, does not mean that Governor-4 is "the point for destiny." Every point, used in the correct context and at precisely the right moment, may restore a lost aspect of self-expression that brings the patient closer to fulfilling his life's potential.

The Nature of Acupuncture Point Function

Each acupuncture point is unique in its ability to touch some aspect of being that has been lost to the individual. By "touching" this aspect of being, the memory of original nature encoded within the point's function may be restored to the patient. Acupuncture points work by harmonizing continuums of unbalanced and extreme expressions into the virtues from which they derive, precisely in the same way that the *chòngqi* is said to harmonize the dualities of heaven and earth into a state of primal unity. An example on a physiological level is the function of Heart-7 ("spirit gate") in its ability to stabilize the pulse. Heart-7 may be used to equal advantage in an individual whose pulse is either excessively fast or excessively slow. In the former case, the function of the point contributes to calming the heart rate, whereas in the latter case, the point helps to raise the heart rate. Hence the function of Heart-7 represents the central point of balance between the extremes of heart function in terms of its rate.

This same principle of harmonizing dualities operates in the realms of psychological, emotional, and spiritual functioning as well. For example, an individual may be excessively belligerent in intimate relationships and at the same time timid in the workplace. These behaviors may be viewed as opposite ends on a continuum representing the unbalanced expression of the wood element. In this instance, the function of Liver-1, "great esteem," may serve to empower the virtue of self-esteem by harmonizing the unbalanced expression of both belligerence and timidity.

The general principle of bringing balance by harmonizing dualities is central to understanding the opposing but complementary natures of Western and Chinese medicine. It is exemplified by the difference between "taking a position" in life and "making a stand." A "position" is always taken relative, and in opposition to, another view. Hence positions often represent "either/or" alternatives to each other and often are taken in habitual and unconscious reaction to a contrary position adopted by another. For example, during the civil rights movement of the 1960s, some African Americans adopted a militant position regarding the bigotry prevalent among white people in America. The two opposing positions of the racist whites and militant blacks were fueled by habitual unconscious motivations on both parts. Rather than adopt a position in opposition to one view or another, Martin Luther King, Jr., made a "stand" between these two unbalanced extremes. Instead of solely advocating for the rights of African Americans, Dr. King advocated for the rights and dignity of all human beings. In this way, he helped harmonize the two extremes of hatred and helped all Americans move closer to the promise and fulfillment of their national destiny.

In a similar fashion, the practitioner must help to continually strengthen the center that harmonizes all forms of unbalanced expression in the patient's being. This center is defined by the patient's constitutional type, and the patterns of unbalanced expression he presents are predicated on his constitutional weaknesses and compensations. These imbalances may be addressed directly by the practitioner's choice of treating acupuncture points and prescribing herbs that speak to the depth of the patient's being.

Access to the inner nature of acupuncture points is only available in the context of treatment whose overall aim is aiding patients to fulfill their destiny. That is to say, we cannot just throw a few of these points into a treatment plan and expect them to empower the virtues discussed here. In the appropriate context, any point may be useful in harmonizing any imbalance in the patient's being. But in order to return the patient to his lost spontaneity and true nature, the sage as healer must be so united with variable circumstances that treatment is based on the functional dynamics of the patient at that moment.

For the practitioner, the patient appears as a pointillist painting. During each treatment, the practitioner uses her diagnostic skills to comprehend the functional portrait that emerges from the patient. The practitioner, in choosing a treatment, is concerned with where in the portrait to place a dot (acupuncture point) and what color to make it (quality of *qi*) so that the picture is complete in the moment. Between therapeutic sessions, the patient's functional dynamic will shift and, on each presentation, manifest a new picture that will have to be reassessed each session anew. The practitioner must herself respond spontaneously to each new presentation and not treat the same points repeatedly. Repeating points in an attempt to "cause" something to happen may be analogous to the practitioner forcing her will on the patient. Continually receiving the same points will cause the patient to stagnate as he becomes habituated to their effects. This is counterproductive because the goal of the highest medicine is to support the patient's evolution. Ideally, the practitioner is able to respond to each new presentation in a way that is unencumbered by her past experience with the patient. Even if a point is effective, avoid the inclination to use it repeatedly—hence Sunzi's warning not to repeat tactics that have worked successfully in the past but to let one's methods correspond to the unique merits of each new situation.[3]

Selecting the appropriate points involves the following process: (1) identify the patient's constitutional type because all treatment is performed in relation to this element and official; (2) identify the functional dynamic of imbalance that exists between the patient's constitutional type and the other elements and officials; (3) identify the discrete aspects of the given functions that the patient is habitually failing to express; and (4) identify the individual points on the relevant meridians most likely to empower the expression of these virtues.

The process of point selection may be informed by input from many sources extant in the life of each practitioner. She must be able to hold her long-term vision of the patient's path of healing while simultaneously responding to the unique circumstances of the therapeutic moment. This process often recedes into the realm of intuition when the practitioner is doing her best work. As in a brilliant musical improvisation, her selection of points expresses truth spontaneously as the rewards of practice mount and the constraints of theory fall away. Of course, we may always go back after the fact and analyze the performance or point selection. In truth, though, the note played or point selected emerges spontaneously out of the harmony of the moment. The practitioner literally has no other choice but to be a vessel for the creative flow of *dao* as expressed through the selection of points.

For the practitioner attuned to the functional relationships represented by the officials, the five-element system offers a method of discovering the deep inner functions of the acupuncture points. Over many thousands of sessions, with proper intention, the practitioner may become increasingly aware of the way each point addresses discrete aspects of human function on all levels of being. Of course, this is a highly individual process as clinical experience reveals to each practitioner truths about the points consistent with her own path, awareness, and belief system. The functions of the points I present here represent truths that are self-evident to me. They are offered only as insights into my own process of discovery and not as ultimate definitions of point function. Hence the information provided here is not meant to contradict any understanding of point functions as they are

presented in other texts. It is my personal belief that the practice of
Chinese medicine as a path means being able to embrace simultaneously apparent opposites and to hold contradictory principles as
reflecting complementary truths. To others who list the functions of
points differently, I would just say, "and that, too."

Listening to the Spirits: Myth, Meaning, and Point Function

Here we examine how the key concepts of destiny, virtue, spirit, and the
evolution of being are present in the names and imagery of various
acupuncture points. My specific intention is to elucidate these aspects of
being as they pertain to the diagnosis and treatment of the human condition and to the quest for the fulfillment of destiny. This journey will
take us around the cycle of five elements as we follow the various stages
in the evolution of *dao*.

The Primal Axis

Located along the central anterior and posterior axis of the body,
the conception vessel and the governor vessel are the seas of *yin* and
yang in the human being. These two meridians form the axes that orient the other twelve principal meridians and functions to the universal
poles of *yin* and *yang*. Embryologically, these two meridians are among
the first to develop.[4] Points Conception Vessel-1 and Governor Vessel-
20 are located on the perineum and vertex of the head, respectively.
Taking a line between them forms the central axis of the human being.

Conception Vessel-1, Huiyin, "Meeting of Yin"

Conception Vessel-1, named "meeting of *yin*," represents the source
of *yin* in the human being. Governor Vessel-20, named "hundred meetings," is the gathering point of the *yangqi*. Governor Vessel-20 may be
taken to represent the North Star as it rises out of the ocean of *dao*, as
represented by Conception Vessel-1. These points together delimit the
central axis of heaven and earth as it occurs in the human being.
Treating them together may help restore the balance between the primordial *yin* and *yang* and provide access to a reserve of these
influences. Interestingly, an alternate name for Conception Vessel-1 is
jinmen, or "metal gate," which recalls the entrance to the kingdom of
the queen mother.[5] In myth, the primordial brother and sister resurrect

the human race after riding the crest of the flood through the "golden gate." Similarly, a key function of Conception Vessel-1 is revival after drowning. The *Nei Jing* states that the conception vessel originates in the uterus[6] and, as in myth, it is the "metal gate" which provides passageway into and out of the womb of *dao*. In discussing the connection between the metal gate (Conception Vessel-1) and the top of the head (Governor Vessel-20), Wang Jizhen (c. late 1200s) writes,

> The right kidney is the Gate of Destiny; it is situated at the extremity of the spinal column. Beneath it is a large bone. The marrow in this bone enters the urinary tract . . . its god is the queen mother. It is called the Metal Gate because it is situated in the West. . . . The spinal column communicates with the Jade Capital: It is the main road to the Jade Capital at the top of the head [GV-20].[7]

Governor Vessel-20, Baihui, "Hundred Meetings"

After quelling the floods, Emperor Yu ascended Mount Mao, convening a meeting of the hundred spirits encountered on his journey. In so doing Yu brought spiritual unity to ancient China, founding the mythic Xia dynasty. However, one of his subjects, Oppose-the-Wind, arrived late to attend the meeting and was thus beheaded for his defiance. Oppose-the-Wind was not a loyal subject but a rebellious influence, one who tried to prevent the communication that was to occur during the ritual.[8] In the microcosm of the body, acupuncture point Governor Vessel-20, located on the vertex of the head, is named the hundred meetings. The Daoist text, the *Dao Cang* (hidden *dao*) states that the head is the meeting point of the hundred spirits.[9] Governor Vessel-20, then, is the place on top of the head (Mount Mao) where the hundred spirits meet.

The traditional function of Governor Vessel-20 in draining wind from the head is implied in the "beheading" of Oppose-the-Wind, the influence that threatens the integrity of the kingdom by opposing Yu's mandate to rule. For it was Yu who established harmony by controlling the rising waters of chaos. In Chinese medicine, wind is defined as any sign or symptom in an individual that changes location and severity quickly. Its general presentation is that of chaos, and it is exemplified by muscle spasms, seizures, violent outbursts of anger, or headaches. Point Governor Vessel-20 can help center on the most basic level, restore control, and marshal the patient's resources to quell the chaos.

Governor Vessel-20 is the point that aligns us with the polestar, to which "all the lesser stars do homage."[10] The polestar, *di* (帝), is the heart of heaven just as the emperor, *di* (帝), is the heart of the nation. The polestar is located at the center of the universe, and the Governor Vessel is the meridian that centers all functions in the human being to the axis of heaven. The dynastic rule of Emperor Yu is associated with the wood element, reinforcing his connection to Governor Vessel-20 that is the apex of the liver meridian. It is Yu's virtue in being a man aligned with heaven's heart that allows him to fulfill his destiny and unify his kingdom.

The Mysterious Pass: Governor Vessel-4, Mingmen: "Gate of Destiny"

Although it is often translated as "life," here I have translated *ming* as "destiny," which I believe is more consistent with the inner function of the point. Usage of the term *mingmen* varies to the extent that the *Neijing* refers to it as the eyes and the *Nanjing* refers to it as the right kidney.[11] The term *mingmen* when used in reference to the eyes at first appears to be an entirely different context than its usage when referring to the *mingmen* associated with the kidneys. This may lead to confusion regarding the meaning of the term *mingmen*.

The quality of *shen* coming through the eyes is addressed by acupuncture point Bladder-1 (*jingming*, "eyes bright"). Yeh Lin, in his commentary on the *Nanjing*, quotes the *Lingshu* and *Suwen*: "The *jingming* [hole is passed by influences that] come from the brain and heart. [The eyes] are therefore the holes where one's life arrives. Hence they are called the "gate of destiny."[12] We may consider the eyes to be an organ for receiving life as it appears to us through light, the spiritual brightness *(shenming)* emanating from heaven. The macrocosmic *shen* of heaven is channeled by the eyes, into the heart, and from there via the will, to meet the *jing* in the kidney. This is one example of how heaven within may be joined with heaven without, as the pure heart, which does not color this interaction with the mind's interpretation, manifests heaven's purpose. Hence, with some analysis, the eyes as the "gate of destiny" may be seen as an outer emanation of the inner "gate of destiny," thus resolving the apparent contradiction. A single term may be applied to different aspects of the same phenomenon, regardless of where that phenomenon is located in space. This is an important foundational principle in Chinese medicine.

Although scholars for centuries have debated the location of *mingmen*, in our discussion we are only concerned with its function. For the function of *mingmen,* like the "mysterious pass," is present in all aspects of one's being. The 36th difficult issue in the *Nanjing* states, "The kidney on the right is the gate of life . . . where the spirit essence *(shenjing)* lodges; it is the place to which the original influences are tied."[13]

Mingmen may be considered synonymous with the *dantian,* or lower cinnabar field found in spiritual alchemy. Here reside the original and authentic *yin* and *yang,* as endowed by heaven.[14] *Mingmen* is the crucible containing the infusion of one's authentic *(zhen)* water and fire. The interaction of authentic water and fire "conforms to the real nature, the deep nature of an individual."[15] Simultaneous with this interaction is the infusion of the inherited constitution (early heaven) with the acquired constitution (later heaven).

The composite term *shenjing* indicates the infusion of the activating influence of *shen* with the potential for manifestation *(jing).*[16] It is the directionality of this interaction, as focused by the will *(zhi),* that determines how well an individual is able to fully express his or her "authentic self" and how much "habitual" behavior occurs.

Establishing *ming,* as defined by Mencius, involves nourishing one's original nature within and accepting heaven without. This results in an alignment of human will with heaven's will. This alignment is synonymous, on an functional level, with the clear infusion of early and later heaven in *mingmen,* unsullied by the accretions of life's experience and habitual, mundane consciousness—hence the imagery from internal alchemy of stoking the furnace of the *dantian* to burn off the refuse of acquired conditioning and return to original nature.

Governor Vessel-10, Lingtai, "Spiritual Tower"[17]

In Daoism, *lingtai* is a term that refers to the heart. Mencius recounts the tale of how the multitudes flocked to wise King Wan as if they were his children and built his "spiritual tower" *(lingtai)* in one day. This is a prime example of the effectiveness of the role of the sage. The people "rejoiced" to do this work because the sage empowered the people so that they took pleasure in aligning themselves with his purpose. Thus by empowering the people, the emperor's own heart was in turn rectified.

This tale of the *lingtai* brings to mind the Daoist folktale of the forlorn governor who could not see over the trees surrounding his residence. So he built a tower to enable him to gain perspective on his kingdom.[18] Like the tower, Governor Vessel-10 is a point that facilitates the perspective and "penetrating insight" of the heart.

神
道

Governor Vessel-11, **Shendao,** *"Spirit Path"*

We may become addicted to the insight afforded by peak states of awareness. If we do not come down "off the mountain" (see GV-10 earlier) and make use of our knowledge in the world, then what use is the wisdom acquired there? The shock of divorce, the loss of a loved one, or even receiving a terminal diagnosis are all occurrences that may shake up our view of reality in a way that provides a glimpse of original nature. This glimpse occasionally produces a "high" or, in other words, a manic reaction. This reaction may be characterized by the momentary experience of an all-empowering vision of the significance and interrelationships of the events in one's life. The vision may be experienced in a way that had previously been hidden by one's mistaken interpretation of reality.

Consider the nature of a significant intimate relationship. The plot of the relationship consists of all the individual events from the moment the two parties meet until they part ways. The theme of the relationship is the nature of the lesson to be learned from the connection. While engaged in the relationship both parties are so involved in the plot of what is happening that the theme often eludes them. Imagine that one party to this relationship becomes dissatisfied and, over time, grows apart from the other party. Eventually, the dissatisfied partner will feel ready to leave the relationship and notify the other person of the decision to do so. By definition the theme of the relationship is what ties together every event from the first moment to the last. Presented with the end of the relationship the partner being left may be shocked out of involvement with the plot. Now that the relationship is over an all-embracing comprehension of the theme may occur in one instant. The implications of all the subtle communications and meanings that previously signaled the other partner's dissatisfaction become painfully clear.

Generally, the individual experiencing this vision appears inappropriately happy, given the seriousness of the life events in which he or she is engaged. This may be interpreted as denial. The source of this "empty joy" results from the all-embracing vision of past events coupled with feelings of unlimited potential for the future. Initially this artificial feeling of joy will fluctuate with depression and, as the person heals, these fluctuations will diminish. I have often used Governor Vessel-11 with Governor Vessel-10 for quieting the heart and sedating tendencies toward mania as well as for uplifting the heart during depression. Note that these are both important points on the governor vessel meridian for addressing the functional relationship between the heart's *ling* and *shen* spirits. These points are located on the dorsal aspect of the body directly behind Kidney-23, Kidney-24, and Kidney-25, whose importance in addressing the balance between *ling* and *shen* is discussed later.

_____

Water

Bladder-52, Zhishi, "Room of Will"; Jinggong, "Palace of Essence"

志 精
室 宮

Acupuncture point Bladder-52 is intimately associated with the relationship between the human heart *(xin)* and the fulfillment of destiny *(ming)* through the recognition and cultivation of inborn potential as stored in *jing* (essence). According to Zhu Xi, "The will *[zhi]* lies in the deepest recesses of the mind *[xin]* and therefore the doctors say the will *[zhi]* belongs to the kidneys."[19] The 34th difficult issue of the *Nanjing* tells us that "the kidneys store the *jing* and the *zhi*,"[20] and that the *zhi* is the spirit *[shen]* of the kidneys. The character *zhi* is present in the name of Bladder-52 *(zhishi)*, which has been translated as "ambition room"[21] and "room of will."[22] Bladder-52 also has the alternative name *jinggong*, or "palace of essence."[23] That the same acupuncture point may be used to simultaneously treat the *jing* and *zhi* points out the intimate relationship between them.

The "authentic" *(zhen)* heart is lost in the individual's inevitable fall from original nature *(de)*. The "memory" *(zhi)* of this true nature is stored in *jing* as a mandate from heaven. It is in directing the mind "down into" the *jing*, the depths of self, via the *zhi* (fixing the will), that the "lost" individual may rediscover heaven's commands, and return to bringing his heart back into the world fully expressed. Hence the function of Bladder-52 is to harmonize the relationship between kidney *jing*, heart *shen*, and human will *(zhi)*. With the careful direction of the practitioner, this point may serve to "soften" an overly "hard" will and protect a depleted *jing* or strengthen the will to focus the *shen* on unused potential.

The Upper Kidney Points

Three points, Kidney-23, Kidney-24, and Kidney-25, are of paramount importance in maintaining balance between the *yin (ling)* and *yang (shen)* of heart spirit.

神
封

Kidney-23, Shenfeng, "Spirit Seal"

Shen is the character for heart spirit and, in a larger sense, the active impulses that emanate from heaven. *Feng* (封) is composed of the character for earth doubled (圭), alongside the character for a hand affixing a seal of authority (寸). Wieger explains the character: "The ancient character first represented a tree upon a tumulus. . . . A knoll, surmounted with a tree, represented the imperial possession of the land. A similar knoll, but smaller, was erected in the fief granted by the emperor to a feudatory."[24] In ancient China, when the emperor invested a noble, a mound of earth would be taken from the imperial altar and placed on the noble's altar as a symbol of the emperor's authority.

The left half of the character is an image of a mound of earth erected for religious purposes. This mound represents the gods of the earth *(she:*社*)* who were worshipped in ancient China. The *she* (earth altar) stood in sacred groves, which themselves may have earlier been the object of the cult. In ancient times, mounds were marked by a sacred tree and a pole. Thus the *she* were quite open to the air. As telluric deities, it was paramount that they remain exposed to atmospheric influences in order to imbibe constantly from the heavenly *qi* and *shen*. To deprive them of power, as in the conquest of a state, it was necessary only to enclose them with a roof and walls, thereby shutting off their access to sunlight and air.[25]

When the Shang empire was overthrown, their *she* was enclosed with an opening that faced north so that only debilitating influences could reach it. Here the potential power of earth *(yin)* had been cut off from the sunlight *(shen)*, the activating influences from heaven. Thus the power of the dynasty dwindled as it lost its mandate from both heaven and emperor. This scenario is similar to what happens in the individual when he receives only influences from the north (water element) and no activating impulses from the south *(shen,* or heart). Cut off from the warmth of his "sealed" heart, the power that stems from his mandate *(ming,* or destiny) diminishes.

In the following passage, Zhuangzi virtually describes the genesis and progress of kidney depletion to which this point speaks:

> Men's little fears are mean and trembly; their great fears are stunned and overwhelming. . . . They fade like Fall and Winter—such is the way they dwindle day by day. They drown in what they do—you cannot make them turn back. They grow dark as though sealed with seals—such are the excesses of their old age. And when their minds draw near to death, nothing can restore them to the light.[26]

This is a person whose heart spirit has been sealed so that the *shen*, the brightness of life, cannot manifest and activate his inborn potential. The patient for whom this point is indicated may show a lack of authority on all levels. Often he may exhibit a sense of being out of touch with his purpose in life and his spiritual identity. "Spirit seal" can help establish the realization that no external confirmation in life is needed to choose a course of action. We need only follow the inner knowing that this direction is present in our heart, placed there by heaven, the highest authority. Ultimately, "spirit seal" may help restore the interaction between the potential present in the kidney official and the mandate from one's own heart and the heart of heaven *(shen)*.

Kidney-24, Lingxu, *"Spirit Burial Ground"* 靈墟

The etymology of the character *ling*, as discussed earlier, relates to the power and potential of the heart spirit to effect change. *Xu* (虛) means emptiness or that which contains nothing,[27] and used as a medical term, it means deficiency or exhaustion. The character *xu* pictures two men on a hill looking in all directions, yet nothing can be seen, for they are in a high upland that is wild and barren. The imperial burial grounds in ancient China were located in exactly such places[28]—hence with the addition of the earth radical (土)we produce the homophone *xu* translated as "burial ground."

Ling appears in the title of the *Lingshu*, the "spiritual axis." Both characters *xu* and *ling* are associated with the potentiality of the empty vortex whirling between heaven and earth. According to the *Dao De Jing*, the *dao's* axis is "empty *(xu)* yet inexhaustible,"[29] and it is precisely this emptiness which gives the *dao* its use.[30]

When the aspect being addressed by Kidney-24 is in balance, an individual may feel connected to the wellspring of *dao*, life's greatest resource, and experience himself as a potent and effective force in the world. Kidney-24 is indicated therapeutically when the potential *(ling)* to manifest in life is exhausted *(xu)*, giving the sense that the *ling* spirit has died. The patient's life may appear like a barren wasteland, scorched by the impulses of the heart's *shen*, with little manifestation of potential. With the *ling* spirit dried up and depleted, the individual may grow sad as he becomes increasingly cut off from his spiritual source and power in life. This exhaustion on a basic level may be predicated on a weakened *jing* and deficient *yin*. The patient evidences an internal spiritual crumbling, which parallels the physical disintegration taking place as his life's resources dry up.

Point Kidney-24 speaks to the spiritual aspect of the imbalance by treating the relationship between the heart and the kidneys in the upper burner. "Spirit burial ground" can help restore the patient's experience of himself as a potent force in the universe by returning him to his spiritual source. The functional quality present in this point may be likened to bringing water to the desert so that life may flourish.

Kidney-25, Shencang, "Spirit Storehouse"   神藏

The first character, *shen*, as in Kidney-23, indicates the heart spirit. The character *cang* means to hide or conceal and also has the meaning "storehouse."[31] Here we are given the image of a reserve of spirit *(shen)*, which is stored in the heart. Thus, when a patient's *shen* is deficient or hidden, Ki-25 can act as a storehouse of spiritual energy.

Cang is a homophone of the character *cang* (藏), meaning compliancy. This character is an image of an official kneeling prostrate before his master whose authority may be symbolized by the halberd.[32] "Spirit storehouse" may not only access a reserve of *shen*, but also help the heart (emperor) enforce its commands with authority and garner the respect it deserves from its officials (the other functions in one's inner kingdom of being).

Analysis of Relationship Among Kidney-23, Kidney-24, and Kidney-25

Acupuncture points Kidney-23, Kidney-24, and Kidney-25 address the *shen, ling,* and *shen* spirits, respectively. Assigning a solid *yang* line to each of the *shen* points (Kidney-23 and Kidney-25) and a broken *yin* line to the *ling* point (Kidney-24) produces the *Yijing* trigram for fire *(li)* (see Figure 13.1).[33] These points lie on the kidney meridian, a meridian associated with water, over the heart, an organ associated with fire in the upper burner, which corresponds to heaven. Hence these points relate intimately to the spiritual alchemy of water and fire, *ling* and *shen*. They address the most fundamental level of balance between the *yin* and *yang* of the human spirit. The functional balance of *ling* and *shen* is essential if life is to proceed effectively and with spontaneity.

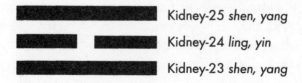

Kidney-25 *shen, yang*

Kidney-24 *ling, yin*

Kidney-23 *shen, yang*

Figure 13.1
LI, THE TRIGRAM FOR FIRE

Wood

Gallbladder-24, Ri *and* Yue, *"Sun and Moon," "Illumination"* 明

After the death of Pan Gu,
his breath became the wind and clouds,
his voice the thunder,
his left and right eyes the sun and moon . . .
– Shu Yi Ji (sixth century)[34]

The name of this point comprises the character for sun *(ri:日)* placed next to the character for moon *(yue:月)*. Together these characters compose the character *ming* (明), which denotes the enlightenment of the sage whose all-embracing vision is able to find the unity in apparent opposites.[35] The tendency of the gallbladder official is to become split, perceiving alternatives as being either good or bad, black or white. This can result in an internal tearing apart that may result in the one-sided symptomatology often associated with the gallbladder official. Judgments of good and bad, beautiful and ugly, split the world apart in a way that does not follow the spontaneity of *dao*. Hence Gallbladder-24 may be useful for empowering a patient to perceive the fundamental unity behind what he imagines are diametrically opposed alternatives in life. In this way we may gain a perspective that harmonizes judgment and constraint. I have also found this point to be useful for treating people who are overly optimistic or pessimistic—able to see only the good or bad in life.

Liver-1, Dadui, *"Great Esteem"* 大敦

As the wood point associated with a wood official, Liver-1 addresses the essence of the wood element. "Great esteem," the first point on the liver meridian, is located on the big toe, which provides our physical root and grounding. This point empowers the specific virtue of self-esteem, which emerges from the vision of those principles that spring from our essential nature, rooting our life. In pruning a plant, we may remove unessential branches so growth may be channeled in a more fruitful manner. However, the roots that anchor the plant into its "ground of being" must not be compromised. When basic principles are compromised, as often happens when intimacy is betrayed, self-esteem erodes. Compromise becomes gradually easier until we may no longer have a vision of our true nature. This imbalance is often evidenced in someone who acts as though any compromise is a personal affront. This point may empower the discernment of those aspects of self that (1) may be compromised (the branches), and (2) those which are fundamental principles (roots) that must be supported and preserved. Note that the character *ben* (本), which translates into English as the words "fundamental" and "basic," depicts the roots of a tree.

Fire

Heart-2, Qingling, "Blue-Green Spirit"

⌒   QING   ⌒

The character *qing* is composed of the character for plants growing [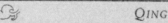] over that of an alchemical furnace [丹] with cinnabar [丶] in it. The image contained in the character *qing* is that of the alchemical transformation and generative power of growth that takes place in plants during spring. The character *qing* is used to represent the "blue-green" color of this growth, and the *Nanjing* assigns the liver the color *qing*.[36]

Alchemy, Ritual, and the King's Heart

The transformative fire of life is found in humans in the cinnabar field, or *dantian* (丹田), the internal alchemical furnace. In medicine, the "life gate fire" seems to take over the role of the cinnabar field in alchemy. Cinnabar is listed in the *Shen Nong Ben Cao* as the first herb in the upper class of those that nourish destiny. According to the *Ben Cao,*

> Cinnabar tastes sweet and is slightly cold, it cures the hundred diseases of the body and the five *cang*. It nourishes the *jingshen,* makes the *hun* and *po* peaceful and benefits the *qi*. It brightens the eyes and kills demons and injurious ghosts. If you take it for a long time you can communicate with the spiritual brightness *(tong shenming)* and you will not grow old.[37]

Cinnabar is considered the strongest herb to calm the heart, bringing stability to the emperor who presides over our inner kingdom of being. Several emperors died of cinnabar toxicity, apparently poisoned by their court alchemists.

The name of Heart-2, *qingling* is the name of the terrace that the emperor went to in order to receive spiritual influences[38]—hence the location of this point on the heart meridian. In reference to the character *ling,* Wieger points out that in ancient China, the shaman's most important role was being able to elicit rain from the heavens. The emperor's role was not so different in that his duty was to be in charge of the performance of rites. In the *Yijing,* hexagram 51 corresponds to the "blue-green dragon," the arrival of spring. The hexagram tells us that even though the thunder may roll and spread terror for a hundred miles around, the ruler remains so "composed and reverent in spirit" that the sacrificial rite is not interrupted. Wilhelm continues, "This is the spirit that must animate leaders and the rulers of men—a profound inner seriousness from which all outer terrors glance off harmlessly."[39]

In this context *qingling* may address the emperor's power to invoke rain from heaven, essential for new growth in spring, through the performing of rights. In general, *ling* may be thought of as the emperor's or heart's potency, as derived from fulfillment of his mandate *(ming)* to rule in an effective manner.

An individual with a heart in which the *ling* spirit is unbalanced may show up as out of synch in life. Symptomatically, this may appear as stuttering, heart palpitations, or insomnia. The individual may also appear shaky and frightened.[40] When the *yin* and *yang* of heart spirit is balanced, then things proceed "as if they were done by no one." Confucius refers to this balance of *ling* and *shen* spirits indirectly when he says that Shun, the great sage king, "merely placed himself gravely and reverently with his face due south; that was all,"[41] for "With correct comportment, no commands are necessary, yet affairs proceed."[42]

King Xuan, in the *Book of Odes (Shijing),*[43] reports to heaven his overwhelming feeling at not being able to perform ritual effectively. He blames his own failure as resulting in a tremendous drought:

The drought is already too extreme!
Scoured, scoured the hills, dried the streams;
The demon of drought exercises his ravages and his oppression.
Like fire burning in the Heart-like fire burning in the hedges—
My lonely Heart is as dried as the heat of summer;
Sorrow in my burning Heart is like the clouds of steam rising from fire;
The many virtuous men of the past!
Its serious consequences they do not hear or understand,
Vast as heaven the above ruler
Be willing to enable me to retire.[44]

The pathology of the emperor's heart is similar to the fate of his nation. With his potency to perform ritual effectively in question, his own heart fire rages and he begs heaven to change its mandate and his destiny *(ming)*. Perhaps a return of spiritual balance, well addressed by the points covered here, would have helped restore harmony to the nation and the heart of the good king.

Small Intestine-19, Ting Gong, "Listening Palace"

聽
宮

> *Don't listen with your ears, listen with your mind.*
> *No, don't listen with your mind, but listen with your spirit.*
> *Listening stops with the ears, the mind stops*
> *with recognition, but spirit is empty and waits on all*
> *things. The way gathers in emptiness alone.*
> *Emptiness is the fasting of the mind.*
> – ZHUANGZI [45]

The function of the Small Intestine-19 is archetypal of the relationship between the heart and small intestine officials. The character *ting* (聽: listen) is etymologically related to the characters, both pronounced *de*, which refer to the rectitude of the heart (悳) and original nature (德).[46] The character *ting* (listen) is composed of the character that stands for the rectitude of the heart (悳) combined with that for the ear (耳) of the disciple (壬) who is listening attentively. The overall sense imparted by this character is that, through attentive listening, one's heart may be rectified. From the imagery of the character *ting*, we might define the ability to "listen" as the ability to hear our heart and the hearts of others without deviation. We who are "listening" in this way are able to know the nature of things immediately in our heart, directly bypassing the analytic faculties of our mind. Therefore, the capacity of listening may be said to empower intuition. The character *gong* (宮) designates the imperial private residence from the Qin dynasty.[47] This allusion to the emperor places further emphasis on the relationship between "listening" and the heart official as emperor in one's inner kingdom.

The Spirit of Listening

Confucius alludes to the importance of "listening" when he describes for us the stages of his inner evolution. He tells us that, "At sixty, my ear was an obedient organ for the reception of truth. At seventy, I could follow what my heart desired, without transgressing what was right."[48] Confucius, in saying that his "ear was an obedient organ for the reception of truth" precisely elaborates the quality of listening that was necessary for the ensuing rectification of his heart.

Hence "listening palace" provides a functional link between the small intestine and heart officials via the "aspect of being" termed "listening." The small intestine is like the emperor's (heart's) closest minister. Its functions are to relay to the emperor (heart official) the essence of what is going on in the nation (the other officials as well as the outside world) and to relate the essence of the emperor's intention to the nation.

Our sense of listening may be affected as we habitually reject momentary reality. Practitioners in the inner tradition should be aware that attentive listening on our part may contribute to the healing of another's heart.

Heart Protector and Triple Heater

> *[A] thousand illuminations, myriad illuminations,*
> *are all two illuminations, inward illumination and*
> *outward illumination, which in totality are one*
> *illumination; therefore it is called fire.*
> *– YIJING*[49]

The heart protector and triple heater may be thought of as the guard stations protecting the imperial city and the borders of the country, respectively. This functional relationship is exemplified in the names of acupuncture points Heart Protector-6 and Triple Heater-5. Termed "inner frontier gate" and "outer frontier gate," respectively, these points regulate the inner and outer aspects of the fires which burn in the "gate of destiny" *(mingmen)*. In fact, the *Yijing* hexagram for fire, *li* (離), appears to depict these two gates (Figure 13.2).

Note that in the names of these two points the character *guan* (關), rather then *men* (門), is used to denote the concept of "gate." The character *men*, as in *shenmen* (Heart-7, "spirit gate"), indicates an ordinary gate such as we might find in a garden. The character *guan*, however, gives the idea of a manned gate at a nation's boundary such as we might find at a customs station. Hence its translation as "frontier" gate is in keeping with the function of the fire officials in establishing boundaries.

Both Heart Protector-6 and Triple Heater-5 are junction *(luo)* points that serve the function of balancing the flow of *qi* between coupled *yin* and *yang* meridians. These two points functionally unite the heart protector and three heater officials in a way that empowers the healthy balance of social and intimate relationships.

Figure 13.2
HEXAGRAM 30, FIRE

*The hexagram for fire (*li, *"the clinging") consists of the trigram for fire doubled and appears to depict the inner and outer frontier gates. The trigram for fire consists of one* yin *line indicating water, bordered by two* yang *lines indicating fire. The image of water within fire recalls the kidney fire associated with the heart protector and three heater officials.*

Triple Heater-5, Waiguan, "Outer Frontier Gate"

One virtue of the *luo* points on the *yang* meridians is that they are able to drain the external pathogen which harms their associated element. Hence Triple Heater-5 relieves exterior and hot conditions. In this respect Triple Heater-5 is like a gate that may vent internal pressure and relieve the entire continuum of function represented by the fire officials. This point may treat a patient whose fire is externally focused as a means for preventing intimacy. This may manifest as excessive social chatter that never touches the heart of the matter. Another example is someone who makes too many social commitments as a means of avoiding intimacy with his or her mate. This point may also empower someone to come out of his or her shell and initiate social contact. Outer frontier gate regulates the external boundary along a continuum of imbalance ranging from an inability to journey up to or past borders to moderating the behavior of one who is habitually driven toward the superficial expression of his or her fire element.

Heart Protector-6, Neiguan, "Inner Frontier Gate"

As the gate to our inner frontier, Heart Protector-6 is an important point for directing our intention into the depths of our heart. Further, this point may evoke the influence of the heart and thus make our experience of our heart a conscious process. I have found this to be a paramount point for calming a restless heart and quieting a mind confused by issues of an intimate relationship. "Inner frontier gate" is a central point effective for treating betrayal of intimacy as occurs in rape, incest, or divorce.

Earth

Stomach-25, Tianshu, "Heavenly Pivot"

The name of this point recalls the earth element as the central pivot around which the seasons and *dao* revolve. Located on both sides of the navel, St-25 addresses the nature of our center as a fixed reference point that may empower stability during transitions. This point empowers the virtue of being able to move dynamically in any direction without excessive deliberation.[50] *Tianshu* is a name for the central star in the Big Dipper constellation, the residence of the spirits *(shen)* who preside over one's destiny.

Spleen-21, Dabao,"Great Enveloping"

The character *bao* reveals in its etymology the image of a fetus surrounded by the womb.[51] Spleen-21 is the great *luo* point that sends collaterals branching around the entire torso and effectively surrounds each person with an enfolding, motherly embrace. The term *baoyi* (包一) in Daoism means to "embrace the one." This evokes the image of the Daoist making the spiritual journey of restoring original nature *(de)* and returning back to the womb by patterning himself on the primal *dao*. The inner nature of Spleen-21 is to empower us to feel surrounded by unconditional nourishment in life as though still within the womb.

Metal

Lung-9, Taiyuan, "Very Great Abyss"

Dao is a whirling emptiness (chong),
Yet in use is inexhaustible.

Fathomless (yuan),
It seems to be the ancestor (zong) *of*
ten thousand things.

– DAO DE JING [52]

The basic movement of *dao* is like a great whirlpool, rising and falling like a bellows, giving birth to all things at its periphery and receiving them back at its center. Lung-9, in being named *taiyuan,* is associated with the whirling abyss situated between heaven and earth. Hence Lung-9 is the assembly point of the pulse whose beating is patterned on the breath of *dao.* An alternate name for Lung-9 is *taiquan* (太泉: great spring), which denotes the origin of a stream.[53] Lu-9 as both *yuan,* the abyss, and *quan,* the source, calls forth the image of the queen mother's metal gate that serves as the womb and tomb for all of creation.

Large Intestine-4, Hegu, *"Joining of the Valleys"*

Here at the entry point of the large intestine meridian, the functions of receiving (lung) and letting go (large intestine) are joined. The image of the valley in Daoism is a symbol of emptiness. The virtue of emptiness is that it empowers us to be receptive to the essential nature of life. The *Yijing* hexagram for modesty tells us that, "the superior man reduces that which is too much, and augments that which is too little. He weighs things and makes them equal."[54] In her comment on this hexagram Anthony states, "To equalize extremes is part of the natural law. A haughty, pretentious attitude stands like a narrow, steep mountain that is constantly being attacked by the elements; as a consequence, it erodes into the valley. The valley, likewise, because it is a depression, receives all that erodes into it"[55]—hence the name, "joining of the valleys."

Water: The Return

Kidney-7, Fuliu, *"Returning Current"*

On the seventh day comes return.

– YIJING [56]

In the Daoist enumeration of being the number seven corresponds to both the loss and return of original nature. The importance of Kidney-7 in breaking the husband/wife imbalance is such that it merits particular attention. Named "returning current," Kidney-7 is the metal point and the tonification point on the kidney meridian.[57] The functional dynamics of the transition from hexagram 23 to 24 as described earlier precisely correspond to the function of Kidney-7. Hexagram 24, "the return," is representative of the reappearance of *yang* within the primordial *yin* and the continual renewal of water that occurs on the winter solstice. The Book of Balance and Harmony states, "The inner medicine is the primordial point of true *yang*, the celestial. It is likened to the center line in the *Yijing* trigram heaven. When it mates with earth, that forms water. The center line [of the trigram for water] represents true inner sense, which is firm and hence symbolized by metal, so it is called metal in water. These are all names for ultimate vitality. When the ultimate vitality is stable, it reverts to generative energy."[58] It is this generative "energy" that fuels another round of evolution as the seasons of life move along the *sheng* cycle. In this same manner Kidney-7, as the metal point within the water element, tonifies kidney *yin* and *yang* so that the integrity of the primordial *qi* remains strong, the fires of *mingmen* are kindled, and the influence of heaven is not exhausted by mundane *yin* influences.

An alternate name for Kidney-7, the key point for helping a patient return, is *waiming* (外命), meaning "beyond destiny."[59] This name indicates that, if one has "failed to return at the correct time," physical illness may have proceeded further than treatment is able to restore. For the illness now has its own life and has gone further than even the fulfillment of destiny can resolve. In this usage Kidney-7 may still help the patient in his transition from life to death as he returns to the primal *dao*.

Summary

Acupuncture points do not exist as discrete anatomical structures. In the physical domain, acupuncture points appear to comprise a unique relationship between nerve, muscle, tendon, blood vessels and arteries, and bones. The relationship that exists between things is not physical, but rather functional, and therefore cannot be directly measured. Similarly, acupuncture point function is neither discrete nor fixed in nature. Rather, acupuncture points address many overlapping domains of being and their effects are purely contextual. Any given point may be used effectively to harmonize any functional imbalance upon which any physical symptom is predicated in a particular person at the right time. Emperor Yu interviewed the spirits of the rivers, mountains, and marshes of China and in so doing received heaven's mandate to unify the nation. By learning the inner nature of the acupuncture points, the practitioner of the inner tradition may receive heaven's mandate to restore unity in the patient's inner kingdom of being.

Questions

1. Would your knowledge of acupuncture point function empower you to contribute to someone's healing if you could not physically touch the point?

2. How much of the efficacy of a given acupuncture point can be attributed to the physical placement of a needle?

3. How much of the efficacy of that point lies in focusing the intention of the practitioner on the functional relationships which are out of balance in a patient's being?

NOTES

1. For ease of reading, in this chapter the practitioner is assumed to be female, the patient male.
2. Note the functional similarity between acupuncture points and the nature of Chinese characters as I discussed earlier. Point function as well as the meaning of a given character both evolve in relation to the development of human awareness.
3. Sun Tzu, 1973, Chapter 6, line 28.
4. Along with *chongmo* and *daimo:* Larre, Schatz, and Rochat de la Vallee, 1986, p. 144.
5. Porkert, 1982, p. 279.
6. Ibid.
7. Lagerwey, 1987, p. 43.
8. Ibid., p. 154.
9. Ellis, Wiseman, and Boss, 1989, p. 344.
10. Wing-Tsit Chan, 1973, p. 22.
11. Unschuld, 1985, p. 200.
12. Unschuld, 1986, p. 385. I have changed Unschuld's translation of the character *ming* from "life" to "destiny."
13. Unschuld, 1986, p. 382.
14. See Homann, 1976, p. 8.
15. Larre and Rochat, 1985, p. 46.
16. The term *shenjing* is assumed here to be equivalent to the more usual appearance of these characters: *jingshen.* See Porkert, 1982, p. 193.

17. Translation mine.
18. Van Over, 1973, pp. 179–180.
19. Munro, 1985, p. 312.
20. Unschuld, 1986, p. 367.
21. Worsley, 1979.
22. Ming, 1982, p. 295.
23. Ellis, Wiseman, and Boss, 1989, p. 180.
24. Weiger, 1965, p. 205.
25. Bishop, 1933, pp. 24–43.
26. Watson, 1964, p. 32. The reference to receiving light brings to mind the point Bladder-6 ("receiving light").
27. Weiger, 1965, pp. 80–81.
28. Fischer, 1930. The burial grounds and mausoleums of many of the emperors contained the character *ling* in their name.
29. Chapter 5; in Chen, 1989, p. 5.
30. Chapter 11; in ibid., p. 82.
31. Mathews, 1931, p. 985.
32. Weiger, 1965, p. 214. Although the characters are homophones and very similar in appearance, they do not necessarily share the same etymology. Nevertheless, the information yielded from their comparison is still interesting.
33. For an explanation of the symbolism of the *Yijing*, see Wilhelm, 1968.
34. As quoted by Girardot, 1983, p. 194.
35. Chen, 1989, p. 123. Another acupuncture point that may address this aspect of vision is GV-24.5 (Ex-HN3, or *yintang*), which is not named in some traditions. Naming creates duality and a "two-eyed" vision of self that is separate from the *dao*. GV-24.5 addresses the function of the "third eye," which grants one the insight that comes from the vision of unity.
36. Unschuld, 1986, p. 170.
37. *Shen Nong Ben Cao.* Cinnabar is the first herb discussed in the *Ben Cao*. This passage can be read to imply that it enables us to be in contact with *(tong)* the emanations of our own heart *(shenming)* and/or the heart of heaven.
38. Lecture with C. Larre (1986). *Ling* not only interacts with our own *shen* but may provide the facility for our communication with heaven. Thus it is our *ling* that attracts heaven's *shen*. In the performance of ritual it is an individual's potency *(ling)* that may summon a response from heaven.
39. Wilhelm, 1968, pp. 197–200.
40. These symptoms may indicate the use of cinnabar therapeutically with formulas such as Tian Wan Pu Xin Wan that treat deficient heart *yin* (*yin* being associated with the *ling* aspect of spirit).
41. Fingarette, 1972, p. 4.
42. Ibid.
43. Ayscough, 1930, p. 111.
44. Ibid.
45. Watson, 1964, p. 54.
46. Weiger, 1965, p. 37. See analysis of the character *de* in the text.
47. Ibid., p. 228. Note that the characters *sheng ren* (聖人), denoting the sage, signify one who has listened to (耳) and understood advice (呈), and therefore became wise (Wieger, p. 211). The character *sheng* is etymologically related to the character *ting* meaning "listen."
48. Legge, 1971, p. 146.
49. Cleary, 1986, p. 126.
50. Similar to the function of GB-30, "jumping circle," but from the orientation of

earth (stability) rather than wood (perspective).

51. Weiger, 1965, p. 144.
52. Chapter 4; in Chen, 1989, p. 61.
53. *Quan* is a spring that gushes out from the ground. "In the middle the bubbles gush up from the earth; on the top, the water expanding; on the sides, the flowing." Weiger, 1965, p. 289.
54. Wilhelm, 1968, p. 64.
55. Anthony, 1981, p. 14.
56. Wilhelm, p. 97. The number seven corresponds to the return or loss of original nature. The seven holes in the human head correspond to the senses and self-awareness. It is in retracing our steps and closing these apertures that we are able to experience the true reality that lies within.
57. Note that the *Bai Wen Bian* (The Hundred Questions), a late eighth-century alchemical text, calls the kidney the "metal radiance" *(jinguang)* and "metal essence" *(jinjing)*. Homann, 1976, p. 48. Homann fixes the time of this text to the school of Lu Dongbin, who was born in C.E. 755.
58. Cleary, 1989, p. 22.
59. Hicks, 1985, p. 16.

14

THE
INTAKE[1]

The Nature of the Diagnostic Process[2]

The goal of the diagnostic process is threefold. First, it offers an opportunity to assess an individual's five-element constitutional type, as well as the important deficiencies, excesses, and stagnations, all of which may be harmonized with acupuncture and herbal medicines.

Second, the diagnostic process involves collecting a detailed patient history that may be used as a reference point for assessing the patient's progress as treatment proceeds. Finally, the diagnostic session should help establish rapport between the practitioner and patient and, most importantly, initiate the patient's process of healing.

One of the most powerful approaches I have incorporated in my practice is helping the patient comprehend the connection between specific symptoms and his beliefs, thoughts, and actions. In the inner tradition, acknowledging those connections is the foundation of true healing, and allows us as practitioners to give patients the greatest gift we can: an opportunity to heal themselves. The first opportunity for directing the patient's attention to these fundamental relationships and initiating him into the process of healing is afforded during the initial diagnostic sessions.

The verbal aspect of the diagnostic process may be divided into outer and inner components. On an outer level, the questions asked by the practitioner are necessary to ascertain specific information from the patient. Additionally, every interaction with a patient offers an opportunity for establishing trust and rapport. Therefore, on an inner level, the practitioner must have clear intention regarding the manner in which each question is asked and be absolutely clear about the nature of the messages she is sending and receiving. The dynamic context for the communication that the practitioner consciously creates is relatively more important than the specific meanings of the spoken words.

Similarly, a patient's responses to the practitioner's questions also consist of an outer and inner component. Superficially, the content of the patient's answers is informational. During the course of the interview each answer contributes to an elaborate story. As in a book, the story changes with every sentence as the interview progresses. However, the main concern of the practitioner is not with the unfolding story, but rather with its theme. For the practitioner, of utmost import in forming a constitutional diagnosis is the way in which the patient relates dynamically to the events described during the telling of his story. Hence one patient may display the theme of loss and grief (associated with the metal element) while discussing his parent's divorce. Another patient may manifest neediness and a lack of sympathy (which establishes a theme associated with the earth constitution) while discussing the same material. Therefore, it is the nature of the inner theme revealed during the diagnostic process that is of primary concern in establishing a constitutional diagnosis and assessing the quality of the patient's unique destiny.

General Guidelines

Ask Open-Ended Questions

Questions must be phrased in a way that allow the patient the greatest liberty in his response. For example, consider the relatively "closed" question, "What is your address?" This offers the patient little latitude in interpreting the question; the practitioner will generally receive only numbers and a street name.

The practitioner whose purpose is directed to the deeper functional aspects of the patient's response is more concerned with how the patient interprets the questions he is asked. The patient's interpretation is dictated by his constitutional type and, therefore, the responses will be deeply revealing regarding the nature of his fundamental imbalance. One may, instead, rephrase the preceding question to, "Where is your home?" Of course, a patient may respond with an address. However, the open-ended nature of the question may evoke a more personal expression of the patient's relationship to the concept of home. For example, the patient might respond, "I haven't had a home since my father died." The elemental expression present during this response could then establish any number of themes relating to constitutional type. For example, a theme of anger and resentment associated with the wood constitutional type might be established.

Every question, no matter how mundane in content, is an opportunity to deepen rapport and to glean information about the fundamental nature of the patient.

Avoid Undue Focus on the Presenting Complaints and Attempt to Ascertain the Patient's Needs Indirectly

Patients often know what they want, not what they need.[3] My clinical experience has made me a firm believer in the general truth of this statement. The specific symptomatic complaint for which a patient comes to receive treatment is often representative of his desire to be comfortable and to be rid of physical pain. This tends to be true to the degree that the patient's life is dictated by unconscious habitual reaction.[4] Because pain is often the result of separation from one's inner nature, in virtually every case, a deeper reason exists for seeking treatment. From the perspective of the inner tradition, this arises from the will of heaven attempting to express itself spontaneously in a way that supports the patient's evolution. To eliminate physical pain without also endeavoring to direct the patient's attention toward his inner purpose may be to perpetuate ignorance. Thus one of the unique features of the inner aspect of Chinese medicine is its ability to promote conscious awareness in people who are drawn to treatment solely for relief from physical symptoms.

In order to glean the unconscious reasons for seeking treatment, during the intake and thereafter, the practitioner's inquiries should not continually focus on the patient's symptoms. When one proceeds in this manner, it may become apparent that patients often will not emphasize their symptoms either.[5] The more one discusses something, the more "real" it becomes. Undue focus on the patient's presenting complaint will tend to reinforce the reality of the condition and does not contribute to a timely healing. In most instances it is more beneficial to help patients understand that the context in which their symptoms occur is defined by their diverse patterns of function in all realms of being.

Observe and Listen Expectantly

In light of my clinical experience, a primary assumption underlying diagnosis may be stated as follows: All of who a patient is manifests in every nuance of personal expression in every moment. As such, every interaction with the patient offers an opportunity for achieving the three primary goals of diagnosis just discussed. A patient's response to any seemingly mundane question may contain the "golden key" that grants the practitioner insight into the patient's depth and path of healing. Therefore, the practitioner must maintain an attitude of open-mindedness to the myriad nuances of the patient's responses. Equally important is allowing the patient time to initiate conversations and questions.

The Intake

The diagnostic process begins with the practitioner's initial experience with the patient. In my practice this frequently occurs when I listen to the messages left on my answering machine.

The Telephone Answering Message

I have often found that I am able to formulate an accurate constitutional diagnosis after hearing the patient's voice on the answering machine. This information may be significant. Consider, for example, (1) the patient's ability to clearly state his purpose in calling; (2) the cadence of his voice; (3) the quality of breath; (4) the capacity to listen and follow directions (e.g., does he have to call back a second time to leave his phone number as requested, or to clarify the previous message?); (5) the sound of his voice in accordance with the five-element associations; and (6) what is happening in the background (for example, Are children screaming? Is someone interrupting? How is he responding to this input?). Hence merely from a simple phone message, with the proper focus, the practitioner may glean a wealth of information.

The Return Telephone Call

Here, again, a great amount of diagnostic information may be available in the form of emotional and elemental responses. Further, the return call presents the opportunity to initiate the process of healing. After identifying myself, I ask, "How may I help you?" This begins to reinforce the notion that help may be available and also requires the patient to make a request for this process to commence. The patient's response to this question may also inform the practitioner about (1) his capacity for speaking up for his own needs; (2) his relationship to hope as reflected in his belief that help may be available; and (3) his clarity regarding the reasons for seeking treatment.

After discussing general concerns regarding the patient's desire for treatment, the conversation then turns toward scheduling an appointment. This part of the conversation offers an ideal opportunity to observe the patient's relationship to time, which may yield insights particularly into the function of his wood element and heart official.[6] One may also note (1) the patient's relative decisiveness and flexibility in determining a specific appointment time, and (2) the patient's response if he must wait for an appointment. I usually schedule 90 minutes for an initial appointment.[7] I conclude the conversation on a positive note by suggesting the prospective patient be optimistic that treatment will be effective.

Initial Meeting

On first meeting the patient, I utilize a wealth of sensory information that has direct bearing on the diagnosis. I often try to catch a glimpse of the patient coming up the walkway. I note possible differences in the patient's comportment when he is not aware of being watched as compared to any changes on entering the office.

Immediately on meeting the patient, I extend my hand in greeting and attempt to make direct eye contact. The patient's ability to sustain eye contact is an important indicator of the overall integrity and quality of his functional state.[8] The practitioner may also note the following from the handshake: (1) the quality of contact; (2) the quality of warmth; and (3) whether or not the patient clings to the practitioner's hand as it is withdrawn.[9] Many other factors may be noted, including the quality and style of the patient's attire, jewelry, facial characteristics, and movement. Such observations may be helpful in supplementing the primary diagnostic criteria for determining a constitutional diagnosis according to five-element associations, which include the patient's color, sound, odor, and emotion (CSOE).

The Treatment Room

The treatment room is a special space and should be made conducive to the process of diagnosis. I always have the patient sit near a window so that available light may help facilitate assessment of his color. I previously arrange my chair and the patient's chair about three feet apart. This distance is close enough to allow me physically to touch the patient at an appropriate time during the verbal intake and potentially glean the nature of his response to this contact. On sitting down, it is always interesting to note if the patient moves his chair closer to mine or farther away.

On entering the room I instruct the patient to "please have a seat in the red chair on the left." I note whether or not these instructions are followed. I then ask the patient how he learned about me. Because virtually all of my patients are referred by word of mouth, this question helps establish rapport through the common bond of someone he knows and trusts. If the patient is wearing glasses, I then ask if he would mind removing them in order to facilitate my diagnosis (of facial characteristics as well as the color emanating from the area of the lateral canthus of the eye). The patient's response may provide information relevant to his (1) vision, (2) ability to trust, and (3) flexibility.

Lastly, I inform the patient what to expect during this session. I explain that I will be asking many questions, that he is free to answer each to any degree he is comfortable with, and that it is fine to notify me if a topic comes up he is not comfortable with. This reassures the patient and helps him feel safe in the diagnostic process.[10]

A chief task of the traditional practitioner is to create the proper context in which healing may occur for each patient. The creation of this context is afforded with every communication prior to and concurrent with the placement of an acupuncture needle. This includes the cultivation of the proper atmosphere in the treatment room, the altar on which the ritual of acupuncture occurs.

The treatment room itself is a sacred space and should be

approached as such. I have discovered that in no other place are my healing abilities as focused or effective as in my primary place of practice. Personally, and in your patients, cultivate a sense of quietude and respect for this special place. Patients have remarked that they feel a sense of relaxation and peace even as they approach my office.

The Interview

The order of the questions is designed to build trust gradually by easing the patient into the examination. The history consists of three sections: (1) The general background appears to be superficial, concerning his family's health history, his job, and his relationships; however, it may contain subtle clues relevant to the patient's diagnosis and specifically regarding his boundaries; (2) The second part involves the patient's reasons for seeking treatment; (3) The third part covers the patient's basic patterns of function as reflected in his lifestyle and habits.

General Background

The first part of the interview has a twofold purpose. On an outer level it eases the patient into the exam with a discussion of his general background and family history. During this part of the exam, a patient often feels he is talking more about others than himself, which helps relax him. However, I find this part of the intake provides some of the most important information relevant to the patient's constitutional diagnosis and prognosis. In my experience, the way a patient relates to his parents and siblings, career, intimate relationships, and/or his own family are key predictors of health and balanced function in all realms.

The family in which we are raised provides both our genetic endowment (early heaven) and our early environment (later heaven). If the patient's relationship to family members plays a significant role in perpetuating patterns of habitual behavior, it will become evident in all aspects of his expression when this topic is discussed. Patients who have major unresolved issues with family members (such as incest or physical abuse) most often carry those issues forward into their intimate relationships with their own spouses and children. Thus the functional theme of a person's life, which is synonymous with his destiny, frequently emerges during the discussion of these significant relationships.

FAMILY
    Q: Where did you grow up?
    Q: Do you still have family there?
    Q: How is your father's health? mother's? sibling(s)?
    Q: Are you close to them?

RELATIONSHIP
    Q: Are you in a relationship?
    Q: For how long?
    Q: How is the relationship for you?
    Q: How is your partner's health?
    Q: Do you have children?
    Q: How is their health?
    Q: Are you close to them?

IF NOT IN A RELATIONSHIP
    Q: How long has it been since you were in a relationship?
    Q: Is not being in a relationship an issue for you?

IF DIVORCED OR SEPARATED[11]
    Q: Why did the relationship end?
    Q: Was it your choice to end it?
    Q: Have you been in another relationship since?

IF MARRIED SEVERAL TIMES
OR WITH A HISTORY OF FAILED RELATIONSHIPS
    Q: Are you aware of any similarities among your various relation-
       ships and the reasons they ended?

In my experience, the degree to which a patient exhibits awareness of his own patterns reflects the degree to which a positive prognosis may be made. It is important for the practitioner to discern between true awareness and mere repetition of a story or interpretation regarding the event. This is particularly important because some patients may have arrived at an intellectual understanding of their life story through assorted therapies, which does not necessarily correlate to the process of deep healing. A traumatic event may still be blocking the patient's progress regardless of the degree of his intellectual understanding. I find that Chinese medicine can be unique in harmonizing the unbalanced *qi* upon which dysfunction is based.

CAREER

   Q: What do you do for a living?

   Q: Do you enjoy your work?

   Q: Is there something you would rather be doing?

Ideally, career choice should be an expression of a person's deepest inner purpose; however, this is not always possible. The time we spend engaged in earning a living represents a significant portion of life. Therefore, I don't believe it is possible to be entirely healthy working in an intensely disliked occupation. The way we relate to our occupation often serves as a potent metaphor for the state of our general health and well-being.

Reasons for Seeking Treatment

When queried about the reasons for seeking treatment, the patient will often not mention his primary complaint or may place little emphasis on it. Rather than continually asking the patient to elaborate on the condition he has already described, I offer him several opportunities to discuss his deeper reasons for seeking treatment. At this point in the exam I often ask, "What benefits would you like to get from receiving acupuncture?" This is an open-ended question that may allow a greater truth to emerge.

To reiterate, the degree of the patient's understanding relative to the deeper nature of his symptoms reflects the degree to which his prognosis may be positive. In my clinical experience, denial is one of the primary bases of illness.

Patterns of Function

I gather information relevant to the patient's general function and daily habits. This information is interpreted in the context of the patient's constitutional type and is not of primary diagnostic value. It may, however, serve as a reference point when assessing the patient's progress and path of healing. Further, this information may influence both herbal prescription as well as acupuncture point selection.

SLEEP

   Q: Do you have difficulty falling asleep or staying asleep?

   Q: What time do you wake up? (to determine the correspondence to the Chinese clock)

Generally, I am most concerned with what the patient is doing when he is not sleeping. A patient with "wood" insomnia will often lie awake either regretting the past or reviewing current emotional material. His mental conversations usually revolve around things he should have done, ought to be doing, or what he is planning to do.[12] I have often found that patients who are awake and working productively and/or whose minds are active and do not fall asleep until after 3 A.M. (the transition of "wood" time to metal) will often sleep more easily if they go to sleep around 10 P.M., before the wood element reaches its high point at 11 P.M.

Earth insomnia presents as a feeling of constraint and worry in which the patient is bound by his own, sometimes obsessive, thoughts.[13] Metal insomnia is often indicated by waking at about 3 A.M. (the transition of the wood to the metal element). Often the patient will be either grieving for what has been lost in the past or experiencing a vague longing for something that seems continually to withdraw beyond his grasp into the future.

I find that water insomnia often presents as a pattern in which the kidney function is not appropriately controlling heart function across the *ke* cycle. In this relationship, the function of the kidney (associated emotion = fear) is unbalanced and is pathologically paired with a continual inappropriate opening and closing of the heart. In my experience, all types of insomnia in some way fundamentally stem from or agitate the heart and, thus, therapeutic attention to the heart in conjunction with other involved organs is appropriate in most cases. Although I have discussed different types of insomnia as being associated with different elements, this information is not of primary significance in determining constitutional type. Rather, it indicates that a particular element is under stress.

ENERGY

Q: When is your energy at its highest level? Lowest level?

Q: When was the last time your energy was consistently good?

The more recently the patient has experienced good energy, the better the prognosis. As in all cases, the practitioner must weigh the patient's response with her own assessment. For example, a patient may report feeling that his energy is good, but mumble in a weak voice while slouching in the chair.

FOOD
APPETITE
CRAVINGS
DIGESTION

BOWELS

URINATION

MENSTRUAL PERIOD
REGULARITY
DIFFICULTIES

Of course, a woman's menstrual cycle is deeply tied to her health and reflected in all aspects and levels of personal expression.[14] Further, menstrual problems may often represent complex relationships between physiological function, sexuality, and intimacy as it relates to the inner function of blood according to Chinese medicine.[15]

PREGNANCIES
DIFFICULTIES
FREQUENCY

Information about pregnancies may yield useful insights into the functional state of a woman's earth element relative to the ability to create a healthy balance between her needs and those of others (her children, partner, etc.). For example, does she ask for sympathy for the pain felt during the birthing process? Or does she downplay what was actually a difficult and painful process that may have involved surgery? Is resentment expressed regarding the pain, indicating possible unbalanced function of the wood element? Or the patient may discuss this material in a balanced way, indicating a healthy-functioning earth element.

The frequency of pregnancies may have some bearing on patterns of *qi*, blood, and, ultimately, *jing* deficiency.

CIRCULATION

SURGERIES

It is often interesting to note if a patient feels somehow changed after undergoing surgery. I recall one patient who, after having his appendix removed, commented that he felt years of bitterness and resentment had been taken from him.

I have not commented at length on the preceding categories relating to the patient's patterns of function. I sense that my interpretation of this material is probably not significantly different from other traditions of Chinese medicine. Paying close attention to the manner in which the patient is relating to his discussion of these and all other topics during the intake is an important aspect of the inner tradition.

HABITS AND MEDICATIONS

Information about habits and medications is particularly relevant in assessing the patient's pulse. All of the following substances may affect the patient's presentation and the pulse in unique ways:

MEDICATIONS

COFFEE AND CAFFEINE-CONTAINING BEVERAGES (E.G., BLACK TEA, COLA DRINKS, ETC.)

TOBACCO

RECREATIONAL DRUGS (TYPES, FREQUENCY, ETC.)

ALCOHOL

VITAMINS, HERBS, AND SUPPLEMENTS

The patient's use of these substances also reflects his overall condition and the degree of concern for his own health. In my experience, habitual reaction is the source of all illness, and as such, addictive behaviors are indicative of deep imbalance. A rule I have found to be true regarding a patient's habits is that patients are generally unaware of many specific patterns of behavior related to their addiction. Of course, being unaware of one's own behavior is a hallmark indicator of habitual patterns of behavior. For this reason, rarely will a patient provide accurate information about the frequency and amount of alcohol, cigarettes, or coffee he consumes. The practitioner will have to pursue the reliability of this information. For example, a patient may state that he drinks only one cup of coffee daily, unless he is "under stress." But knowing that the patient is an air traffic controller, for example, may lead the attentive practitioner to suspect her patient's consumption may be somewhat higher than stated!

Of course, the usage of any of the substances just listed may diminish the value of diagnostic information gleaned from the pulse. However, I have found that substance abuse and medications do not often negatively impact the ability to determine a patient's constitutional type by his color, sound, odor, and emotion (CSOE). Given the percentage of people using these substances and the degree to which they alter the pulse, I consider this to be of significance when comparing an assessment of the pulse with that of the patient's CSOE. It is important to be aware of the vitamins and herbs a patient may be taking because these may interact negatively with the practitioner's own prescriptions.

PREFERENCES

Information regarding preferences is of secondary importance and may support a diagnosis of a specific constitutional type. Additionally, the patient's clarity regarding his preferences may also be significant.

SEASONS
LIKES, DISLIKES

COLORS
LIKES, DISLIKES

ADDITIONAL TOPICS
Q: If you could change anything about your life, what would it be?
Q: Where would you like to be in ten years?
Q: Is there anything that we haven't discussed that is important to you?

This last question is phrased in such a way that it ends the interview leaving the patient with a feeling of being "taken care of," yet being in control of the current process.

Pulse Diagnosis and General Physical Considerations

The shift from the interview to the physical exam marks an important turning point in the diagnostic process. During the interview, the patient's mind has been engaged with his responses. However, these demands are suspended during the physical exam, which is usually conducted with the patient quietly lying down or sitting. This phase of the intake offers the practitioner an opportunity to assess how the patient responds to physical contact in contrast to verbal communication.

Generally, I ease the patient into this part of the exam by talking in a quieter and less direct tone of voice. I endeavor to create an environment in which the patient's mind becomes quiet and receptive. It is at this point that I ask specific questions I may have saved until this time. For example, if I suspect that a woman has received some form of sexual abuse, I may wait until an appropriate moment during the pulse diagnosis to ask if she has such a history. I find it helpful to be in direct contact with the pulse while asking and receiving responses to such potent questions.[16] I make it a practice not to suggest to patients that they were sexually abused. Rather, I pose the possibility as a question that may be easily dismissed depending on the content of, and quality of expression in, the patient's answer. It is always better to allow emotional material to emerge on its own. If an issue is relevant therapeutically, patients will bring it up as they are uniquely ready to deal with it.

Concluding the First Session

Upon completion of the interview, tongue and pulse diagnosis, and evaluation of general physical considerations, I briefly explain the fundamental ways in which Chinese medicine is complementary to Western medicine.

This explanation entails a discussion of how Chinese medicine views health and well-being. I describe the nature of destiny and individual purpose according to the themes which have arisen during the interview within the framework of the patient's constitutional type. I then discuss the patient's specific health concerns within this context. This part of the exam affords the important opportunity of helping the patient to make specific connections between his illness, lifestyle, beliefs, and behavior patterns.[17]

Note that I rarely perform acupuncture or prescribe herbs during this initial meeting; I do so only if the patient is in acute distress. My focus is on establishing rapport with the patient, while gathering information necessary to formulating a diagnosis. Generally, I prefer to allow the patient to assimilate, on its own merits, the quality and nature of the contact made during this session before receiving treatment, so he has a clear understanding regarding his commitment to treatment.

I always leave the patient with a warm handshake, reaffirming once again that he be optimistic about receiving the help he is seeking through treatment.

Assimilation of Diagnostic Information and the Cultivation of Intuition

The process of diagnosis too often involves compiling long lists of observations, which are then categorized according to the limited theories of a diagnostic system. This is often done at the expense of creativity, the cultivation of intuition, and trust in one's own "knowing." It occurs to me that this is perhaps rooted in modern models of standardized education based on an analytic, causative thought process. Generally, I find that my practice of Chinese medicine proceeds best according to a delicate balance of theory and intuition.

During all parts of the interview the practitioner must listen attentively to several "voices" simultaneously, keeping them distinct. Externally, you must distinguish between the superficial information and the deeper thematic messages emanating from the patient's heart that are striving for expression. Internally, you must be aware of two other levels of your listening. The loudest inner voice generally represents the function of your own mind as it organizes the incoming material according to whichever system(s) you have learned. However, you must also listen attentively for the messages that spontaneously arise through the intuitive function of your own heart.

For example, while you touch the pulse during diagnosis, listen to what your intuitive voice is saying, rather than only attending to the formalities of interpretation. When appropriate, follow up on your intuitions by substantiating the accuracy of insights you have gained in this manner. In this way you may remain grounded by verifying your intuition.

If you touch any position on the pulse and sense an inner voice suggesting the patient is considering a divorce, for example, then you might ask the patient how his relationship is going and note the quality of the patient's response. Only in being willing to miss the target will you ever be rewarded with a bull's eye. Over time, your aim will become increasingly accurate with the result that, as the spontaneity of your practice gradually increases, you will become less and less burdened by the constraint of theory. Hence each session provides you with the opportunity to cultivate the highest aspect of diagnosis, which is merely to "look and know."

Formulating a Diagnosis and Treatment Plan

In general, my process of formulating a diagnosis involves first identifying the patient's constitutional type. This process is usually rapid and occurs within the first few minutes after meeting the patient. Unless compelling information to the contrary arises during the exam or later treatment, I generally stay with my constitutional diagnosis indefinitely. Constitution is the thread that joins together all observations regarding the relative balance of all functional relationships. The patient's constitutional type may, therefore, guide the practitioner's intuition in interpreting diagnostic clues as the interview unfolds. Arriving at a constitutional diagnosis allows me to identify the virtues that are trying to emerge spontaneously. In part, these virtues define specific inner changes that will occur as healing proceeds, thus allowing for the close monitoring of progress in treatment.

Having established a five-element constitutional diagnosis, I then proceed to evaluate how the patient's physiology is expressing itself in relation to his constitutional type. This is done by comparing my observations of the pulse, tongue, and eyes with the dynamics of the constitutional diagnosis. I then proceed to formulate short-, intermediate- and long-term therapeutic goals.

The short-term goals usually involve achieving relative stability in the patient's life by first dealing with the most obvious aspects of habituated functioning. This phase may involve addressing obvious behaviors such as addictions (e.g., coffee, drugs, tobacco) or other self-destructive habits. In terms of the pulse, this means addressing the larger issues such as stability of rhythm, rate, and intensity. I often think of this stage of treatment as taking a person out of "shock," defined here as habituated behavior that keeps a person from self-discovery. At this stage, acupuncture may be used to clear the therapeutic field by addressing specific "blocks" to balanced functioning. Blocks which need to be cleared include aggressive energy, akabane imbalances, husband/wife imbalances, exit/entry blocks, and possession.[18] These blocks all have the potential to prevent sustained improvement in function if they are not attended to. Conversely, clearing any of these blocks may initiate a return of the constitutional influences as the guiding force in a patient's life with a corresponding improvement in any and all symptomatology. In terms of herbal treatment, this stage of therapy often entails administering formulas that are clarifying and stabilizing.[19] If no blocks are determined to be present then the primary strategy usually involves a direct focus on integrating the functioning of the *yin* and *yang* officials associated with the patient's constitutional type.

As an intermediate and often secondary goal, I generally address the patient's main complaint. Of course, this may be done simultaneously with the short-term plan at the beginning of treatment. As habituated behavior decreases, there is often more authentic *qi (zhenqi)* available for healing. Thus this phase of treatment generally involves harmonizing the functional dynamics of the constitutional officials with the other officials involved in the pattern of dysfunction. For example, if lung (metal) is primary and heart protector (fire) is secondary, this stage of treatment might involve the harmonization of the balance between metal and fire across the *ke* cycle. During this stage of treatment I may introduce formulas that are constitutional in nature, in addition to formulas that are resolving or harmonizing.

My long-term strategy generally involves integrating the function of the constitutional organs with the functioning of the rest of the officials around the *ke* and *sheng* cycles. Hence, if a person is constitutionally metal, over time I would integrate the function of the associated organ systems (lung and large intestine) with the element's mother (earth), child (water), grandmother (fire), and grandchild (wood) in an order appropriate to the functional dynamics of the situation. This stage of therapy often involves administering one or two long-term herbal formulas that are constitutional in nature.

Of course, these are only general considerations, and you must assess the merits of each individual case. If there are signs of impending serious illness such as cancer or heart disease, you need to address them directly and aggressively in the initial stages of treatment. Furthermore, with occasional patients I sense that if they do not experience quick symptomatic relief, they may not return for further treatment. In such instances, constitutional points always serve as the basis for whatever local or symptomatic points I may treat.

Treatment Schedule

Generally, I see patients once each week for six to eight weeks. I find that this is enough time for people to have a sense they are receiving benefit from the treatments. After that, I see the patient every other week, once every three weeks, and then monthly. In serious cases involving aggressive and debilitating illnesses such as rheumatoid arthritis or multiple sclerosis, I may see a patient initially up to three times each week.

I find that an initial interval of one week between appointments affords me the opportunity to assess the effectiveness of a particular treatment as well as the patient's ability to sustain the effects of that treatment. After the first session it is not unusual to have the patient report having felt better for one or two days and then reverting to the state they were in before the session. As treatment progresses the duration of benefit should increase in proportion to the patient's degree of awareness of the patterns of dysfunction which propagate his symptoms. As the benefits of treatment begin to last an entire week the frequency of treatment is then moved to two weeks. In this way the patient's inner resources are empowered to guide the process of healing as dependency on treatment diminishes.

My goal is that each patient should derive sufficient benefit from treatment that they consider it worthwhile to continue coming at a rate of about every six to eight weeks. For most people, I consider the first six months to a year of treatment to be a time of "leveling the playing field." By the end of one year, most patients are receiving treatment at the longer intervals just mentioned. Once progress has been made with the initial complaints, and grosser levels of addictive behavior (tobacco, alcohol, etc.) have been removed, I find the opportunity arises to directly pursue the preventive and evolutionary aspects of therapy offered by Chinese medicine.

Ultimately, I find that three years constitutes sufficient time for most patients to restore a deep lasting balance whereby the patient is not likely again to lose contact with "original nature," regardless of the magnitude of challenging events in his life.

My treatment regimen is in contrast to the practice of acupuncture therapy in modern China. There, patients typically receive acupuncture every day for an extended period (perhaps ten days in a row), with a short break of a day or two, followed by another course of ten days treatment if needed. I believe that this frequency of treatment is imposed by the state-run health care system whose main interest is the symptomatic relief of pain so that people may return to work quickly. I also believe this approach represents a practice of acupuncture that is governed by principles more suited to herbal medicine. Here acupuncture point "prescriptions" are given daily in much the same way as a patient would be expected to take herbs.

Interestingly, in the ancient Chinese medical texts describing acupuncture therapy, there is virtually no mention of acupuncture frequency or overall duration of treatment. The role of the acupuncture points are discussed, and specific treatments (point selections, methods of inserting, stimulating, and withdrawing needles) are mentioned for particular ailments. However, overall treatment plans are never elaborated. In my view, this suggests that each acupuncture treatment stands alone as it is based on the unique merits of each clinical encounter.

Questions

1. What tools exist in your own tradition of practice to help you see past the plot of a patient's story to the theme?

2. Once you have discerned the theme of a patient's life does it seem to relate more to acquired or inherited characteristics?

3. What diagnostic tools would be necessary to ensure that you were considering an equal balance of these two influences?

4. To what degree does your specific diagnosis of a patient contribute to the outcome of the treatment?

5. To what degree do the parameters that you use to assess a patient's progress limit your view of how the patient's health might be improving?

6. What would happen if you never mentioned the patient's symptom by name unless the patient brought it up?

NOTES

1. For ease of reading, in this chapter the practitioner is assumed to be female, the patient male.

2. The style and principles of diagnosis discussed here are based on those taught at the Traditional Acupuncture Institute (TAI) in Columbia, Maryland. I elaborate this information as it is consistent with my own style and clinical experience.

3. A goal central to my practice is promoting the patient's ability to know what lies in his own heart. There is always a quality of objectivity available when the patient is receptive to input from a practitioner who has been empowered to guide one's process of healing. Knowing oneself is not mutually exclusive of receiving direction from others regardless of the degree of conscious awareness that one has obtained.

4. Many people are not aware that Chinese medicine is capable of addressing deeper issues. Therefore, if a patient is focusing solely on physical issues during the intake, I often inform him that Chinese medicine is capable of addressing many aspects of function which affect health and ask if there are any nonphysical issues that he wishes to address in treatment.

5. Through a multitude of diagnostic procedures, the practitioner may, of course, monitor the progression of the patient's symptoms in many ways less explicit than directly asking about them. It can be equally important, however, to direct a patient's attention to the subtle ways that his symptoms are improving. The practitioner needs to direct her own attention toward striking a reasonable balance between these two approaches.

6. Liver function is associated with planning and gallbladder function with decision making. As emperor, the heart is responsible for clear insight and the performance of ritual (being in the right place at the right time).

7. Generally this is divided as follows: 35 minutes to gather information verbally, 40 minutes for the pulse diagnosis, and 15 minutes to explain my findings and answer questions.

8. Inability to sustain eye contact may be indicative of the existence of "shock" that has disintegrated the balanced functioning of the fire officials, thus disturbing the delicate balance of the heart's *shen* and *ling* spirits. This observation, along with other signs of chaos, may also be indicative of "possession."

9. A patient who clings to the practitioner's hand may be manifesting a need for contact and warmth. Note that "clinging" is the translation of the *Yijing* hexagram for fire.

10. Ultimately, the patient must be conscious of the fact that he is in the office of his own volition, having extended his own initiative in asking for help. Only occasionally do patients seem especially uncomfortable with particular questions

regarding their personal life. Most people seem pleased that I take the time to discuss their concerns with them. However, the nature of the material that a patient wishes not to discuss may be as revealing as any answer he might have given.

11. I use the term "divorce" here to signify that a long-term relationship to which the partner had made a major commitment has ended.

12. It is as though the patient is haunted by ghosts of regret and indecision that keep him awake. I have found GB-44 [Gallbladder-44], the metal point on the GB meridian, to be ideal for this type of insomnia. The metal within wood may empower the wood to "let go," thus empowering the healthy balanced control of metal over the wood element.

13. It is as though the patient is like a plant that is constrained and being choked by its own roots. In this regard I have found Spleen-1, a point often used to treat insomnia, to be most useful. As the wood point on an earth meridian, Spleen-1 may help to reestablish a balanced relationship between the wood and earth elements. Its effect may be likened to taking a root-bound plant and transplanting it into a larger pot so that it may thrive. My interpretation of this point's inner function was gleaned from a set of old lecture notes attributed to J.R. Worsley. When using Spleen-1 in this fashion I generally pair it with Stomach-43 (wood point) and Stomach-8, whose name may be translated as "head tied," for one who is bound by his own thoughts.

14. I find that the menstrual cycle provides a type of outlet valve that may allow women to express pent-up feelings on a regular basis so they do not accumulate. I have seen PMS completely disappear in women after merely suggesting that their feelings of anger or frustration were real and should be attended to rather than being dismissed as "just being PMS." In general, I think that the outlet provided by women's menstrual cycle tends to make them more emotionally healthy than men. Compare, for instance, a woman who becomes emotional once each month for a few days with a seemingly "emotionally stable" man who may be diagnosed by his physician to be "in good health." For lack of an outlet, however, the man may eventually go into a sudden rage that appears to "come from nowhere."

15. See Jarrett, 1995a, 1995b.

16. The pulse may afford the practitioner with an opportunity to receive immediate feedback from specific officials and organ systems pertaining to the quality of the question and the patient's response. The ability to extract this information from the pulse is a diagnostic skill that I plan to elaborate on in future writing.

17. On occasion, practitioners of other traditions have expressed their concern about intervening at the level that I access in treatment when a patient has only come for a sore shoulder. In this regard, I explain to each patient my view of his or her condition and what treatment will entail. Hence each patient has a clear view of the agreement he or she is making when receiving treatment. I must also emphasize my belief that patients often know what they want and not what they need. If they had known what they needed, and had had the will to take the appropriate actions, they would most likely be well and not be seeking treatment.

18. The presence of an akabane imbalance suggests that one or meridians are unbalanced in the relative quantity of qi available to the left and right channels of the meridians involved. For example, it may be determined that the gallbladder meridian has a relative excess of qi in its channel on the right side of the body and a relative excess of qi in its course on the left side of the body. Such imbalances are usually associated with one-sided symptomatology and are generally treated using the involved meridian's *luo* points.

19. See Jarrett, 1995b (pp. 132–134), which covers herbal therapy utilizing Yunnan Paiyao, Meridian Passage, and Sheng Mai San in this regard.

15

CASE
STUDIES

THIS CHAPTER PRESENTS TWO DETAILED CASE STUDIES
using the constitutional perspective discussed in Chapter 9. I have
included the first eight to ten acupuncture sessions with each patient,
along with my point selection, herbal prescription, and assessment of
progress. These applications offer a broader perspective of the theory
set into practice. It goes without saying that each clinical case is unique
and must be assessed on its own merits. In each case study, I have provided enough background information to allow the inquisitive reader
to follow the logic of my point selection process.

CASE 1: KATHRYN

I have treated Kathryn since April 1994. Only her initial treatments
are included here in order to convey the essential components of her
case and to offer a glimpse of my approach.

Sex/age: Female, age 33

Height: 5' 4"

Weight: 144 pounds

Reasons for seeking treatment: (1) cervical carcinoma in situ;
(2) concerns about emotional stability.

Color: Yellow

Sound: Singing

Odor: Fragrant [1]

Emotion: Excess sympathy

Constitutional type: primary—earth (spleen);
secondary—fire (heart)

General Impression

First Telephone Communication

The message Kathryn left on my answering machine was short, yet her voice clearly had the singing tone associated with the earth element. During our first conversation, she informed me that she was scheduled for a cone biopsy, subsequent to a positive Pap smear and punch biopsy. She was interested in knowing if acupuncture and herbs could help her avoid the procedure. I suggested that it would be best to have the procedure and to schedule our initial appointment for a time shortly afterward. I assured her that her concerns were within the scope of my practice, and in addition to addressing her physical concerns, she could look forward to feeling better overall. She seemed quite open to this suggestion and welcomed the reassurance. Her general openness to what I had to say was a positive sign.

First Meeting

Kathryn greeted me with a warm smile as she entered my office. She was dressed neatly and colorfully and wore several silver rings and an ankle bracelet. Very attractive, she appeared about twenty pounds overweight for her height. Her face and body were round and full, and her color was clearly yellow. Her odor was fragrant. The warmth and quality of her smile and overall presentation were "enveloping," engendering a welcoming quality that gave the impression of a deep desire both to nurture and be nurtured. This tendency corresponds to the emotion of sympathy associated with the earth constitutional type. Throughout the process of diagnosis, I allow myself to free-associate names and functions of acupuncture points that match the patient's momentary dynamic, and in this instance, the names of Spleen-21 ("great enveloping") and Stomach-9 ("people welcome") came to mind. My initial impression of Kathryn, which was verified throughout the diagnostic process, was of an earth constitutional type, specifically spleen.

Highlights of Intake Interview

General Background

Parents

Kathryn's parents were divorced when she was 9 years old, and she was raised by her mother. When she mentioned the divorce, she exhibited a rapid fluttering of her eyelids, which I identify with dissociation.[2] This behavior immediately alerted me to the possibility of problems, perhaps "shock," related to her parents' divorce.

Father

Response: Kathryn gave very little information about her father's history, except that he had developed psoriasis at age 20 while in military service. As she said, "He's in agony," her eyelids fluttered rapidly. At this point, her yellow color became vibrant and the singing tone in her voice changed to a monotone. (Both signs are associated with the earth constitution. I associate the monotone with a type of barrenness that is the opposite, or absence, of the singing quality. The monotone quality can be likened to the dull drone of insects during late summer.)

Impression: The flatness of Kathryn's voice was present simultaneously with what appeared to be repressed anger and the lack-of-shout quality associated with liver disharmony. This fluctuation suggests that the earth element was under immediate stress in response to the material being currently discussed and that the wood element might have been overcontrolling earth across the *ke* cycle. The image of her father in agony with an aggravating skin condition suggested that some inner emotional issue may have been "eating away" at him. The pairing of the father's agony with his daughter's repressed anger and its undermining effect on the stability of her earth element suggested to me that, in some essential way, the relationship between Kathryn and her father was a key factor in her dysfunctional dynamic.

Mother

Response: Kathryn mentioned her mother's physical condition, including an unspecified seizure disorder and angioedema.

Impression: There was no specific waver in Kathryn's functional balance as she discussed her mother that suggested any emotional content worthy of deeper analysis. Her mother's disorders suggest unbalanced functioning of the nervous system.

Overall impression: Both parents' health problems are consistent with unbalanced function of the nervous system.[3] This suggests that Kathryn may be contending with a genetic (and possibly karmic) background of nervous system disorder. If there is a karmic component, Kathryn may be able to resolve the issue in this lifetime, a possibility having direct bearing on the fulfillment of her destiny.

Marriage

Response: Kathryn has been settled for six years in what she describes as a "good" marriage. While answering this question, she exhibited ambivalence, a quality I often associate with a dysfunctional relationship between the small intestine and spleen officials.

Impression: When Kathryn described her marriage as "good," her ambivalence became apparent in a hesitancy in her voice; her response seemed much more like a question than an assertion of fact. Her ambivalence suggested several diagnostic possibilities: First, emotional pain from her past may be affecting her marriage in the present; and, second, she may have a tendency to portray outwardly things as all right when, in fact, they are not. This tendency to be ingratiating is a strong indicator of the earth constitutional type. (An observation of this type, essential to constitutional diagnosis, emphasizes the importance of discriminating between the patient's story and the functional dynamics or theme underlying the story.) At this point, I chose not to press Kathryn further on the nature of her marriage, preferring instead to allow this information to surface at her own pace during the interview.

Children

Response: Kathryn said she had no children and that the wisdom of having children in the future was a big question in her mind. Because of her own psychological instability, she was concerned she might not be a good mother. She also feared becoming overwhelmed by the responsibilities of caring for children.

Impression: Her response indicates a good degree of awareness of the issues involved in having and caring for children and the seriousness of the decision. (As discussed earlier, the degree of the patient's awareness of issues indicates the degree of likelihood of a positive prognosis.) On this issue, Kathryn revealed an ability to be introspective and honest with herself. Her concerns about her own needs relative to the needs of a child and about being a good mother evoke the imagery of an unbalanced earth element. A sense of reciprocity, a virtue associated with the earth element, must emerge between mother and child if the relationship is to nourish both parties.

Career

Response: Kathryn is employed as an American Sign Language interpreter. She enjoys her work, whose nature suggests a desire to assist and serve others (again, characteristic of the earth type).

Impression: This is an example of how the constitutional theme of an individual's life often manifests in the chosen field of work. Given that a major life task for Kathryn lies in gaining awareness of her habitual tendency to be ingratiating and in cultivating the ability to speak up for herself, it is interesting that her work empowers others to communicate without using the spoken word.

Reasons for Seeking Treatment

Cervical Carcinoma in Situ

In response to receiving a positive Pap smear test several months before, Kathryn had a conization in which carcinoma in situ was excised from her cervix.

She reported that her menstrual cycle had begun at age 14 but lasted only one day. She became so distressed by the appearance of her period that it did not recur for another two years.

Impression: This finding suggests a strong link between her emotional state, her emerging sexuality, and vulnerability associated with blood. It is likely Kathryn experienced some traumatic event during that time of her life. Currently, her menstrual cycle is regular because of the birth control pill she has taken daily since age 19 (over fourteen years). However, before taking the pill, her cycle had always been irregular. She still has some pain with cramping, and her menstrual blood is dark and clotted. She reported usually feeling "depressed and on edge" for one week before each period.

Concerns About Emotional Stability

Kathryn reported that she experienced a "complete break with reality" in 1991 that occurred after using a nicotine patch to quit smoking. Over four consecutive nights, she developed nightmares and insomnia, leading to treatment and counseling in an outpatient psychiatric unit. She exhibited episodes of paranoia that included "imagining triangles of relationships with other people." Having been left by a previous boyfriend who had an affair with another woman, Kathryn was constantly worried that her husband was also in love with someone else and would eventually leave her too. This quality of worry is an extreme example of the obsessive thoughts that I associate with the earth constitutional type.

Kathryn reported that she had also been hospitalized for cocaine addiction and alcoholism in 1986. Her cocaine use occurred over a seven-year period; during the final several years, she used the drug three to four times weekly and also drank alcohol heavily. When she stopped using these substances simultaneously, Kathryn experienced a severe withdrawal reaction. However, in an attempt to protect her father, who had been selling the drugs to her, she failed to mention her drug use to her physicians, who proceeded to diagnose her as psychotic and treated her accordingly. (This is a classic example of the tendency of the earth constitution to take care of others' needs rather than their own.) It was at this time that Kathryn was able to admit to herself that she was an addict, and she began the process of recovery.

At the time of our interview, Kathryn had been drug-free and sober for seven years. She attributed her addictions to an attempt to avoid the pain of the relationship that had ended with such difficulty. But in actuality the use of drugs had begun before the end of the relationship, and I guessed that the emotional pain from the breakup was just one of several factors contributing to her habitual behavior.

In response to my question, "What would you like to see for yourself five years from now?" Kathryn answered, "I want to feel at peace and feel connected to spirit." Kathryn's awareness of her spiritual journey began during participation in twelve-step programs after her hospitalization for drug addiction. She had read *A Course in Miracles*,[4] a text frequently used by groups focusing on addictive behavior, as well as studied Native American spirituality.

It is important to note that Kathryn did not mention her presenting symptom of carcinoma in situ during the portion of the interview focusing on her reasons for seeking treatment.

Patterns of Function

Sleep

Kathryn has experienced no sleep problems.

Exercise

Kathryn lifts weights and uses a treadmill two to three days weekly.

Energy

Her energy level has been "average"—high in the mornings and dropping in the afternoon about 3 P.M.

Appetite

"My appetite is okay. I try to eat good food. Eating fruit in the morning helps my energy. I try to avoid eating protein and starch together. My digestion is all right now but has been bad historically."

Cravings

Pasta and sweets.

Bowels

"My diet now helps, but I tend toward constipation. In the past, my bowels fluctuated between constipation and being loose."

Surgeries

In 1992 a swollen lymph node was removed from her breast. She reports feeling ongoing breast tenderness.

In 1994 a cervical conization for carcinoma in situ was performed.

Substance Use

Coffee: One cup daily

Alcohol: No consumption for seven years

Tobacco: No use for two years

Recreational drugs: No use for seven years

Medications: Birth control pill

Preferences

Colors: Likes blue and purple; dislikes yellow.

Seasons: Likes fall and winter.

Analysis of the Interview

Constitutional Analysis: Destiny and Virtue

My initial assessment of Kathryn's color, sound, odor, and emotional state was substantiated throughout the interview, confirming her as an earth constitutional type. Other findings were consistent with the manifestations of the earth type, including (1) high energy in the morning, which is earth time (stomach: 7–9 A.M.; and spleen: 9–11 A.M.) according to the Chinese clock; (2) poor digestion and fluctuating bowels, indicating deficient spleen *qi* and a weak digestive system; (3) cravings for sweets, associated with the earth constitution; (4) a dislike of the color yellow, associated with the earth constitution; (5) insecurity about becoming a mother, a role requiring full exercise of all virtues of the earth type; (6) dysplasia and carcinoma of the reproductive organs, which are the physical bases of reproduction and mothering and associated with the earth element; and, finally, (7) mucus on the tongue, suggesting deficient spleen *qi*.

Kathryn's unbalanced relationship to nurturing and sympathy was apparent in a dynamic that emerged during the interview. Each time I offered concern and support while discussing her symptoms, addictions, and hospitalizations, she would relax, becoming more grounded and centered as worry momentarily subsided. However, my nurturing did not seem to have a lasting effect on shifting her expression away from the themes of the earth element (a need for more sympathy and support) to which she continually returned.[5]

I was continually impressed by Kathryn's empathy. She often seemed to be on the verge of tears, which gave me the sense of her desire to give to others and to have others know how much she cares. Her need to take care of others was also evident in the apparent compassion she displayed for her father. She was apparently suppressing her natural instincts toward anger in an attempt to take care of him instead of herself. This dynamic is inherent in the earth constitutional type, whose destiny is to transform ingratiating behavior into the virtue of integrity, manifesting as a balanced relationship between fulfilling one's own needs and the needs of others.

Kathryn's tears were accompanied by a brightness in her eyes, suggesting that she was overwhelmed by both joy and pain in her heart. It was as if she were frustrated by never feeling sated in either giving or receiving nurturing and support. These qualities immediately called to mind several acupuncture points. Her quality of earth neediness, combined with her heart sorrow, suggested the functional dynamic contained in the exit/entry combination of Spleen-21 and Heart-1.[6] The constant welling up of tears called forth the image of Stomach-1 ("receive tears"), and her display of and need for sympathy conjured up the function of Stomach-9 ("people welcome").

As stated, the virtues associated with the earth element are sincerity and reciprocity. In the course of treatment I expected Kathryn would exhibit more balance in her ability to trust that her sincerity and heart are felt by others. Concurrently, she would manifest greater ability to stay grounded and centered within herself, rather than constantly spilling out emotionally in the form of tears. I also expected that the virtue of reciprocity would progressively emerge, strengthened as her need to give and receive constant support subsided.

The Issue of Betrayal

Throughout the interview, Kathryn exhibited numerous signs of betrayal, suggesting to me that she may have been a victim of incest perpetrated by her father. I noted these, but chose to wait until I could evaluate the pulse for signs consistent with this diagnosis before broaching the subject with her. As detailed later, the pulse itself reflected a great deal of instability and other qualities that further suggested she had received an emotional shock of great magnitude. At an appropriate moment during the pulse exam, I quietly asked her if she had ever been sexually abused. Tears welled up in her eyes as she revealed several episodes of incest with her father, beginning when she was 14 years old. Although clearly upset, she was unable to express anger; but it was apparent she needed to be comforted. She again displayed compassion for her father even when tearfully discussing the pain of incest.

The following findings, when taken together, alerted me to the possibility of betrayal as an etiologic factor in Kathryn's imbalanced condition. The dissociation evidenced by the rapid flickering of her eyes when discussing both her parents' divorce and her father's skin condition provided my initial clue that she had received a substantial shock to her heart. The dynamic between her suppression of anger and the instability of her constitutional element (earth) was strongly present while discussing her father's skin condition. This indicated to me that perhaps her relationship with him was the primary factor in her functional imbalance. That her father was supplying her with cocaine, and she attempted to protect him during her hospitalization for withdrawal, was objective evidence of the dysfunctional nature of this relationship.

Kathryn's hesitancy in stating that her marriage was good, along with her obsessive fear that her husband would leave her, suggested that perhaps habitual patterns from the past were preventing her from having a fulfilling relationship in the present. Although it was true she had been hurt in a previous relationship, it was my assessment that her pattern of behavior and emotional instability predated that particular incident.

Her addictive behaviors began during her mid-teens, strongly suggesting that, even at that early stage, she was already struggling to avoid some great emotional pain. Particularly telling is that she became so emotionally disturbed at starting her menstrual period that it did not return for another two years. From the perspective of Chinese medicine, we can only wonder what sort of functional insult could contribute to this dysfunction. My assessment is that the intensity of suppression of both her sexuality and the function of her associated organ systems contributed to her presenting symptom of carcinoma in situ. This condition may be seen as a direct physical correlate of damage to the spiritual aspect of blood (a congealed blood pattern), which can occur as a result of betrayal. That the quality of her blood was compromised is also suggested by the presence of dark, clotted menstrual blood and a finding of engorged purple veins under her tongue (see later).

The presence of congealed blood may be viewed as a separation of oneself from pain that is too threatening to integrate into one's conscious awareness. I believe that the "complete break with reality" Kathryn experienced when she quit smoking represented a turning point and the beginning of a process of integrating the emotional material generated by her experience of incest. My findings on the pulse further confirmed my suspicion of "shock" associated with betrayal.

Pulse Diagnosis and General Physical Considerations[7]

Tongue: Kathryn's tongue showed a bit of mucus. The veins underneath were purple and engorged.

Pulse: I begin every patient's diagnosis by taking the pulse on all six positions simultaneously. This allows me to quietly orient myself to the larger picture on the pulse while creating an atmosphere of stillness in the room. My observations of Kathryn's pulse follow.

General Pulse Findings

Rate (BPM): Beginning: 75; end: 70; with movement: 72

The overall quality of Kathryn's pulse showed continuous changes in intensity, rate, and amplitude. This finding indicates a condition of "chaos" predicated on compromised heart and attendant circulatory function. The heart is the emperor presiding over our inner kingdom. Instability of the magnitude found on Kathryn's pulse may indicate that heart function is so compromised, it provides little foundation for stability in the other organ systems. I interpret this condition to be a response to an emotional or physical shock, or both.[8] In view of my assessment of Kathryn's constitutional type, I suspect this imbalance lies in the dysfunctional relationship between the spleen and heart officials.

The *qi* depth of the entire pulse was tense, indicating the presence of a nervous system tense condition. This condition is predicated on a heightened sense of vigilance. Its presence suggested possible factors in Kathryn's past that caused her to habitually respond to life as if she were in danger. The entire pulse also revealed a hesitant quality, indicating a tendency toward obsessive thoughts and worry.

Individual Pulse Positions

Upper burner: (1) Both distal pulse positions exhibited inflated and tense qualities, suggesting that *qi* and heat had stagnated and were trapped in Kathryn's upper burner. Upon questioning, she revealed that, in fact, she did experience tightness in her throat. I immediately associated this stagnation with her frustration, difficulty in communicating, breast tenderness, and neediness, and with the function of acupuncture point Stomach-9 ("people welcome"). The stagnation also suggested using the herbal formula Pinellia and Magnolia (Ban

Xia Hou Po) to circulate the *qi* in the chest, help to remove frustration, and empower appropriate communication of needs in a similar way to Stomach-9. (2) The left neuropsychological pulse was present, indicating involvement of the *shen* as it manifests through the function of the nervous system. (3) The right distal pulse position exhibited a vibration at all depths, indicating compromised function of the lungs. This finding was supported by the presence bilaterally of the special lung pulse. These pulses manifested with a tight quality and vibration, indicating *yin* deficiency of the lungs and compromised organ function.

Between upper and middle burner: The diaphragm pulse was present bilaterally, suggesting that the painful conclusion of Kathryn's previous relationship was still negatively affecting her. This finding also indicated that separation may still be an issue in her present relationship. The herbal formula Pinellia and Magnolia again seemed appropriate to recommend here. Further, the exit/entry combinations of Liver-14 and Lung-1, and Spleen-21 and Heart-1, offered an ideal way to move the stagnant *qi* through the chest.

Middle burner: Both middle pulse positions exhibited changing qualities, indicating that the middle burner as a whole was experiencing great disharmony, perhaps predicated on the separation of *yin* and *yang* in the organ systems involved, in this case, the liver and spleen. These positions particularly showed changes from tight (*yin* deficiency) to spreading (*qi* deficiency) to empty (severe deficiency of *zhenqi*).

Lower burner: (1) Both proximal pulse positions exhibited tight and pounding qualities, suggesting *yin* deficiency resulting from overworking the nervous system and overtaxing the kidney in her system's attempt to overcome stagnation. Hence the excess heat generated from overwork and overstimulation had produced a condition of *yin* deficiency. (2) Both the large and small intestine pulse positions were tight and exhibited a biting quality, together indicating *yin* deficiency, stagnation, or pain. In these positions, the tight and biting qualities also suggest the presence of fulminating emotional states as discussed in Chapter 8. (3) The pelvis and lower body pulse position was present and tense bilaterally, indicating the stagnation leading to her gynecological problems.

Interpretation of Pulses

The most significant pulse finding in need of immediate attention was that of chaos. I believe the presence of chaos, expressing as instability in Kathryn's heart (official) function, was predicated on an emotional shock stemming from the betrayal by incest. It is likely that the habitual use of cocaine also greatly contributed to the instability of her pulse.

The presence of the neuropsychological pulse suggested an involvement of heart *shen*. The presence of the hesitant quality of her pulse also indicated compulsive thoughts and worry. This implicates the involvement of not only the heart *shen*, but also the *yi* (thought, ideation), which is the *shen* of the spleen and the emissary of the heart spirit as it is present in that organ. In this case, the emotional shock to the heart exacerbated the functional weakness in the constitutional organ, the spleen.

Another fundamental contributing factor to the chaos on Kathryn's pulse was the imbalance exhibited in the middle burner. This condition of unraveling *yin* and *yang* suggested the dysfunction in the middle burner was a functional "hole" that was depleting the entire system of *zhenqi*. This finding was consistent with the diagnosis of her constitution as spleen. Little stability was furnished by the earth element, whose function is to empower a sense of being grounded and centered in all aspects of being. Further, with liver function so compromised, the virtues of vision, planning, and self-esteem had been eroded. Because spleen (earth) is Kathryn's constitutional type, it was imperative to focus on balancing its function and reestablishing harmony of function in both the heart and the liver.

The presence of chaos on Kathryn's pulse, the effects of drug use, emotional instability, and her inability to feel secure in her present relationship because of a habitual reaction to past emotional pain provided strong confirmation that the shock of sexual abuse was an etiological factor contributing to her patterns of dysfunction. It was important, therefore, to clear the shock caused by this unwelcome intrusion into her life, so a foundation of stable functioning could be established. In this way, her emotional pain could be confronted directly so the inner wound could be healed and no longer dictate her actions in life.

Therapeutic Strategy

The emerging overall picture indicated that Kathryn's spleen was not fulfilling its task of nourishing, grounding, and creating a strong physical and emotional center. In turn, the weak earth was not supporting the function of the liver, which constantly invaded the earth in a desperate attempt to "put down roots" and stop the physical and emotional erosion

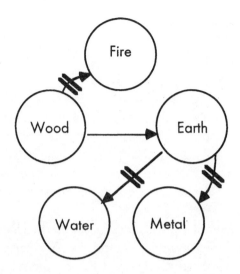

Figure 15.1

KATHRYN'S FIVE-ELEMENT CONFIGURATION

The double bars indicate pathways of restricted qi flow. Kathryn's weak earth provides an inadequate center, and therefore the function of all elements and organ systems suffers. The metal element is disempowered in its "letting go" function, evidenced by her constant mental vigilance, constipation, and failure to grieve and move past the loss of her previous relationship. Her earth element also fails to control the water element across the ke cycle, a condition that manifests as constant fear and anxiety as the nervous system overworks. Because of an insubstantial earth element, the liver does not support the function and stability of the heart, but instead attacks the spleen across the ke cycle. This manifests as poor digestion and a constant knot and burning in the area from Conception Vessel-12 to Conception Vessel-16. Finally (not depicted), the spleen (the twelfth meridian) is not nourishing the heart (the first meridian and the next meridian after the spleen) in the direction of qi flow according to the Chinese clock. The failure of her heart to be nourished could help explain both her emotional instability and the instability on her pulse.

that was occurring. Further, the function of the heart was not being supported by either the creative *qi* of the wood element or by the nourishing functions of the spleen (see Figure 15.1). In light of this diagnosis, the primary therapeutic strategy was first to stabilize the function of the organ systems responsible for this situation (spleen, heart, and liver). Improvement in the overall stability of the pulse would be a strong indication that stability of the organ systems was being restored.

Toward this end, I recommended discontinuing the birth control pills, which I consider to have a significant detrimental impact on women's health.[9] I had Kathryn wean herself from coffee, which tends to overstimulate the nervous system and undermine the function of the heart, liver, and kidneys. Finally, I suggested restricting the intake of dairy products, which may create dampness and were contributing I believe to her overall damp condition as reflected in the tongue mucus, digestive problems, excess weight, and obsessive thoughts.

Suggestions and Imagery

1. *Self-esteem:* Kathryn's fear that her husband could leave her at any time was partially based on her low self-esteem. That she had been previously hurt by a man who had "dumped" her suggests that her past experience is currently limiting her ability to be spontaneous and to assess her new relationship on its own merits. Functionally, the connection between wood and earth across the *ke* cycle was relevant here. The wood was not appropriately controlling the earth. Her constant state of worry was literally like an erosion of earth; her foundation was being washed away, leaving no solid ground beneath her feet. Just as we might plant trees on a hillside so their roots might prevent this kind of erosion, the practitioner might strengthen the wood element, specifically liver function, so it appropriately controls the earth element across the *ke* cycle. The additional step of strengthening the weak earth element may create sufficient grounding to anchor the tree and keep it from continually "falling over" in the face of adversity. Kathryn's self-esteem was also supported in treatment by suggesting images associated with point functions that are congruent with the message of respect and esteem.[10]

2. *Facing death:* Kathryn's fear of her husband's leaving their relationship may reveal the death of her self-image and ego. When applicable, it can be useful to remind patients that, in fact, they have lived through worse before. It was essential to point out to Kathryn that her interpretation of the event was "made up in her mind" and therefore had no actual basis in "reality." I worked with her on this issue by taking her through a series of mental exercises. Her fear of being "left for another woman" was based on her interpretation that if her husband did leave her, it would confirm her poor self-image and her feeling that she was indeed not good enough for him.

Over the course of treatment, I continually pointed out whenever she was making interpretations that undermined her inner stability. I suggested an alternative interpretation of the possibility of her husband leaving: "If he leaves, he doesn't deserve a woman as beautiful and loving as you are. If he leaves, it's his own fault for failing to value and to be nurtured by you." After I made this suggestion, the atmosphere in the room became very still. Kathryn had arrived at a state of mind in which she could not interpret the incoming data in a way consistent with previous experience. This state represents a significant moment of potential receptivity and offers the practitioner an excellent opportunity to remain silent in order to reinforce the suggestion and state of openness with specifically selected acupuncture points.

Herbal Treatment

Short term: My first strategy was to harmonize the overall condition of chaos and to mend the functional imbalance in Kathryn's middle burner. To establish stability on the pulse, I initially prescribed Yunnan Paiyao. This herbal preparation was expected to ease the shock to her heart, heart protector, and circulatory system that were impacted by the sexual abuse.

Long term: To balance the functional relationships between the liver and spleen, I prescribed Xiao Yao Wan (Bupleurum sedative pills). Gui Pi Wan (restore spleen pill) was also prescribed to nurture the relationship between the spleen and heart. These formulas were continued for three months. After that period, I discontinued the Xiao Yao Wan and replaced the Gui Pi Wan with Gather Vitality, a more potent form of the same formula.[11] Note that Gui Pi Wan both addresses spleen *qi* deficiency, a source of the imbalance in the middle burner, and nourishes the heart blood. On a psychospiritual level, this formula is greatly "centering" and addresses the overall dynamic between the spleen and heart. Its function is similar to the point combination of Spleen-21 and Heart-1.[12]

Acupuncture

SESSION 1
Acupuncture points: Check for "aggressive energy." Spleen-3, Liver-3, and Heart-7.[13]
Kathryn showed no signs of aggressive energy. I selected the three

earth and source points to assist in gently grounding her and helping to establish an initial balance of the officials most involved in her functional dynamic.

Herbs: Yunnan Paiyao: one pill, three times daily.

SESSION 2

Report from last session: Kathryn felt generally relaxed after the first session.

Acupuncture points: Stomach-36, Spleen-4, Large Intestine-11, and Heart Protector-6.

The earth point on the stomach meridian was treated in conjunction with the *luo* point on the spleen meridian. These points were selected together to integrate the functions of the earth officials in order to continue supporting the constitutional basis of the imbalance and heal the source of the imbalance in the middle burner. Large Intestine-11 was selected as the earth point on the meridian; this point is the child of the earth constitutional type. According to traditional Chinese medicine, one function of this point is to clear blood heat, which I found to be present in the pulse diagnosis. It may also empower the large intestine to eliminate stagnation resulting from "undigested" past experience. Symptomatically, this could help ease Kathryn's complaint of constipation and possibly also her throat tightness, which may result from harboring undelivered communications from the past.

Heart Protector-6 was treated to bring *qi* into her heart and to support the process of relaxing the tightness in her chest. Note that Heart Protector-6 and Spleen-4 are also the master and couple points of the *Chong Mai*. Needled together, these points are deeply nourishing to the womb and heart and grounding in their overall effect.[14]

SESSION 3

Report from last session: Kathryn again mentioned feeling relaxed and "centered" after the session. She noted that a skin outbreak from touching poison sumac had been bothering her, and the rash had cleared up immediately following that treatment. In general, Large Intestine-11, needled in the last session, is ideal for draining heat from the blood and might be expected to have a positive effect in helping to clear a rash.

Acupuncture points: Stomach-40, Stomach-8; Spleen-4, Spleen-6; and Heart-7.

With this selection, I continued to support the integration of the functions of Kathryn's constitutional organ systems, stomach, and spleen.

Stomach-40 ("abundant splendor") was needled with several intentions. As its name indicates, this point helps the patient feel supported and nourished by life. As the *luo* point, Stomach-40 drains dampness, which in this case is an accumulation of what should have been transformed into nourishment, but became a burden instead. Kathryn's dampness manifested as excess weight and worry. Stomach-8 ("head tied") was paired with Stomach-40 and treated as a local point to ease Kathryn's mental constraint. I have found Stomach-8 to be an excellent point for someone whose mind is "tied in knots," constrained by excessive thoughts. By needling *luo* points Spleen-4 and Stomach-40 simultaneously, the functions of these two officials are brought into balance with each other. Spleen-6 was treated here as a reunion point of the spleen, liver, and kidney officials. The selection of Heart-7 continues to establish the balance between the fire and earth element.

SESSION 4

Report from last session: Kathryn again reported feeling well for one day after the session. She noted that her moods were fluctuating up and down, as opposed to remaining down as they had before. This indicated to me that the function of the earth was stabilizing. As the functioning of earth element continued to improve, I expected Kathryn's moods would stabilize at a generally healthier and happier level.

Herbs: Gui Pi Wan and Xiao Yao Wan: 8 pills each, three times daily.

Acupuncture points: Spleen-4, Heart Protector-6, Kidney-16, Conception Vessel-14, and Liver-3.

Spleen-4 and Heart Protector-6 were treated again to open up the *Chong Mai.* This time, however, I channeled the *qi* through Kidney-16 up to Conception Vessel-14, both points for nourishing heart function.[15] I find the combination of these four points to be extremely potent for this purpose.

SESSION 5

Report from last session: Kathryn reported that her energy was increasing, digestion was improving, and craving for sweets was subsiding. These results may be attributed in part to the function of the herbal formulas. I have found that Gui Pi Wan can be quite helpful in treating cravings for sweets in persons who are earth and fire constitutionally.

Acupuncture points: Stomach-42, Spleen-3, and Heart Protector-7.

The source points were selected on the meridians of Kathryn's constitutional type: spleen and stomach. The functions of the heart protector and spleen were joined along the *sheng* cycle by needling the earth point on each meridian. The intention of this gentle treatment was to continue to establish a connection between the mother (fire) of the earth element and its child (earth).

Session 6

Report from last session: Kathryn returned complaining of tension in her chest, with an intense "stabbing" pain directly behind her heart and between her shoulder blades that prevented her from taking a deep breath. She also reported that she had begun perspiring, which was unusual for her even with strenuous activity.

This session represented the turning point in Kathryn's healing. I associated the pain that she felt in her chest and between her shoulder blades with her heart. Our efforts to remove the stagnation and strengthen the middle burner were beginning to pay off. Her pain indicated to me that her heart was struggling as it was being "asked" to open and to begin addressing the past pain that had been suppressed.

Acupuncture points: Bladder-14, Bladder-43 (38); Spleen-2, and Heart Protector-8.

Bladder-14, the *shu* point of the heart protector, was treated in conjunction with Bladder-43, which supports the spirit level of function of the heart protector. This combination of points was selected to support the continued opening of the heart protector and to ease the tension between the shoulders and in the diaphragm. Heart Protector-8 ("palace of weariness") was treated as a distal point to ground Bladder-14 and Bladder-43. As the fire point on the heart protector, it is particularly effective in strengthening and stabilizing a weary heart. Spleen-2, the fire point on the constitutional meridian of the spleen, was treated in conjunction with Heart Protector-8 to continue integrating the function of these officials.

Session 7

Report from last session: Kathryn reported that she felt less tension and pain in her chest and between her shoulder blades and that her "heart had improved." This was validated by the increased stability on the pulse, indicating that the condition of chaos was beginning to subside. She reported still having pain between her shoulder blades radiating up her neck. She also reported having a sore throat. In retrospect, considering the following two treatments and their results, her sore throat might have been the embodiment of her liver discharging old pain and resentment as she was becoming increasingly empowered to speak her inner truth.

Acupuncture points: Governor Vessel-10, Governor Vessel-11; Heart-8, Spleen-2, Bladder-20, and Bladder-21.

Governor Vessel-10 and Governor Vessel-11 were selected as the points that bring perspective to the heart. These points align the function of the heart with the governor vessel, the central axis of *yang* in the body, and itself aligned with the center of centers, the North Star. Here Spleen-2, the fire point on the constitutional meridian of the spleen, was treated in conjunction with Heart-8 in a continued effort to integrate the functioning of these two officials. Bladder-20 and Bladder-21 are the *shu* points on the spleen and stomach meridians associated with Kathryn's constitutional type. As powerful reserves of *qi,* these points were treated in order to ground and support the functioning of their associated organs. I typically treat *shu* points after I feel the basic functioning of an organ system has been integrated and stabilized using distal points.

After inserting the needles, I suggested to Kathryn that she imagine bringing her heart up into a tower to allow it to gain perspective. This visualization reminds us of the stories associated with the functions of Governor Vessel-10 and Governor Vessel-11 in Chapter 13.

SESSION 8

Report from last session: Kathryn felt very relaxed after the last treatment and reported that her heart pain was gone. However, she also felt very emotional and reported this with tears welling up in her eyes. She also reported feeling pain in her lower back from gardening.

Acupuncture points: Stomach-9, Stomach-42; Bladder-10, Bladder-40; and Governor Vessel-3.

Although Kathryn's pulse continued to indicate increased stability, the distal positions bilaterally (corresponding to the heart [on the left] and lungs [on the right] officials) manifested an inflated and tense quality. The bilateral presence of these qualities indicated that *qi* and heat were trapped in the upper burner. Very often, this finding is associated with throat tightness, suggesting that constraint is inhibiting the communication of emotionally significant material.[16]

For this condition, I have treated Stomach-9 ("people welcome") in conjunction with the meridian's source point, Stomach-42, in order to provide grounding.[17] Stomach-9, as the "window of heaven" point on the stomach meridian, provides access to the deepest spiritual dimensions of the stomach official's realm of function. I often use this point to empower the patient to communicate needs appropriately, often a key issue for the earth constitutional type. This point is ideal for people who are ingratiating, always trying to please others. These individuals swallow a little bit of resentment every time they ignore their own needs in deference to another's, until, finally, they have "had it up to here." (The patient will often gesture toward the throat while saying this.) This point is also effective for people who are overly self-sufficient, as it may empower them to bring others into their "process."[18]

After treating points Stomach-9 and Stomach-42 on the front of the body (the front corresponding to *yin*), I treated paired points on the back (the points corresponding to *yang*). In Kathryn's case, these points were treated to empower her resolve, allowing her to access deep levels of spiritual strength. Bladder-10 ("heavenly pillar") is the "window of heaven" point on the bladder meridian. Located at the top of the trapezius muscle,[19] this point may empower one to access deep sources of inner strength. I grounded this point with Bladder-40 ("equilibrium middle"), the earth point on the bladder meridian. This point allows the earth element to control the water element across the *ke* cycle. Its function is qualitatively similar to bringing earth to build dikes along a river that is overflowing its banks. This is a good metaphor for the earth element, providing the inner stability needed to control the fear associated with the water element. This function is underscored by the location of this point behind the knee (in the middle of the crease within the popliteal fossa), a joint essential for providing balance and stability to the body. Finally, Governor Vessel-3 is treated to enhance the effectiveness of Bladder-10 and Bladder-40 by strengthening the lower back. I occasionally use these three points together to empower patients to "stand up for themselves."

After needling the points, I wait for an indication that the patient has reached a moment of receptivity, as indicated by positive changes in breathing, color, sound, odor, emotion, pulse, and other general indicators of relaxation. Then I deliver the specific suggestion that I want the patient to receive. In Kathryn's case, I suggested this treatment would put her in touch with a deep reserve of spiritual strength that would empower her to speak the truth and communicate her needs appropriately to others.

SESSION 9

Report from last session: Kathryn reported that she had decided to confront her father for sexually abusing her as a youngster. She would soon be with him at a family gathering and had asked her sisters to be present for emotional support. Note that Kathryn is manifesting the virtues of self-expression and inner strength addressed by the previous treatment. The recruitment of her sisters is evidence of the empowerment enabled by the earlier treatment of Stomach-9. She was understandably nervous and quite emotional about the upcoming discussion.

Herbs: Women's Palace[20]: sixteen drops, three times daily.

Acupuncture points: Stomach-36; Large Intestine-11, Large Intestine-17; and Conception Vessel-22.

Both Stomach-36 and Large Intestine-11 are earth points on their respective meridians. The two points were treated to empower the integration of these functions and to support Kathryn in letting go of everything that no longer served her. I consider Large Intestine-17 to be similar in function to a "window of heaven" point. I associate the function of this point, *tianting* ("heavenly vessel"), with the functional dynamics described in *Yijing* hexagram 50, *ting* ("the cauldron").[21] Large Intestine-17 empowers the pristine clarity that comes from letting go of the old in order to receive the new.

Finally, Conception Vessel-22 ("heaven rushing out") is needled as the "window of heaven" point on the conception vessel meridian. Located at the center of the throat, this point may empower communication "centered" by the conception vessel, the central axis of *yin* in the microcosm.

In this session, I prescribed the herbal formula Women's Palace to assist Kathryn in clearing out the past residue of betrayal manifested as dysplasia and general stagnation in the uterus.

SESSION 10

Report from last session: Kathryn returned for this session after confronting her father. She reported finding a "centered place," and although there were many tears, he had been open to hearing what she had to say. She had felt a tremendous reserve of strength from the last session and reported that the knot in her stomach (Conception Vessel-12 to Conception Vessel-16) was completely gone.

Discussion

As a result of these sessions, Kathryn was able to unleash a profound undelivered communication, confronting her father for having sexually abused her. She was able to stand up for her needs and to take care of herself rather than stifling her own expression because of her constitutional tendency to be overly sympathetic toward the feelings of others. Hence the virtues of the earth element, sincerity and reciprocity, have become increasingly established as her habitual behavior has subsided.

One year after the last session, Kathryn began successful counseling with her husband and had two negative Pap tests, indicating no further evidence of the carcinoma in situ. Her heart function was increasingly stable, and she has reported no tension or stabbing pains in her chest since.

In a subsequent session Kathryn reported, "feeling on the fence about needing to forgive her father." This was said with sadness and judgment against herself for "being stuck" and being unable to move on in life. I suggested that forgiveness is not a onetime event, but a process, and that throughout her life she will experience progressively deeper levels of forgiveness. A feeling of "being stuck" is her interpretation of the emotion that arises each time she is about to experience a new level of forgiveness.[22] Often patients interpret the reemergence of old feelings and emotional material as stalled progress in their treatment or in their lives. It is important to direct their attention to the real progress they have made and the deeper levels of understanding they have reached.

The treatments in sessions 7 and 8 demonstrate an important principle about the role of the practitioner's knowledge and intention and the function of acupuncture points. In session 7, Governor Vessel-10 and Governor Vessel-11 might have been treated by a practitioner of any tradition to alleviate the pain that Kathryn was feeling between her shoulder blades. In session 8, Stomach-9 and Stomach-42 similarly might have been treated solely to relieve the "tightness" in her throat and her digestive complaints. In the same session, Bladder-40, Bladder-10, and Governor Vessel-3 might have been treated just for her lower back and neck pain. When I select these points, I am certainly taking the physical symptoms of the patient's condition into consideration. However, because I am familiar with the broader capabilities of these acupuncture point functions, I am able to use them to direct the patient's awareness to the inner virtues empowered by the point and thereby pursue as therapeutic goals the fulfillment of destiny and alignment with the primordial *dao* made possible by the practice of the inner tradition of Chinese medicine.

Summary

If the practitioner's awareness is confined to the physical effect on symptoms of point functions, then many opportunities for supporting the patient's deeper healing processes may be missed. Although patients treated strictly symptomatically may report improvement, there may be no discernment or acknowledgment of the quality and direction of this feeling. One of the most significant opportunities for healing afforded by the inner aspects of Chinese medicine lies in the practitioner's capacity to guide patients to comprehend the functional relationships between their physical complaints and unbalanced thoughts, attitudes, and belief systems. When these connections are acknowledged and firmly reinforced, a process of healing may commence that embraces all aspects of personal expression.

CASE 2: BRIT

Sex/age: Female, age 37

Height: 5' 8"

Weight: 160 pounds

Reasons for seeking treatment: (1) pain from severe endometriosis, which has spread and attached itself to various organ systems, and (2) secondary infertility.

Color: White/Red

Sound: Weeping

Odor: Rotten/Scorched

Emotion: Grief

Constitutional type: primary—metal (lung); secondary—fire (heart protector)

General Impression

First Telephone Communication

During my first conversation with Brit, I was immediately struck by the soft, breathy quality of her voice, which suggested the weeping tonality associated with the metal constitutional type. Apparently she had talked to another practitioner, who informed her that Chinese medicine could not treat her endometriosis. I told her that treatment was possible, and a sense of relief was immediately discernable in her voice. Again, it is important that the practitioner create a context for healing by giving positive suggestions to the patient from the very first contact.

First Meeting

Brit's initial presentation of herself seemed somewhat guarded and nervous. As I began the interview, I immediately detected a slight fluttering of her heart *qi* and shallowness of breath. Her *qi* seemed weak to the point of failing in the upper burner in the area between Conception Vessel-17, Lung-1, Heart-1, and Conception Vessel-22. This flutter of heart *qi* was quite responsive to the degree of force in my own presentation. If I raised the intensity of my voice or leaned forward, her *qi* immediately became unsettled on subtle levels of expression associated with the organ functions (heart, heart protector, and lung) in this region.

The quality of her nervousness reminded me of a greyhound racing dog I had once known who had been abused by a previous owner. Each time he approached me for affection, he would retreat if I made the slightest move toward him. The only way to make contact was to remain still and let him come to me. Observing this dynamic throughout the exam, I intuited a history of abuse as a possible etiological factor in Brit's pattern of dysfunction. Her element, as expressed through the indicators of color, sound, odor, and emotion, strongly suggested a constitutional type of either metal (lung) or fire (heart protector). My initial impression was of a person with a delicate heart spirit obscured by clouds of grief.

Highlights of Intake Interview

General Background

Parents
Response: Brit's parents were divorced when she was 22 after what she described as "five years of warfare." When asked where she grew up, she responded, "I grew up all over the East Coast. We moved constantly because of my dad's work."

Impression: Her response to my first question about her family background was enough to confirm my initial suspicions and constitutional diagnosis. I must emphasize that it is not so much the content of the answer which is relevant to making the diagnosis, but the way the patient relates to and expresses the content. Brit responded to my question about her family by immediately establishing the theme of grief over her losses. This theme emerged relative to constantly having to move when young and its connection to her relationship with her father. When she mentioned her father, the white color next to her eyes intensified, as did the weeping sound in her voice. The metal element became so strongly present during this discussion that I suspected her father represented an important loss in her life and the possible source of abuse.[23] My initial impression that familial abuse is a primary etiological factor in a patient's makeup often comes from the quality of his or her response to my first few questions about family.

Family Health

Father

Response: "He has had high blood pressure his whole life. He's in massive denial."

Impression: Here Brit gave another hint that my assessment of abuse is correct. She evidenced judgment and anger rather than sympathy for his condition. I feel that this anger, although perhaps appropriate, has a component of resentment, which I view as unhealthy. I did not push Brit further on this sensitive topic at this time, preferring instead to ask her directly about her father later in the interview after trust has been established between us. As we discussed her parents' divorce, the theme of loss in life again became strongly apparent.

Mother

Response: Brit reported that her mother is diabetic and hyperthyroid.

Impression: As soon as Brit mentioned her mother, her tone and presentation changed as she relaxed and smiled. She evidenced a genuine warmth and lightheartedness, indicating a clear source of *qi* residing in her heart spirit.

Siblings

Response: Brit's older brother, 39 years old, has severe bipolar illness.

Impression: The absence of a strongly negative functional shift when she discussed her brother made me feel that he was not the source of the possible abuse. This was reinforced by her expression of genuine concern for his well-being.

Response: Brit has two younger sisters. The 35-year-old sister is hypothyroid; the 30-year-old has high blood pressure, which is managed through diet and exercise.

Impression: The existence of two parents and three siblings, all of whom are manifesting notable physical symptomatology, paints a picture of a weak genetic background. It also suggested the possibility that a dysfunctional family environment early in life contributed to the manifestation of Brit's difficulties.

Marriage and Children

Response: "I've been married six years, but we've been together for fifteen. It's good most of the time. I have a 5-year-old boy and love being a mother."

Impression: A genuine joy, lightheartedness, and brightness of *shen* was evident in Brit's eyes when she discussed her child. This made it clear that her heart spirit held a reserve of clear *qi* to cultivate and to tap, and therefore a good prognosis was likely. The presence of a long-term commitment to an adult relationship she enjoys also suggested that the functioning of her heart had not been too badly damaged and supported a good prognosis.

Career

Response: "I'm a floral designer. It's my outlet for everything I keep inside."

Impression: Here the theme of guarding tender feelings associated with her heart and lungs was further developed in the imagery of flowers as an outer expression of her inner feelings. This brought to mind the point Conception Vessel-20, translated as "flower canopy," that refers to the lungs as they cover the heart. This added weight to my sense that her heart represents a clear source of functional strength that could be tapped for healing.

Reasons for Seeking Treatment

Pain Relief from Endometriosis

Brit had evidenced some symptoms of endometriosis before giving birth to her son. They became significantly worse one and a half years after childbirth (three and a half years prior to the consultation). She had toxemia during pregnancy and problems with her blood pressure and blood sugar levels, all requiring bed rest for three months during pregnancy. One year prior to the interview, she had a laparoscopy and laser surgery to diagnose and treat severe endometriosis. Her pain improved for six months and then returned to previous levels. After trying to become pregnant, again unsuccessfully, for four years, Brit was given hormones for her supposed infertility, which made the pain worse. At the time of our interview, her physician had offered the options of a repetition of her previous surgery or a chemically induced menopause.

Brit's presenting symptoms included an extreme stabbing pain traveling from her left rib cage near Liver-13 down to her groin along the inguinal ligament. This pain was also present to a lesser degree on the left side of her back from Governor Vessel-4 to Bladder-25. She described her symptoms as improving several days before and after ovulation, then a continual building of the pain as her period approached. She commented, "It feels like my pelvis is going to crack." Her pain was helped by soaking in hot water and exercising. Ginger compresses offered some relief. However, she said, "I try to suffer through the pain. Taking aspirin leaves me feeling like junk is in my body. I like to clean everything out."

Impression: Brit understood the importance of addressing the issues underlying her poor health rather than opting for the choices offered by her physicians. This demonstrated a good degree of consciousness and an ability both to stand up for herself and to take care of her own needs. Again, this finding suggested a good prognosis.

The fixed nature of Brit's stabbing pain suggested the presence of congealed liver blood. The location of Brit's pain suggested that this symptom was following the course of the liver meridian. Her feelings of being "unclean," associated in this case with the use of aspirin, are typical of the metal constitutional type, who often evidences themes of functional imbalance around the issue of purity. The stoic notion of hardening one's self and suffering through pain is also associated with the metal element. These relationships between metal and wood evoke the function of Liver-4 ("middle seal"). As the metal point on the liver meridian, Liver-4 can help the liver detoxify the blood by empowering the metal virtues of purity and letting go within the wood element.

Other Health Concerns

Response: Brit reported that for quite a while she had been waking up with night sweats. However, these symptoms had stopped once she eliminated dairy foods and meat from her diet.

Impression: The presence of night sweats suggested deficient *yin* as a therapeutic issue.

Hair Loss

Brit's fine blond hair was thinning and falling out. Tests for lupus and thyroid condition were negative. I often associate very fine hair on both the head and body with the metal constitution. I also consider hair loss to be a sign of blood deficiency, a finding later confirmed on Brit's pulse.

Breast Milk Production

Brit reported that her right breast was still producing milk even though she had not breast-fed in over four years.

Impression: I interpreted this as a possible sign of holding on to the experience of childbirth and early motherhood. It added weight to the theme of grief, loss, holding on, and longing demonstrated throughout the interview.

Patterns of Function

Sleep

Response: Brit's normal pattern of sleep was disrupted by pain associated with endometriosis.

Impression: The functional basis of endometriosis could in part be attributed to congealed blood. Her sleep disturbance indicates the involvement of her heart *shen* in this dynamic.

Circulation

Response: Brit reported that her hands and feet were always cold.

Impression: Cold hands and feet often signal an inhibition of circulation attributable to a counterflow of liver *qi*. Brit's symptom suggested to me a possible exit/entry blockage between Liver-14 and Lung-1.

Energy

Response: Brit reported that since her surgery the previous winter, her energy had been lower and that she often became very tired between 3 and 4 P.M.

Impression: According to the Chinese clock, 3 P.M. is the high function time of the bladder official and the low function time of the liver official. The function of the bladder is to store reserves of *qi* and to regulate their expenditure. Brit's reserves were generally quite low, and she often used the force of will to push beyond her limits. However, at 3 P.M. the bladder's function of storing reserves increases to the point that it actually empowers her to slow down so she is forced to rest. At the same time, her liver, now at its functional low, relaxes long enough to stop driving her.[24]

Appetite

Brit's appetite has been good.

Cravings

Brit craves chocolate, but because it is bad for her condition, she does not eat it.

Digestion

Brit reported her digestion as generally good; however, she has difficulty digesting dairy foods.

Bowels

Response: Brit's bowels have been moving normally.

Impression: The absence of any difficulty with bowel movements highlights that an imbalance can exist functionally in an official and manifest on emotional and spiritual levels but not manifest on physical levels. In Brit's case, the large intestine official, as part of the metal element, was a significant factor in her constitutional makeup, but never showed itself in any physical symptoms.

Urinary Elimination

Response: Generally, Brit's urination has been good, other than occasional bladder infections. She reports having kidney stones in the left kidney and a kidney infection at age 28.

Impression: Bladder and kidney symptomatology may be interpreted as the mother (metal) manifesting in the child (water). The presence of kidney stones suggested that metal (calcium) was being inappropriately condensed in the kidneys (water).

Surgeries

Brit's sinuses were surgically enlarged at age 13.

A fibroid tumor (one-inch diameter) was removed from the end of her uterus.

During pregnancy, Brit's uterus hemorrhaged on the left side at a site of her presenting pain. Subsequently, she had a Cesarean section and delivered her baby one month prematurely.

Impression: Early sinus surgery suggested a block in the pathway and associated function of Brit's lung official and large intestine official, which terminates at the Large Intestine-20 ("welcome fragrance") at the outside of the nose. The fibroid indicated the inappropriate accumulation of waste material that should be eliminated. This again suggested a possible imbalance in the function of the large intestine, the *yang* official associated with the metal element.

The metal element was again suggested with the reappearance of the theme of premature loss with Brit's inability to carry her pregnancy to full term. The metal element is the last stage of the *dao's* movement on the *sheng* cycle before the return to water. The transition from metal to water is paramount in the processes of both birth and death.[25] Brit's hemorrhaging likely contributed to the blood deficiency evident in pulse diagnosis and to the attendant blood stagnation evident in her menstrual period, her symptomatology, and her tongue.

Substance Use

Coffee: Quit one month ago

Alcohol: Usually one glass of wine with dinner but recently quit to assist in her healing

Tobacco: None

Recreational drugs: Some marijuana when younger

Medications: None

Impression: Brit had stopped consuming coffee and alcohol on her own volition, indicating a strong motivation and commitment to improve her health. This observation improved the prognosis considerably and signified that she would be quite receptive to therapeutic suggestions.

Menstrual Period

Response: Brit reported that her periods are regular, lasting about twelve days. The blood is very clotted.

Impression: The clotted blood was further evidence of blood stagnation as a primary physiological basis of Brit's pain. The length of Brit's period was also excessive as is often the case in severe endometriosis.[26]

Preferences

Colors: Likes blue and green; dislikes red.

Seasons: Likes cold; uncomfortable in summer.

Impression: Summer and red are the season and color associated with the fire element that is overcontrolling her metal element across the *ke* cycle.

Other Questions

Relationship with Father

After establishing trust during the interview, I asked Brit about the nature of her relationship with her father. She told me that she was subjected to physical abuse, which she described as "very bad." Her father had beaten, choked, and kicked her and her siblings "in moments of explosive temper." She had tried to establish a relationship with her father in recent years, but he was "in complete denial" and refused to take responsibility for his part in their dysfunctional relationship. Much anger, sorrow, and grief was evident during her discussion of these matters.

Eyes and Tongue

Eyes: The whites of Brit's eyes evidenced a blue hue, indicating a liver and gallbladder imbalance. The membranes inside the eyelids were quite red; all vessels were confluent, indicating heat.[27]

Tongue: A narrow line, containing a little phlegm, ran the full length of the tongue. The tip was very red, and the material was pale with a purplish tint. The veins under the tongue were quite purple.

A line in the tongue indicates an inherited heart imbalance. The presence of phlegm in this "heart crack" indicates that the orifice of the heart is obstructed: in Brit's case, one more physical manifestation of the clouds of grief obscuring the heart.[28] The red tip indicates heat trapped in the heart. This heat may be interpreted as a sign of unexpressed emotion and desire. The paleness of the tongue indicates a general blood deficiency, and its overall purple hue and purple veins suggest blood stasis. These observations suggest again, in Brit's case, the involvement of the heart and heart protector as they contribute to her functional dynamic.

Analysis of the Interview

Constitutional Analysis: Destiny and Virtue

Throughout Brit's interview, grief resulting from loss was a continuous theme. Constant moving from one location to another as a youngster and her parents' divorce were two major sources of loss early in life. In truth, her relationship with her father had been lost long before the divorce, when trust had been broken as a result of his physical violence. Having identified Brit as a metal constitutional type, I hypothesized that her destiny is to learn to harmonize the issues of gain and loss. As treatment progressed, I suspected she would evidence less longing and that past losses would have a diminishing influence on her self-expression in the moment. Over time, the virtues associated with the metal element—righteousness and justice—would gradually emerge. I believed that Brit's heart *qi,* although weak, is very pure and would provide a strong source of healing influence to be cultivated and tapped. I would liken my overall approach to treatment to a clearing away of clouds of grief (lung) that obscure the sun (heart). My general assessment was that Brit is metal constitutionally and her fire element is secondarily involved because she was greatly affected by her father's betrayal.

I interpreted Brit's endometriosis as tears of grief manifesting physically in the lower burner. The sharp, stabbing nature of her pain and the clotted blood during her menstrual period indicated to me that her guardedness of her vulnerable aspects (blood and sexual organs) were manifesting as a congealed blood pattern. Congealed blood, in general, may be viewed as a "separation from self" that occurs as emotional material that is too painful to integrate is hidden from consciousness.

Many of the physical expressions of Brit's illness were manifesting through the wood element and the liver, in particular. Notable signs of liver involvement were (1) a history of mononucleosis, (2) a blue hue in the whites of her eyes, (3) a stabbing pain along the liver meridian from Liver-12 to Liver-13, (4) the presence of resentment, which is a "toxic" emotion that affects and emanates from the liver, (5) cold hands and feet, (6) low energy from 3 to 4 P.M., and (7) systemic blood and *qi* stagnation for which the liver is partially responsible. Her color, sound, odor, and emotion did not substantiate the presence of liver as a constitutional issue. Therefore I interpreted the liver involvement as a secondary compensation arising from her life experience.

Pulse Diagnosis

General Pulse Findings

Rate (BPM): Beginning: 72; end: 75; with movement: 80

The overall quality of Brit's pulse was deep at all positions and typified by a thick, cotton quality. The pulse also evidenced continuous changes in intensity and was feeble or absent in many positions. Generally, the right side of her pulse was more tense and stronger in quality and quantity than the left side, which was deeper, thinner, and ultimately feeble or absent.

Individual Pulse Positions

Upper burner: Both distal positions were feeble or absent bilaterally. There was a special lung pulse, which was tight with a bilateral vibration.

Middle burner: There are no qualities in common in the middle positions on the left and right hand. This indicates that any qualities found in these positions are unique to particular officials and are not shared by the middle burner as a whole.

Lower burner: There are no qualities in common. The pelvis/lower-body pulse was muffled bilaterally. Because of the thickness of the cotton quality and the general thinness and depth of the pulse, many of the complementary positions (such as gallbladder, large intestine, duodenum, etc.) could not be discerned.

Interpretation of Pulses

The presence of the massive cotton quality on all positions of Brit's pulse indicated a profound resignation from an early age. This suggested that an unbalanced functional relationship was likely present between the heart, heart protector, and lung officials.[29] For Brit, this quality indicated a child who has closed her heart and suppressed her lung function in an attempt to avoid emotional pain.[30] My interpretation that a constitutional dynamic existed between her lungs and heart was reinforced by the feeble/absent quality present on both distal positions that correspond to the upper burner bilaterally. Long-term suppression of life force, combined with a constitutional vulnerability, had led to severely compromised function of the officials in the upper burner.

Physiologically, the finding of the feeble/absent quality in both distal positions corresponds to deficiency of heart and lung *qi,* blood, and *zhenqi.* The constant change in the intensity of Brit's pulse indicated a heart *qi* deficiency and, in general, a severe depletion of *qi,* blood, *jing,* and *shen.* In this case, the poor function of the heart was affecting the function of the circulatory system as a whole. The tight qualities found in the special lung position bilaterally indicated a chronic lung *yin* deficiency, and the vibration there suggested a deep level of organ dysfunction. The presence of these qualities confirmed for me a picture of the organs of the heart, heart protector, lung, and the functional state of the upper burner in general as being the major etiological factors in Brit's pattern of dysfunction.

The presence of the feeble/absent quality on the whole left side of Brit's pulse indicated a suppression of the *yang* evolutionary force, which manifests on this side of the pulse. This suggested to me a classic husband/wife imbalance, a fairly serious condition in need of immediate attention. The overall depth of her pulse suggested both a *qi* and a blood deficiency; the withdrawal of her life force deep into the interior indicated a deficiency of *yang.* This finding was consistent with her guardedness, which was generally and thematically present throughout the diagnosis. In general, the depletion on the left side of the pulse, relative to the right-side pulse, indicated a condition in which *yin* and *yang* were moving toward a terminal point of separation.

Upon questioning, Brit revealed that she had not been allowed to donate blood because of "weak blood." This finding was consistent with the overall depth and thinness of her pulse. The bout with mononucleosis in her teens, a disease that can affect liver function, may have contributed to the feeble/absent quality of her left middle pulse, the left side of the pulse, and the general amount of *qi* stagnation present in all areas of expression. Liver disharmony was also evident in the bluish color of the whites of her eyes.[31]

The tense quality on Brit's right proximal position indicated *qi* stagnation in the lower part of her body, its severity suggested by its muffled quality. This muffled quality may also indicate blood stagnation.

It was present bilaterally in the positions that correspond to the pelvis and lower body, suggesting a serious condition, such as tumor formation, was possibly imminent.

Therapeutic Strategy

Aside from the psychospiritual issues involved in Brit's case, I was very concerned about the possible development of serious physical illness in Brit. First, the massive cotton quality on the pulse suggested the possibility of slow tumor formation over the next ten to thirty years. The presence of the muffled quality bilaterally in the lower burner, paired with the presence of an already diagnosed and possibly precancerous condition (endometriosis), emphasized the seriousness of dealing with the *qi* and blood stagnation locally in her uterus and the *weiqi* stagnation. Second, the overall blood, *qi,* and, ultimately, *jing* deficiency, plus the presence of the husband/wife imbalance, indicated the basic organ functions sustaining her life were compromised. This emphasizes the need to tonify as well as to move the stagnation that resulted from her overall deficient condition. The presence of the husband/wife block suggested an urgency to reestablish the functional connection between the metal and water elements.

My initial treatment strategy for Brit was to use acupuncture to access the spiritual influences that would be the reservoir of strength to support Brit's commitment to life and healing. Acupuncture would break habitual patterns of function manifesting as deficiency and stagnation and whose physical correlates were tumors and endometriosis. The *weiqi* stagnation, present on the pulse as a cotton quality and in the psychospiritual domain as resignation, would be addressed using acupuncture, with every treatment aimed at correcting the constitutional imbalance between her metal and fire elements. Suggestions and imagery based on the names and functions of the acupuncture points would also be employed to support this process. Herbal medicine would be prescribed to promote the function of the organ systems and to move stagnation.

The chronology of the treatment plan was to treat aggressively the stagnation in the lower burner in order to address the impending seriousness of the condition there and to provide some initial pain relief. After moving the local blood stagnation and building up the associated organ functions, herbs would be given to both tonify and move blood stagnation systemically. Progress on these two fronts should address Brit's secondary complaint of infertility.

Suggestions and Imagery

At the end of the intake session, I gave feedback to Brit on my general assessment of her condition and my general approach and concerns. I emphasized that healing her relationship with her father was essential to improving her condition. In response to this suggestion, she became somewhat defensive and guarded. She explained that she had tried unsuccessfully to develop a healthy relationship with her father and had cut off all communication with him six months before. I countered that the primary healing of this relationship had to occur inside her. In essence, her father had caused her pain in life that was beyond her control. Because she could not heal the relationship itself, she might need to remove herself from that source and threat of pain. However, it is primarily the pain she causes herself over the loss of this relationship that needs healing. We cannot avoid pain in life, but we can avoid making that pain worse through habituated patterns of behavior, thought, and belief. I explained that whatever course she chose with her father, she must make peace with the relationship so it no longer creates pain or prevents her from manifesting her own purpose in life. She was quite receptive to this idea, so I assigned her daily meditation on the affirmation that she would let go of any pain and burden in life that no longer served her. This can be a particularly effective image for people of metal constitution because it relates directly to the function of the large intestine official.

Herbal Treatment

Short term: My herbal treatment strategy was to stabilize pulse intensity, relieve shock, strengthen the heart protector, and clear away feelings of betrayal. The presence of physical and emotional abuse, paired with changing intensity on the pulse, attendant circulatory problems, and blood stagnation indicated an initial course of Yunnan Paiyao, two pills daily for eight days.[32] This formula was prescribed on the second visit, corresponding to the first acupuncture treatment. It was to be repeated periodically as needed.

Long term: My treatment strategy was to tonify any underlying deficiency and to move the related blood and *qi* stagnation in the lower burner. My intention was to empower the virtue of being free to choose to be vulnerable from a position of strength, a quality inherent in the function of blood in its spiritual aspect. For this purpose, I prescribed Wu Chi Bai Feng Wan, six pills, three times daily. I find Wu Chi Bai Feng Wan to be a highly effective formula to both tonify blood and *yin* deficiency in the lower burner and to move blood stagnation due to *yin* deficiency. The ginseng and astragalus in the formula make it an excellent *qi* tonic for women who are also deficient in kidney and liver *yin*

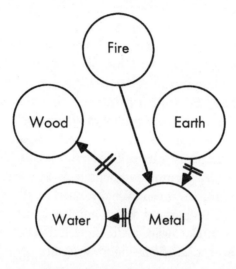

Figure 15.2
BRIT'S FIVE-ELEMENT CONFIGURATION

Double bars indicate pathways of restricted qi flow. Brit's five-element functional dynamics are depicted. Her primary dynamic involves a weak constitutional element (metal) acted on across the ke cycle by the fire element. Further, the weak metal cannot control the wood element appropriately, as evidenced by her difficulty in letting go of the pain and anger associated with her father. The seriousness of her condition is underscored by the failure of her metal element to generate water. This is evidenced on the pulse as great depletion on the left half of the pulse relative to the right half, suggesting a husband/wife imbalance and the possible terminal separation of yin and yang. As in all treatment, the primary therapeutic strategy involves harmonizing these relationships so that the elements create each other following the sheng cycle and control each other appropriately across the ke cycle. The most efficient way of creating this balance is to harmonize the functioning of the metal element, which is constitutional, and to balance its relationship to the secondary element, fire. The presence of a husband/wife imbalance indicates that serious attention must be paid to continually supporting the functional connection between metal and water.

and blood. It may also help to break a husband/wife imbalance by supporting the function of the kidneys and the liver. I consider it to be deeply nourishing in nature. This formula was prescribed on Brit's first visit, after the intake.

As a companion formula, I prescribed Women's Palace, sixteen drops, three times daily. This formula is excellent for *qi* and blood stagnation in the lower burner. It is particularly effective in cases where stagnation results from abuse or betrayal of trust. The formula was prescribed on the fourth visit after the third treatment.

Finally, I prescribed Turtle Shell Tablets. This formula is quite effective for the treatment of endometriosis by moving congealed blood in the lower burner, a condition evidenced by the muffled quality found bilaterally on the pulse positions corresponding to the lower body and pelvis. Blood stasis as a systemic condition was also reflected in the purple color of Brit's tongue. The formula prescribed consists of turtle shell, amber, and rhubarb. The presence of rhubarb in the formula requires monitoring the patient's bowel movements because of its tendency to loosen the stool. The formula was prescribed on the first visit after the intake.

Acupuncture

Although many meridians were selected to treat Brit, the intention of each treatment was always to support the function of the organs associated with her constitutional type.

SESSION 1

Acupuncture points: Check for aggressive energy; Lung-9, Heart Protector-6, and Triple Burner-4.

Aggressive energy was found to be mildly present on all points tested on Brit. This treatment can be powerful in taking the edge off a patient's *qi* when the toxic emotions of bitterness and resentment have accumulated. This "draining" of the system helps therapeutically to level the playing field by balancing the *zang* organ system and draining perverse *qi*.

The *luo* point on the heart protector meridian (Heart Protector-6) and the source point on the triple burner meridian (Triple Burner-4) were selected to integrate the functioning of these two fire officials. Lung-9 touches the constitutional influence of metal. In this context, these three points combined empowered Brit to surrender her heart's pain and grief to the abyss. By harmonizing the imbalance of fire and metal across the *ke* cycle, the natural functioning of the *qi* flow inherent in the *sheng* cycle was reinforced. This simple treatment was aimed at first touching the constitutional influences so that I could measure Brit's initial response to a gentle treatment.

SESSION 2

Report from last session: Brit felt very calm after the treatment, but she was concerned because she went home and slept for twenty hours. She reported dreaming that she was trying to piece together pipes, and the water kept flowing in the wrong direction. By the end of the dream, the water was flowing correctly. The dream took place in "a basement that was dark and had bad things in it, but I could see the sun." The imagery of the basement with "bad things in it" may represent the diseased state of Brit's lower burner. Her ability to see the sun through the darkness suggests the return of healthy *qi,* as does her feeling of having the water *(qi)* finally flowing in the right direction.

Brit also reported that the pain in her side increased after taking the herbs. I interpreted this as a positive sign that the herbs were likely beginning their work in moving congealed blood.

Acupuncture points: Conception Vessel-17, Lung-1; Kidney-24, Heart Protector-2; Heart Protector-4, Lung-6; Kidney-3.

This treatment was designed to synchronize the rhythm of the heart and lungs (Conception Vessel-17, Lung-1), to awaken the heart spirit (Kidney-24, Heart Protector-2), and to move stagnation in the heart protector and lung channels (Heart Protector-4, Lung-6). Kidney-3 was treated to tonify the kidneys and to gently moderate the effects of Kidney-24, a strong point. Note that the lung and kidney points in the upper burner addressed the husband/wife imbalance by deeply integrating the spirit-level functioning of these organs.

SESSION 3

Report from last session: Brit reported feeling better, with less pain. Usually, her pain was very bad one week before the start of her menstrual period, but this time, it was much less. However, pain was still present under her left rib.

Acupuncture points: Liver-8, Liver-13; Kidney-1, Kidney-16, Conception Vessel-15; Small Intestine-19, Bladder-1.

Liver-8 tonifies the liver and increases the quality of *qi* flow. *Qi* was directed to the site of the pain using Liver-13. Liver-8 draws *qi* from the kidney, just as Kidney-1 pushes *qi* to the liver. Kidney-1, Kidney-16, and Conception Vessel-15 were needled in combination to tonify the heart essence. Kidney-1 empowers rootedness and permits tapping into the source of *qi*. I channeled Kidney-1 up through Kidney-16 bilaterally (a point that tonifies heart essence) and then to Conception Vessel-15, which, as the heart protector *mu* point, tonifies the heart protector. Small Intestine-19 and Bladder-1 are not treated here as an exit/entry block, but rather as points to "open the orifices," so that the fires of *mingmen* may be fueled with an accurate perception of reality rather than the false interpretation of the habitual mind.

SESSION 4

Report from last session: Brit experienced a little leftover pain around her groin and pubic bone but much less pain around the ribs. She reported "saying good-bye to the male presence who has been a sort of spirit guide during this pain." Both the patient and I interpreted this as a sign of lightening of the spirit and lessening of the symptoms.

Acupuncture points: Seven Internal Dragon points: The "master" point between Conception Vessel-14 and Conception-Vessel-15, Stomach-25, Stomach-32, Stomach-41[33]; Heart-7; and Conception Vessel-3.

The imagery of Brit's spirit guide left me feeling the need to establish protective boundaries around her and to chase away negative influences and possibility of "possession." The idea of possession in several Chinese medical traditions suggests that the person has become so deeply habituated in one form of emotional expression that no room is left for any other form of personal expression. The Seven Internal Dragons were needled to help release this form of stuckness. Heart-7 was needled to reaffirm Brit's control as a force in her own life after clearing out the "demons." Conception Vessel-3 was needled to continue empowering functional improvement in her lower burner.

Herbs: Women's Palace, sixteen drops, three times daily.

SESSION 5

Report from last session: Brit's menstrual period was much improved, lasting 5 days and with significantly less pain. Menstrual blood was red with no sign of clotting or brown color. She had contracted a cold with sinus symptoms; despite her condition, she felt very well for two days of that week.

Acupuncture points: Small Intestine-19, Bladder-1; Large Intestine-20, Stomach-1; Heart Protector-5, Lung-8; Spleen-4, Heart Protector-6.

The exit point of the first two pairs—Small Intestine-19 and Large

Intestine-20—were needled together for fifteen minutes each and then entry points Bladder-1 and Stomach-1 were needled with a quick insertion and removal.[34] Heart Protector-5 and Lung-8 were also left in during this fifteen-minute period. These needles were then removed, and the last pair—Spleen-4 and Heart Protector-6—was needled for fifteen minutes. The first two pairs are the exit/entry points of their respective meridians. They move stagnation and harmonize excess and deficiency along the course of the meridians as well as stimulate the dynamic functions of the corresponding officials.

Heart Protector-5 is the metal point on its meridian that is joined functionally here with Lung-8, the metal and horary point on the lung meridian. With this combination, a functional path is made across the *ke* cycle between Lung-8 (the transmitting point) and Heart Protector-5 (the receiving point). Using this technique, the virtues of the lung official are empowered within the heart protector. This pair addressed Brit's constitutional type directly and served to further integrate the functional relationship of the heart protector and lung officials.

Spleen-4 and Heart Protector-6 are the master and couple points for the extra meridian known as *chongmai,* or "sea of blood." This meridian helps nourish the womb and move stagnation present in the reproductive organs.

SESSION 6

Report from last session: Brit was feeling signs of a cold with sharp pain over the right eye in the vicinity of Gallbladder-14. She woke up every day with nausea, which usually faded by 2 P.M. Her right side was bothering her a bit, but still it was much improved. She reported feeling cold all the time. Her hair was still thinning. She had a feeling of a heavy weight on her chest in the vicinity of Conception Vessel-17, something "like a lump." On the day following her last treatment, she'd had a bloody vaginal discharge that was clotted and dark in color.

Acupuncture points: Kidney-22, Heart Protector-1; Heart Protector-8, Conception Vessel-15, Lung-3, Lung-9; Gallbladder-14.

Kidney-22 and Heart Protector-1 were selected to move *qi* across the chest through the heart.[35] Heart Protector-8 ("palace of weariness") was selected for its psychospiritual properties. As the horary point on the heart protector meridian, Heart Protector-8 may rekindle the fires of a heart that has grown weary from the pain of past disappointments and betrayals. When treated at the appropriate time, Heart Protector-8 can induce a state of bliss, which may restore the patient's memory of the safety and joy that lies buried in the depths of self. Needling this point may touch the source of the heart's function and influence that always lies beyond any pain experienced in later heaven. I have found this to be one of the most profound points for reawakening the heart's fire and capacity for joy. Heart Protector-8 was selected as the distal point. Conception Vessel-15 was selected as the *mu* point of the heart protector to give a central focus to the *qi* moving through the chest. Lung-3, the "window of heaven" on the lung meridian, was grounded with Lung-9, the meridian's source point. With this point selection, I again addressed Brit's constitutional dynamic between fire and metal. Gallbladder-14 was selected as a local point for her headaches. I view this as a point to address the function of the eyes as they relate to deeper aspects of vision. By choosing this point, I intended to empower Brit with a perspective that may engender forgiveness toward herself and her father so she can move forward in life unencumbered by regrets and resentments from the past.

SESSION 7

Report from last session: Brit reported, "I felt wonderful for four days. I felt very joyful and like a little girl again. Was happy to get up and would run to look out the window to greet the day. A lot more energy now, can stay up and work late, like I used to be able to. I feel like I have my old self back." Brit experienced some stomach bloating and pain in the groin as her menstrual period approached. Her right breast had stopped producing milk. This finding may be significant evidence of the efficacy of the point combination Kidney-22 and Heart Protector-1 needled in the last session.

Acupuncture points: Kidney-13, Kidney-3; Liver-8, Liver-11; Conception Vessel-4.

Kidney-13 ("door of infants") was used here with multiple intentions. This point, used in its psychospiritual aspect, addresses deeper issues from infancy to 3 or 4 years of age. Of course, its name and location in the lower burner suggest a relationship to the womb and gynecology. Indeed, this point addressed Brit's infertility and endometriosis while at the same time touching on the deeper, older issues related to these symptoms. Liver-8, as the water point on a wood meridian, empowers the quality of flexibility during growth. This point enables *qi* to flow around obstacles in the same way that a seedling grows around a rock, blocking its path as it breaks through the soil toward its goal, the sun. Liver-8 was paired with local point Liver-11 to assist the flow of *qi* through the sexual organs. Lastly, Conception Vessel-4 was added to focus the treatment in the lower burner.

Session 8

Report from last session: Brit's menstrual period had begun. Dark clots were present; however, the overall quality of the blood was bright red. Although she felt some pain, overall the period was much improved. Her spirits were still high. Brit reported a dream about her father in which she was responsible for him missing a train. She felt bad in the dream because he was crying.

Acupuncture points: Bladder-25, Large Intestine-4; Bladder-13, Bladder-14, Bladder-43 (38), Bladder-53 (48); Kidney-3.

The first point combination consists of the large intestine *shu* point (Bladder-25) paired with the source point of the large intestine (Large Intestine-4). These points are treated constitutionally as a deep reserve of strength to support the large intestine official and its associated functions. Located in the lower burner opposite the uterus, they may empower the letting go of grief stored in this part of the body, manifesting symptomatically as endometriosis and infertility.

The second combination of points treats the lung *shu* point (Bladder-13) with the heart protector *shu* point (Bladder-14) and its associated point on the outer line of the bladder meridian (Bladder-43). These are also constitutional points, addressing the relationship between the fire and metal element. Point Bladder-43 addresses the deep spirit level functioning of the heart protector.[36] Bladder-53 (Womb and Heart Diaphragm) was used for its ability to harmonize the relationship between the function of the heart protector and the sexual organs.

Lastly, I used both moxa and a needle on Kidney-3 as the meridian's source point. Brit's kidney pulse exhibited extreme weakness, which I interpreted as the mother (metal element), which is constitutionally weak, not feeding the child (water element). While the moxa was burning on Kidney-3, I continually monitored Brit's left proximal pulse (a kidney position) for an increase in strength. Because her response to this final point was strongly positive, I focused future treatments on reestablishing the balanced relationship between the metal and water elements and attempted to harmonize her husband/wife imbalance. In the near future, I planned to have a female colleague treat Brit on Conception Vessel-1 and Governor Vessel-1 to bring up the overall quality and quantity of *qi* on the pulse, to move stagnation, and to tonify *qi* in the lower burner.

Summary

Brit's initial response to treatment, both constitutionally and symptomatically, was excellent. Her spirit appeared lighter and her attitude became increasingly positive. Physically, her pain subsided and her first menstrual period after initiating treatment was much improved. In the early stages of treatment, she had several colds, which I interpreted as a sign of grief clearing from the lung official. Her report of feeling "like my old self" after the sixth treatment is the hallmark of success during the initial stages of constitutional treatment. Although these results were excellent, I was concerned that they might represent her subjective response to being given access to deeper reserves of spiritual strength. I emphasized to her that things tend to feel better long before they are better and warned her about the importance of conserving and cultivating her resources during this most important turning point in her path to healing.

Brit's health continued to improve, and after several months she became pregnant, suggesting a deep balance had been achieved in her reproductive organs. Consistent with this was a significant improvement in her endometrial pain. Only one period before becoming pregnant had been difficult, with heavy cramping, which she did not associate with the quality or severity of pain she had previously attributed to her endometriosis. In March 1996 Brit gave birth to a healthy baby girl.[37] In my clinical practice, I have always considered aiding in the creation of new life as my greatest reward. With the birth of Brit's daughter, heaven had fulfilled its promise of eternal new beginnings.

Questions

Things to consider while conducting a diagnosis:

1. Forgetting all technical skills, what is your major impression just sitting with a patient?

2. What are the most significant moments during the intake?

3. How are these moments thematically related and how does this theme emerge as an expression of the five elements?

4. Given each weakness and strength the patient exhibits, what is its polar opposite?

5. What group of up to four points and what herb formula most succinctly characterize this patient's functional dynamic?

6. What element are these points or herbs associated with?

7. What are the virtues associated with that element?

8. What virtue could the patient embody that would help integrate and balance his or her entire system of functioning?

9. What emotion is the patient habitually seeking to avoid or indulge in?

10. What evidence is there for the patient's relative level of ignorance and/or awareness?

11. To what degree does your prognosis limit the patient's capacity to heal during treatment?

NOTES

1. Patients are advised not to wear perfume or cologne to their sessions in order to facilitate diagnosis by odor.
2. See Jarrett, 1995a, p. 46.
3. I am making the inference here that her father's psoriasis resulted from heat in his blood, which in turn resulted from *yin* deficiency, itself predicated on overactivity of the nervous system.
4. Foundation for Inner Peace (1975).
5. A hallmark of constitutional type is the form of functional expression habitually exhibited. During the interview, the practitioner may interact with the patient purposely to activate each emotion in the present. This allows him to assess how easily the patient is able to move through each form of elemental expression. During Kathryn's interview, she moved fairly easily through expressions characteristic of the other four elements. However, she continually returned to the expression of an excessive need to give and receive sympathy characteristic of the earth type.
6. See Jarrett, 1994.
7. My analysis of the pulse represents my own synthesis of nineteen years of experience in the Worsley five-element system of *Nanjing* pulse diagnosis and eleven years of study with Dr. Leon Hammer. Although much of my pulse nomenclature is taken from Dr. Hammer, my interpretation of pulse qualities of any specific patient often occurs within the context of constitutional diagnosis and does not necessarily correspond to Hammer's associations of these qualities in all cases. See Hammer (in press).
8. This interpretation of "chaos" and the importance of stabilizing the pulse is consistent with the teachings of both the Traditional Acupuncture Institute, Columbia, Maryland, and Dr. Leon Hammer. For a discussion of this topic, see Hammer, 1993a and 1993b.

9. By imposing on the body's natural hormonal processes, birth control pills often artificially mask imbalances that otherwise would manifest symptomatically in a woman's reproductive system. Illnesses become more difficult to diagnose and treat. I am inherently suspicious of any drug that intrudes on a function so vital to the body's balance and health.

10. As an example of giving the patient an image associated with a point function, when treating Liver-1, I affirmed to Kathryn, "This treatment helps empower you with the ability to discern what roots you into the ground of existence and cannot be compromised." The manifestation of this deep vision in life is the basis of self-esteem and a primary function of Liver-1. For greater detail on the inner nature of the acupuncture points, see Jarrett, 1995b and my Web page at http://www.spiritpathpress.com.

11. Formulated by Jade Pharmacy, Eugene, Oregon.

12. Jarrett, 1994, pp. 21–22.

13. Acupuncture point designations separated by a comma are located on the same meridian; designations separated by a semicolon are located on different meridians.

14. Each of the eight extra meridians has a master and couple point, which when needled open up and initiate the function of that meridian.

15. The use of Kidney-16 to nourish the heart is taught by Dr. Leon Hammer. In my experience, this point is ideal for empowering communication between the kidney and heart. I often use it as the central focus of treatments to balance the functional relationship between these two organs.

16. I often treat these qualities and this condition with the herbal formula Pinellia and Magnolia, which effectively circulates the *qi* of the chest.

17. "Grounding" here refers to the process of selecting a distal point that will root the treatment and determine its overall elemental quality.

18. Stomach-9 is both a window point and a confluent point for the divergent channels of the stomach and spleen meridians. Divergent channels are a mechanism by which emotional material that is too painful to assimilate may be sublimated away from conscious experience. Treating a window point may help reunite the head and heart and thus bring past pain into consciousness, allowing it to be processed and let go. This material is my interpretation of notes taken in a lecture with Jeffrey Yuen.

19. The trapezius muscle may be thought of as the "pillar that holds up the head (heaven)."

20. Formulated by Jade Pharmacy, Eugene, Oregon. For a discussion of this formula, see Jarrett, 1995b, p. 149 n. 26.

21. Wilhelm, 1967, p. 193.

22. A virtue associated with the earth element is the ability to move easily through transitions. This is explained in some five-element charts that place earth at the transition point between the other four elements. Hence "being stuck" is a common attribute ascribed to the earth constitution and may be interpreted as the stomach and spleen failing to perform their function of processing and transformation of life.

23. Whereas the earth element connects through the umbilical cord to the mother, the metal element connects through the virtue of inspiration to the father.

24. See Jarrett, 1994.

25. See the discussion of the husband/wife imbalance in Chapter 7.

26. Typically, a woman's period lasts about 5 days.

27. From my studies with Dr. Leon Hammer.

28. Phlegm that obscures the heart may be likened to clouds obscuring the sun. It is the lungs' function to digest vapor, and the emotion associated with the lungs is

grief. When the lungs engender grief and fail to descend the fluids, then moisture (clouds) builds in the upper *jiao* and may affect the heart, which resides there along with the lungs.

29. The cotton quality can occur in a person of any constitutional type. In Brit's case, I believe the stagnation resulting from the closing of the functions empowered by the officials in the upper *jiao* caused the secondary collapse of the liver function, which in turn was manifesting many of her symptoms. The creative flow of liver *qi* is stifled here as the functioning of the heart and lung is suppressed, leading eventually to the collapse of the entire left side of the pulse.

30. This concept was introduced to me by Dr. Leon Hammer.

31. This concept was introduced to me by Dr. Leon Hammer.

32. Although this formula addresses peripheral circulation, in the five-element tradition, peripheral circulation falls under the functional domain of the heart protector, termed alternately the circulation/sex meridian. I have discussed the use of Yunnan Paiyao for this purpose in Jarrett, 1995b.

33. The Seven Internal Dragons comprise a point on the conception vessel between CV-14 and CV-15, which is palpated for, and three bilateral points, adding up to seven points.

34. See Jarrett, 1994, pp. 19–30.

35. Acupuncture point Heart Protector-1, located one inch lateral to the nipple, has historically been "forbidden" to needle on women largely because of social taboos and the physical sensitivity of the point's location. In my opinion, it is feasible for experienced practitioners to needle this point in women with small-sized breasts. Because of its position, male practitioners must be sensitive to the woman's feelings and observe appropriate boundaries. This can be a most potent point in empowering the overall spiritual well-being and function of the heart protector official. Note that I used Heart Protector-2 in the second session with Brit and here wanted the stronger effect of Heart Protector-1.

36. Generally, points located on the outer bladder line address spiritual aspects of function that correspond to points on the inner bladder and governor vessel located at the same level. For example, Governor Vessel-4 addresses the "gate of destiny"; Bladder-23 addresses the kidneys, Bladder-52 the *jing*, and the spirit of the kidneys, the *zhi* (human will).

37. After Brit gave birth by Caesarian section, I prescribed a ginseng nutritive formula that is excellent for systemic *qi* and blood deficiency and was particularly suited to address her constitutional dynamic by tonifying both the heart and lungs. I have found this formula helpful for mothers regaining strength after childbirth. After Brit's recovery began, I prescribed the formula Dang Gui Si Ni Tang to establish boundaries and to harmonize the constitutional dynamic between the lungs and heart. The use of this formula is supported by my observations of a fine, deep, barely perceptible pulse (particularly on the left-hand side), cold hands and feet, dysmenorrhea, infertility, *yang, qi,* and blood deficiency, and the metal/fire constitutional dynamic. Note that Brit's timidity described earlier suggested an imbalance of the *yingqi* (interior) and *weiqi* (exterior), which also may be well addressed by this formula. The formula was expected to empower Brit to express her heart spirit and fire *(yang)* more freely externally (thus warming her), rather than hiding them (because of counterflow or suppression) internally.

The Complementary Natures of Chinese and Western Science and Medicine

"No indeed!," said Jo of the North Sea. "There is no end to the weighing of things, no stop to time, no constancy to the division of lots, no fixed rule to beginning and end."
– ZHUANGZI[1]

Before we can speak of coarse or fine, however, there must be some form. If a thing has no form, then numbers cannot express its dimensions, and if it cannot be encompassed, then numbers cannot express its size. We can use words to talk about the coarseness of things and we can use our minds to visualize the fineness of things. But what words cannot describe and the mind cannot succeed in visualizing—this has nothing to do with coarseness or fineness.
– ZHUANGZI[2]

At the beginning of institution names come to be.
Once there are names, one must know when to stop.
One who knows when to stop does not become exhausted.
– DAO DE JING[3]

Without stepping out the door, know the world.
– DAO DE JING[4]

Introduction

At the time I began to take seriously the notion of a career in Chinese medicine, I was pursuing a Ph.D. in neurobiology at the University of Michigan. Having invested a lot of time and identifying myself with this path, I did not find it an easy decision to leave the program with a master's degree and enter what, at that time, could hardly have been called a profession in the United States. In retrospect this was a great moment and turning point in my life, although not so easy at the time.

Chinese medicine appeared to me to comprise the other half of everything I had been taught as a science student. I felt a deep yearning for any and all information on Chinese medicine I could find so that I could feel complete inside myself. Because of my training in the analytical sciences, it was essential for me in changing my life's direction to understand Chinese medicine as a rational mode of scientific inquiry and not just as an art form or folk medicine.

The work I present here represents the understanding that I have arrived at regarding the complementary natures of what I consider to be the two predominant scientific views in the world today. For the purpose of this discussion, I refer to the practice of acupuncture and herbal medicine as set forth in this text as "Chinese medicine," and I refer to the practice of the predominant style of medicine found in Western hospitals as "Western medicine." I hope to show here that the assertions and assumptions regarding health, healing, and the nature of existence found in this text flow directly from the very core of the theoretical foundations on which Chinese medicine is based, inasmuch as they represent a complement to the predominant mode of scientific inquiry developed in the West.

Complementary Modes of Inquiry

All models of medicine are based on sciences which, in turn, are based on an underlying worldview that reflects the values and beliefs of the society in which it was formulated. The fundamental assumptions on which a scientific view is based must ultimately define the weaknesses and strengths of the medical system built on it. Here I discuss the theoretical foundations of Chinese medicine as it complements Western medicine. Please note that this material has been well covered in the past by Porkert. I merely extend his ideas and hope to make the material more approachable.[5]

For the practitioner, understanding Chinese medicine as it complements the practice of Western medicine is important for several
reasons. Unless practitioners of both Chinese and Western traditions
understand the theoretical weaknesses and strengths of their own systems, it is unlikely that either will appreciate the appropriate
applications of complementary systems of medicine. When practitioners of a given discipline see a deficiency in their own system, they are
often tempted to coopt a technology from a complementary system in
order to compensate for the deficiency. When this occurs without
understanding the theoretical model on which the technology is based,
then both systems become compromised. This is happening in the West
today as physicians, unhappy with the perceived limits of Western
medicine, are rapidly adopting technologies such as acupuncture without sufficient understandings of the theory and worldview that give
acupuncture its efficacy. Further, practitioners of Chinese medicine
with insufficient understanding of their own model try to incorporate
pseudo-scientific technologies into their practice, such as electrical
point locators and stimulators, to make up for deficiencies in their own
diagnostic capabilities.

Practitioners of healing arts and sciences must recognize that the
models on which they organize their perceptions of the world are
merely stories made up by human beings and do not constitute "reality." Individuals grounded in the Western scientific framework often
find it difficult to make the paradigmatic shift necessary for understanding the scientific basis of Chinese medicine or other
complementary healing arts. Offering vague notions of causality and
cloaked in seemingly esoteric language, Chinese medicine holds little,
on first inspection, for the analytic mind to grasp firmly.

Students of Chinese medicine know that the healing modality they
are learning is very different from that of "Western" medicine, yet they
may only have a vague sense of the theoretical basis for these differences. Medical students and physicians may also be aware of
deficiencies in the approach of Western medicine, yet may not be aware
that these are implicit in the very heart of the theoretical model being
used. Often the inclination of practitioners of any discipline is to imagine that limitations in efficacy are merely "problems" which will
eventually be solved with further study and clinical experience, or the
advent of newer technology or scientific discovery. Practitioners need
to understand the limitations of the model on which their medicine is
based; *there are certain realms of efficacy in life that a given model
cannot attain based on theoretical considerations alone.*

The Complementarity of Chinese and Western Medicine

If we were to reduce all of Western science to an absolute principle, it might be expressed in this way: "If you can't measure a thing, then it does not exist. The degree of accuracy to which a thing can be measured is the degree to which we can know and make factual statements about it." Although this may appear to be an extreme position, it is a direct quotation from a professor, made during the introductory remarks to a course in clinical neurology I attended while pursuing my graduate degree in the neurosciences.

The fundamental assertion of Asian philosophies found in many Daoist, Hindu, and Buddhist writings might be summed up in this way: "Whatever can be measured is the most superficial and transitory aspect of a thing. Material reality is an illusion that must be transcended in order to feel the depth of spirit inherent in a thing."

At first glance these two viewpoints appear to be diametrically opposed and, in fact, do serve as opposite and absolute poles around which the Western and Eastern sciences are respectively built. Using these two assertions as building blocks, we arrive at two worldviews and two medical models, both valid and useful, but only over a limited range of life's experience.

Comparison of Models

Western science may be said to be a system that proceeds by the quantitative measurement of things. The emphasis on measurement as a mode of inquiry in the West limits its scope of study to physical structure or, in other words, that which is materially real. Hence the utilization of machines that can measure things with great accuracy is central to the diagnostics of medicine based on this model. Many diagnostic statements are expressed in terms of numbers such as pulse *rate*, triglyceride *level*, blood *pressure*, bone *density*, cell *count*, and lung *capacity*, for example.

Chinese science proceeds according to the qualitative assessment of function. It does not study *things*, but rather the functional relationship between things. Chinese medicine focuses on the qualities and movement of *qi*, and the diagnostics of Chinese medicine are limited to what can be directly perceived with the senses. Rather than relying on technology, practitioners spend a lifetime developing their ability to interpret and perceive the patient's color, sound, odor, emotion, pulses, and all other sensory data. In effect, practitioners become finely tuned instruments. Diagnostic statements are made, not in terms of *quantity*, but rather in terms of *quality*. Qualities attended to may include patients' emotional expression, physiological function, social and intimate relationships, and, ultimately, their quality of life.

Western science is termed "reductionist" because of its tendency to reduce its view of the things it studies to their most elementary structures. Its strength lies in providing a great understanding of the hierarchy of structures that constitute life. For example, Western science can tell us about the liver, the cells in the liver, the components in the cells (organelles), the proteins that make up the organelles, the amino acids that make up the proteins, the atoms that make up the amino acids, and finally, the charges and components of the atoms themselves.

The strength of any system of thought always defines its corresponding weakness. A weakness in the reductionist model is that as analysis penetrates to increasingly smaller levels of structure, it becomes difficult to integrate observations back to the higher order of what one initially set out to study. For example, when discussing the structure of an atom in the liver it is difficult to relate this information in a meaningful way back to liver function, let alone the function of another organ system or the organism at large. This limitation is depicted in Figure A.1.

Psychoneuroimmunology is currently receiving a lot of attention in Western medical science. The major insight of this field is that the emotions, nervous system, and immunological systems are somehow related. In the holistic model that is at the core of Chinese medicine as a complementary science, the view that these systems, so vital to the integrated function of the human being, might not be intimately related is implausible.

Figure A.1 illustrates the fundamental differences between a structural and functional approach to the study of life. At the lowest level of the hierarchy, the study of the material universe generates data that are easily generalizable from one atom to another. For example, the properties of a given carbon atom may be assumed true for any other carbon atom. As we proceed up the structural hierarchy of life, observations become increasingly ungeneralizable within categories and unintegratable between categories. The sheer number of things that exist, coupled with the Western emphasis on reductionism, results in the phenomena of "specialization" in research, scholarship, and medicine. Unable to grasp all the information available, each practitioner specializes in one aspect of medical practice. Hence each physician and

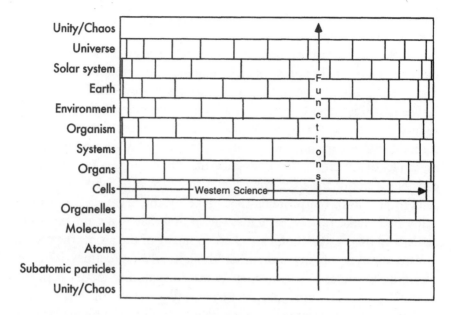

Figure A.1

STRUCTURE VERSUS FUNCTION

This figure depicts the increasing structural complexity of life as we travel up the hierarchy of scale from atoms to solar systems and beyond. Note that the extremes beyond both the largest and smallest imaginable physical manifestation in life may be represented as unity. Western scientific study proceeds laterally according to field of specialization. The organ functions in Chinese medicine span this hierarchy vertically, however. Therefore Chinese medicine more easily integrates observations regarding functional relationships across various levels of existence as life becomes more structurally complex.[6]

researcher specializes in the study of a particular physical manifestation of life. This tendency toward specialization is indicated in the figure by the horizontal arrow. Western science and medicine proceed laterally as each participant learns increasingly more in life about his or her narrow field. For example, a researcher may spend a lifetime learning about the structure of one group of proteins found in a small mass of cells in the brain. In turn, a physician may specialize in illnesses that affect only one organ or organ system.

In contrast, the practice of Chinese medicine proceeds vertically (vertical arrows): The functions that compose the officials span all levels of the physical hierarchy. This allows the traditional practitioner to incorporate any observation about patients and their lives into the diagnosis, prognosis, and treatment plan. For example, the function of the large intestine may be said to empower the letting go of all that no longer serves a person. On the physical level, this function is, in fact, most strongly represented by the large intestine. However, the capacity to let go of the by-products of metabolism is equally present at the cellular, organ, and even the systems level.

For example, the nervous system discharges its waste into the cerebrospinal fluid. On an emotional level, the function of letting go is represented by the presence of the emotions grief and longing. The function of letting go continues past the individual human being and into society, ecosystems, and perhaps even into planetary systems. Hence the individual functions transcend the distinctions both among mind, body, and spirit, as well as the distinction between self and not-self, the larger ecological and social context within which the individual exists.

I have found it to be an interesting exercise to apply the concepts of Chinese physiology to the environmental condition of our planet. We may consider fossil fuels to represent the planet's *jing*. Oil is, in fact, the remains of our ancestors. Our emphasis on production in the world has combusted and thus depleted our reserves of oil. Correspondingly the protective layer of ozone, which may be considered to correspond to the earth's *weiqi* (protective *qi*), has been eroded. This process has resulted in a general increase in the earth's temperature, which may be thought to correspond to a *yin*-deficient state. Correspondingly, we see humanity suffering from autoimmune diseases and an increase of skin cancer due to an increase of radiation associated with the decreased protective shield of ozone.

At the point of development where systems exist in the evolution of the biological hierarchy, consciousness emerges from the cells of the nervous system. It is here that the mind/body duality emerges in the Western scientific paradigm. It is also approximately at this point that observations become no longer generalizable between categories. The body/mind duality is easily overcome by Chinese medicine because functions transcend all levels of body/mind/spirit (a separation that cannot be communicated in the classical language of Chinese medicine). Hence, at precisely the level where Western inquiry is most effective (atomic and molecular level), Chinese medicine is at its limit of resolution. Conversely, at exactly the level that Western science begins to break down (the level of physical structure at which consciousness emerges), Chinese science becomes quite effective.

All scientific systems have a core of applicability. As we move away from this core, the application of the Western causal and reductionist paradigm is stretched to the point where it is no longer useful. The

Western scientific paradigm, ideal for the study of atoms and the smaller building blocks of life, degenerates when it is applied to more complicated levels in the hierarchical structure such as organ function, organisms as a whole, and social systems. The efficacy of the Western scientific method is therefore inversely proportional to the density of substrata that constitute the manifestation of life being studied. In contrast, the greater the density of substrata, the greater the functional basis that supports the officials studied in Chinese medicine. The science of function begins to be effective at the cellular level, exactly that point at which the science of structure begins to be compromised.

In accord with its reductionist view and corresponding focus on the individual parts of organisms, Western medicine may also be called "mechanistic." This mechanistic view springs directly from the underlying views of Newtonian physics in which the universe is understood in terms of the mechanical interactions of its components. Western medicine views the body as a complicated machine that may be understood through the quantitative analysis of each of its discrete structures. Consider, for example, its use of machines to replace body parts and its modeling of human consciousness using computers.

Chinese medicine is termed "holistic" because it studies the important functional relationships present in the whole. Practitioners of classical Chinese medicine can tell us nothing about the actual structure of the liver, but they may have a lot to say about the relationship between the liver, the emotion of anger, digestion, the quality of the left middle pulse position, our ability to formulate plans, and many other qualities of personal expression. Instead of seeing humans and nature as complicated machines made up of discrete parts, practitioners of Chinese medicine see them as a living whole whose natural processes and functional relationships extend from the workings of the heavens to human physiology.

The difference between reductionist and holistic thought is illustrated in the following example. If we imagine that a human being is like a pointillist painting, then the two sciences have quite different ways of interpreting this painting. We could say that each specialist in Western medicine has information on only a part of the picture. There are doctors who specialize in red dots at the center of the picture and ones who specialize in blue dots in the upper right-hand corner, and so on. However, each physician has only a small part of the picture, and difficulty may exist when physicians practicing in different specialties try to communicate with each other about the nature of the painting. For no one of them has an integrated view of the whole. Patients are consequently often overtreated as each practitioner treats the subsystem in which he or she specializes. Serious implications may ensue for the patient because medications prescribed by various specialists can have adverse reactions when combined.

Practitioners of Chinese medicine, in contrast, do not focus on any one detail of expression but stand back to synthesize a view of the entire picture that is emerging. This does not give the practitioner detailed structural information on each subsystem, but does yield an overall sense of the functional dynamic that is emerging newly in each moment. As opposed to specializing in a given aspect of treatment, practitioners are able to treat whole patients in a more integrated and natural way. It has occurred to me that due to specialization, a Western scientist learns more and more in life about less and less. In Chinese medicine, in contrast, one tends to learn less and less about more and more!

A dietary and exercise regimen, acupuncture, herbs, attitudes, and core belief systems may be addressed. Instead of the conflicts that often occur between the multiple prescriptions given to a single patient by various medical specialists, all therapy is given with the same clear intention of affecting the primary underlying functional imbalance. Hence the notion of specialization is particularly ill-suited and at odds with the fundamental theoretical strengths inherent at the heart of Chinese medicine. Note, however, that specialties are beginning to develop in the practice of Chinese medicine in the West. I see this as an unfortunate development predicated on the attempt to emulate the prevailing model in Western medicine. Unfortunately the net effect is to move away from the core that defines Chinese medicine as a complementary modality and thus undermine its efficacy.

Quantity versus Quality

Experimentation is not a criterion of a scientific method.[6] What is needed is the ability to integrate observations, using a set of standards, into a system that yields repeatable, predictable results. Western science references all its observations to the CGS (centimeter, grams, seconds) system of quantitative standards. Chinese medicine references its observations to qualitative systems of standards such as the five elements and eight principles. When an object of study is described by the methods of Western science, we are always left with a list of its components and corresponding numbers. The differences between quantitative analysis and qualitative assessment are illustrated by the following example. If we were to describe a pen using the methods of analytic science, we might generate data similar to that in Figure A.2.

Analysis of a Ballpoint Pen					
Component	Length	Weight	Density	Melting Point	Boiling Point
Spring					
Ink					
Plastic					
Metal					

Figure A.2
ANALYSIS OF A BALLPOINT PEN

Although the data we might enter in Figure A.2 certainly tells us in detail about the pen's physical structure, it tells us nothing of its function. To describe this pen using qualitative Chinese science we might say, "This object is held in the hand and used to write with on paper so that ideas may be symbolized and remembered and/or communicated to another person." This statement may be true, but none of it can be directly verified through measurement. In reality I have not described the pen at all but the functional relationships that exist among the pen, paper, thought, the hand, memory, and so on. Chinese medicine does not study "things" but rather the functional relationships that define the context within which things exist. However, relationships do not exist in things, but between things, and therefore do not exist materially.

Relationships can only be described qualitatively and cannot be directly measured. For example, if I ask you to describe the most significant relationship in your life, you will respond, not with a numerical analysis, but with an assessment of the qualities inherent in the relationship. Further, the relationship is only what you and the other person involved say about it, or whatever anybody else says about it, and all are correct, as each individual perceives the relationship through his or her own interpretive filters. The relationship is not static in nature but changes with every heartbeat of the two individuals involved. Hence the ways of knowing devised in ancient China emphasized understanding dynamic processes of change rather than the fixed and static manifestations of individual things.

Five different individuals might use very different words to describe the pen in the preceding example, yet each description would only enhance the others by filling in more detail. The Chinese recognized early on that the nature of reality depended in large part on the perceiver. They chose the number five to represent the directions on earth, the fifth direction representing the center or position of the observer. It is quite possible in the practice of Chinese medicine that different practitioners might generate an altogether different diagnosis of a given patient. However, these would not be seen as invalidating each other, but would represent each individual's unique quality of connection with that patient. In Chinese medicine it must be understood that a practitioner's diagnosis is always of the nature and quality of his or her relationship to the patient and not of a property ascribed to the patient alone. The patient is viewed as a complex diamond that may be entered through any of its facets, all of which lead to the same basic inner truth. It is thus quite conceivable that practitioners with very different functional diagnoses could equally help a patient because of the unique qualities which define each person's relationship to that patient.

In order for a Western scientific analysis to be considered correct, however, the same data must be arrived at regardless of who is doing the measuring. For example, if ten scientists set out to weigh a rock, their independent measurements are expected to yield the same results. If one individual obtains results that differ from the other nine, it is assumed either that person is a bad scientist or his or her machine malfunctioned. Western science values objectivity and seeks to discern that the properties of what is being studied exist solely in the object, independent of the individual making the observations and the object's surroundings. For this reason, Western science proceeds to learn about the world through controlled experiment. When studying a thing, it is important to isolate it completely from its natural environment in order to rule out all effects on it that might be attributed to nonspecific factors. This contrasts with Chinese science, which strives to observe how a thing functions in relationship to its natural environment. Traditional Chinese medicine's emphasis on our intimate connection to the environment affords an ecological perspective vitally important in the world today. In contrast, the reductionist method of Western science perpetuates feelings of separation between humans and nature and thus contributes to the environmental problems that compromise our health and threaten our very existence.

Prevention

Chinese medicine is unique in its ability to assess, based on patients' momentary presentation, both the events in their past that have brought them to their current state and the future course of events should nothing be done to alter their path. This is done in much the same way as meteorological prediction is done in the West. Meteorologists do not conduct experiments but merely make observations in the moment and interpret them based on past experience. For example, in predicting the weather, they may take into account the present direction of the wind, cloud formations, relative humidity, and temperature. They then may compare these observations with recent patterns and the entire database of their past experience. In this way they may formulate an educated estimate of the direction the weather is about to take. In the same way, a practitioner of Chinese medicine may be able to predict accurately the direction in which a patient's health is proceeding. The orientation of Chinese medicine toward prevention is in direct contrast with that of Western medicine, which only treats illness after it has manifested. Although this approach is appropriate when treating acute trauma, it lacks applicability in treating the long-term functional relationships on which health is predicated.

Specialization

To a man who has a hammer, the whole world looks like a nail.
– Source Unknown

Because of its emphasis on constancy of numerical data, Western science is unable to integrate viewpoints that differ when studying the same subject. Differing viewpoints on the same phenomena are not able to be integrated because Western science pursues ultimate truth. This is another factor that leads to specialization as people in different fields attribute the etiology of any given condition to their area of interest. Hence many different physicians treat each aspect of physical functioning, psychotherapists treat the mind, and the spirit is left to the domain of religion. Each practitioner sees the cause of imbalance as emanating from the aspect of being that they study, and no language exists for them all to communicate with each other in a meaningful way. The physician may thus diagnose a condition of abnormal behavior as the consequence of unbalanced brain chemistry, a geneticist may attribute the same problem to an inherited genetic defect, and a psychologist may view it as a learned behavior.

Chinese science does not ask questions about life to which it seeks concrete answers. Instead, it inquires into the nature of things, not expecting ever to reach an end point at which the inquiry is complete. Chinese medicine emphasizes evolution and change rather than the static nature of life. Western science, in focusing on the material world, places its emphasis on the fixed nature of life's manifestations. This orientation leads it to search for concrete answers to questions about the structure of the material world.

The Role of Emotions and Spirit in Illness

At some point in the structural hierarchy that comprises a human being, the phenomenon of mind begins to emerge. Mind, however, cannot be identified in any of the components that make up the hierarchy. That is, it is not found by the physicist, cell biologist, or even the neurobiologist. True, disciplines exist in the West such as psychology that seek to understand the role of the mind in illness, yet these disciplines often stretch to its breaking point the usefulness of the Western scientific model on which they are based. Fields such as behavioral psychology and sociology attempt to apply the tools of quantitative analysis to nonmaterial human and cultural phenomena. Humanistic clinical psychologies, still in an early stage of development, do entail concepts relating to function. But they cannot be said to be truly holistic because they contain only elementary schemes for integrating physiological data and are not based on an ecological worldview.

In contrast we can see examples of the theoretical foundations of Chinese medicine being pushed to their breaking point under the auspices of "holism." For instance, some practitioners utilize electrical devices, including computers, in both diagnosis and treatment. The recommendation has also occasionally been made that it is necessary to develop computer models that can be used to substantiate and develop Chinese pulse diagnosis. For every development in technology another human virtue and ability has eroded. Placing a machine between the practitioner and patient is in direct conflict with the very theoretical principles on which Chinese medicine is predicated.

The materialistic focus of Western science limits its ability to comprehend the contributions of the emotions to health and illness. It is unable to study meaningfully the role of the spirit or emotions in illness because they are not quantifiable. Hence Western science is unable to diagnose or treat effectively a wide range of conditions to which it gives the pseudo diagnosis of "psychosomatic" (involving mind and body). When patients' tests reveal no diagnosis, they are often told their illness is "in their head," having no material basis in reality.

Comparison of the Concept of Diagnosis

The concept of diagnosis in Western and Chinese medicine is substantially different. Diagnosis in Western medicine aims at determining the physical manifestation of an illness and therapy focuses on altering that manifestation. Hence a typical diagnosis of the cause of an individual's back pain might be "a ruptured disk between the fourth and fifth lumbar vertebrae is placing pressure on the sciatic nerve." Therapeutic intervention then attempts to alter surgically the physical relationships between the herniated disk and the affected nerve. Chinese medicine is much less concerned with the purely physical aspects of illness and seeks instead to discover the functional basis that underlies the manifestation of the given symptom. From the standpoint of Chinese medicine, many of the so-called diagnoses of Western medicine are not diagnoses at all, but rather terms that merely describe the physical manifestations of an illness. Western diagnoses often consist of language that reiterates the patient's complaint in medical terminology. A woman complaining of "burning in her muscles" may be told she has "myofibrositis," a term that only informs her there is inflammation in her muscle tissue, yet says nothing about the functional etiology of such inflammation.

In the practice of Western medicine, individuals who share the same physical diagnosis receive the same treatment according to whatever the current standard of practice is at the time of their diagnosis, regardless of the differences in the functional etiology behind the disorder. For example, the individual diagnosed with myofibrositus receives a course of anti-inflammatory agents for the condition. The Chinese medical practitioner, however, would seek to determine and then harmonize the underlying dysfunctional physiology that is generating this condition. Ten individuals, each experiencing similar physical sensations and having the same Western diagnosis, could be determined to have entirely different diagnoses according to Chinese medicine. In Chinese medicine, people with similar functional imbalances may receive similar treatment regardless of the symptomatic expression and

Western diagnosis. For example, a patient with migraine headaches might receive similar treatment to one whose primary complaint was arthritis if the two patients had similar functional imbalances. In truth, however, the possible combinations of acupuncture points and herbal prescriptions are nearly infinite, and it is highly unlikely that any two individuals would receive identical treatment.

In Chinese medicine, the correct diagnosis of a patient is the one that restores a proper balance of functioning most efficiently. This can never be absolutely known, however, as only one treatment protocol can ever be tried on a given patient at a given moment in time. The Chinese emphasis has always been that what works is the confirmation of diagnosis. In the West the confirmation of diagnosis comes before treatment is attempted, and as long as the tests yield the same results, the diagnosis will not change, even if the patient shows no improvement. An extension of this principle is that the illness is often seen as a "thing" being studied, independent of the patient who has it. This often leads to alienation from self and a decreased responsibility for healing on the part of patients who turn their well-being over to a health-care professional. In the Chinese view, illness is a direct emanation of functional imbalance that permeates every aspect of a patient's being. Patients are held responsible for consciously intervening in those aspects of their life in which they can effect positive change.

The Complementary Nature of Treatment

The two main tools of intervention available to the Western medical practitioner are surgeries and drugs, which are aimed at suppressing the expression of physical symptoms. Chinese medicine, instead, focuses on harmonizing the dysfunctional state on which the presence of physical symptoms is predicated. From the point of view of the inner tradition, the suppressing of physical symptomatology in chronic conditions is to perpetuate ignorance and is seen as contrary to the highest purpose of medicine as presented in this text. The presence of pain is often the result of having lost touch with some fundamental aspect of self. Pain may be interpreted as heaven's attempt to draw our attention toward the aspect of self-expression that has been lost. To suppress pain predicated on our suppression of true self, without simultaneously educating patients regarding the relevance of this pain to their life, is to perpetuate the underlying habitual patterns on which the pain is based. Heaven will always find a way to express its will, and pain suppressed in this way will always manifest elsewhere in the body and usually in a more serious way.

The dangers inherent in symptomatic treatment are illustrated in the following example. Suppressing physical symptomatology may be likened to driving a car and putting a bandage over the oil light when it comes on (like medicating an illness) so we cannot see it. When the temperature gauge indicates the car is overheating, we might proceed to cut all the wires going to the dashboard (surgery) in a further attempt to avoid the warning signs of imbalance. Of course, the oil light was merely a warning sign, and the car will now break down sooner rather than later.

From the point of view of Chinese medicine, we must read the signs of imbalance before they manifest physically in order to determine the functional cause of the problem (in this case the car needs oil) and thus prevent the illness. Symptoms, such as the oil light coming on, must be attended to immediately to prevent the manifestation of a deeper level of imbalance. Whenever the expression of a symptom is blocked therapeutically, the expression of imbalance will manifest at another, perhaps deeper level, of illness. This is true regardless of whether the modality used to suppress the expression of the symptom is acupuncture, herbal medicine, homeopathy, or surgery.

The Limits of Materialism in the Study of Function

Western medicine, although it embraces the concept of function, is limited to the study of only those aspects of functioning that have clear physical, measurable correlates. It is not possible to measure a function directly. We can only measure a physical reality correlated with a function. If, for example, we assess liver function by a given enzyme level, it is not actually liver function that is being measured but rather the level of an enzyme. We can therefore only study the physical correlates of function scientifically to the degree that current technology is capable of measuring them. Hence untold aspects of human expression lie unstudied and are not able to be integrated into diagnosis. Western science's study of function is as limited as the study of anatomy was in ancient China. Ancient Chinese medical texts include drawings of the different organ systems, yet these functional diagrams are quite crude by modern standards. The study of function by Western science would appear similarly crude to the practitioner of Chinese medicine.

In Chinese medicine, clinical effectiveness is only inherently limited by the resolution of the individual practitioner's sensitivity and knowledge base. Views on the causality of illness change in the West as new technologies are invented. As anatomy became a highly developed science, illness thus was seen as emanating from individual organs, and surgery became the therapy of choice. With the advent of technologies that give us access to the study of molecules, such as radioimmunoassays, the current vogue claims illnesses are a result of biochemical imbalances. In Chinese medicine the theories regarding the cause of illness have not changed appreciably since the writing of the *Nei Jing Su Wen*. Illness is always seen as caused by incomplete self-expression resulting from an underlying functional imbalance.

Acute versus Chronic Care

In acute cases of illness and traumatic injury, Western medicine's emphasis on quantity allows it great efficacy because it can stabilize vital signs (numbers) and save life. However, in most chronic illness, where the quality of life has been affected and the important functional relationships of the body's systems have been compromised, holistic medicines are better able to restore balance. Chinese medicine specializes in long-term care for chronic imbalances that involve the functional interrelationship of many aspects of being, physical and otherwise. Chinese medicine also works preventively because the practitioner can sense functional imbalances and harmonize them before they result in organic pathology. In the realm of acute care, Chinese medicine offers little that can rival the reattachment of a severed limb using microsurgical techniques. Of course a tradition of acute care exists in Chinese medicine, but it developed not as a strength but rather as a historical necessity. In terms of chronic care, Western medicine is effective in replacement therapies such as providing insulin to a diabetic. However, in a real sense these treatments represent acute care that occurs over the long term. For if diabetics do not receive their insulin, the consequences are grave.

Western medicine concerns itself with the survival of the material body. The concern of Chinese medicine is not with survival but with evolution. Although it is true that the practitioner of Chinese medicine must deal with the realities of physical illness, ultimately he or she is concerned with helping patients transcend imagined limitations and helping return them to the full self-expression that is synonymous with health.

Summary

The complementary natures of Chinese and Western science presented here represent absolute poles that define the relative strengths and weaknesses on which each medical model is based. Each of the models has a core of efficacy that is compromised as one's practice moves increasingly far from it. In Western medicine the practice of lifesaving medicine in trauma units defines the highest pinnacle that Western medicine can theoretically achieve. But as one moves away from this core applicability toward managing chronic conditions with surgeries or medications, the foundations of the model are compromised and the patient is not well served. Similarly, the heart of Chinese medicine resides in assisting the restoration of original nature and fulfillment of destiny as described in this text. As one's practice moves away from this center toward the symptomatic suppression of pain, the efficacy of Chinese medicine is compromised.

No medicine or technology is in and of itself either holistic or reductionist independent of the intention of the practitioner utilizing it. Although a model of medicine may have its theoretical strengths and weaknesses, the human capacity to heal is not ultimately limited by such constraints. Practitioners of medicine each bring their own unique capacities to their practice. Compassion in touching another's heart and the wisdom to offer patients the most effective care is within the grasp of each practitioner regardless of their tradition of practice.

Questions

Models of medicine are based on scientific models that have cores of theoretical applicability. As clinical practice moves away from the theoretical core of the science it is based on, the strengths of whatever healing model being used is compromised.

1. Is this statement true?

2. What is the relationship of a system's capacity to promote healing to science?

3. What is the relationship of one's capacity to heal oneself or another to scientific or medical theory?

NOTES

1. Watson, 1964a, p. 98.
2. Ibid., p. 99.
3. Chapter 32; in Chen, 1989, p. 133.
4. Chapter 47; in ibid., p. 166.
5. See Porkert, 1983, pp. 1–15.
6. Porkert, 1983, p. 7.

GLOSSARY OF CHINESE TERMS

This simple glossary will provide the reader with the most common usage of the included terms as they occur throughout the text.

BAI HU DONG *(Discussions of the White Tiger Hall)* (79 B.C.E.) 白虎堂 A work by scholars interpreting the writing of Confucius in which the Confucian virtues were first paired with the five elements.

BAI WEN BIAN *(The Hundred Questions)* 百問篇 Alchemical text that focuses on the functional correspondences between humanity and the microcosm. Possibly dates as far back as the Tang dynasty (618–906 C.E.).

BAOYI 包一 To embrace the one. Refers to the sage's ability to follow the principles of *dao*.

BEN MING YUAN SHEN 本命元神 Primordial spirits of fundamental destiny. The ascended spirits who live in the center of the Big Dipper and assign a destiny to each individual commensurate with personal merit at the moment of conception.

BULE 不樂 Literally, not joy, sorrow.

CHANG 常 Everlasting, eternal.

CHANGDAO 常道 The eternal virtue and nature of the unnamed *dao*.

CHENG 成 Completion. Characteristic ascribed to the eternal *dao* in the *Dao De Jing*. Suggests that the *dao* comprises totality.

CHONGMAI 衝脈 The sea of blood. Refers to the third of the eight extra meridians. As the *chongqi* blends heaven and earth, so too does *chongmai* blend the *yin* and *yang* of the human being as they are mediated by the conception and governor vessels, respectively.

CHONGQI 沖氣 Whirling abyss situated between heaven and earth. That which perfectly blends the qualities of these two universal poles so that duality is returned to unity.

CHONGXU 沖虛 The void.

CONFUCIUS, OR KONG FU ZI (551–479 B.C.E.) 孔夫子 Philosopher and educator.

DANTIAN 丹田 Cinnabar field. Located below the navel. The furnace that empowers alchemical transformation. Functionally related to the concept of *mingmen*.

DAO 道 Life's motivating force.

DAODE 道德 In the Daoist trinity signifies the manifestation of potential.

DAOXIN 道心 Consciousness; contrast with *renbuzhi*. Literally, "path of the heart."

DAOYONG 匋熔 To fuse, as in the smelting of metals.

DE 德 Original nature; virtue. Suggests intuition, or the ability to spontaneously comprehend truth uncolored by the mind's interpretation.

DE 惠 Rectitude.

DEQI 得氣 To attain *qi*; the sensation associated with the needling of an acupuncture point.

DI 帝 Emperor; the North Star or polestar.

DOU 豆 Sacrifical vessel.

ER 二 The number two.

FAMING To invent; to produce a thing by illuminating it from the void of *dao*.

FANG 反 To return.

FANGMING 方命 To neglect one's orders or destiny. Refers to Gun's inability to quell the floods.

FENG 豐 Two plant shoots; vitality and abundance.

FU 復 *Yijing* hexagram 24, "return." Termed by Liu Yiming "the door of life."

FU 付 To give.

FU 符 A deed in two halves; a Daoist talisman, believed to protect the possessor.

FU 府 Treasury, storehouse; the *yang* organs (腑).

GAOHUANG 膏肓 Area located between the diaphragm and the heart.

GONG 宮 Palace.

GU 痼 Chronic; a deeply rooted illness or habit.

GUAN 官 "Official." The sum total of an organ's sphere of influence.

GUAN 關 Border pass or customs station. Found in the acupuncture point names of Heart Protector-6, *neiguan*, and Triple Burner-5, *waiguan*.

GUI 鬼 Ghost; demon.

GUI 歸 To return.

GUN Father of Emperor Yu. Mythological figure who failed to quell the floods.

GUQI 穀氣 *Qi* derived from alimentation.

HAN FEIZI (280?–233 B.C.E.) 韓非子 Philosopher of the Legalist school who wrote the text bearing his name.

HOUTIAN 後天 Later heaven; all positive influences that we acquire in life after drawing the first breath. The period of time between the first breath and death.

HU 忽 Literally, "change." The emperor of the North Sea in the myth of *hun-tun*.

HUAINANZI 准南子 Early Daoist text written in the Han dynasty (122 B.C.E.) by guests of the court of Liuan, the prince of Huainan.

HUANGDI 黃帝 The Yellow Emperor.

HUI 會 Assembly, meeting.

HUN 魂 The *shen* associated with the liver official. In Daoist philosophy, the *hun* comprises *jing, qi,* and *shen,* termed the "three treasures." The *hun* governs the human ascension in life represented by the officials in the left half of the *sheng* cycle. It is the influence that allows for the evolution of the spirit through physical being (contrast with *po*). Upon death, the *hun* is said to leave the body through acupuncture point Governor Vessel-20 and ascend to heaven, where it reports on the relative merits of the individual accrued through fulfillment of destiny.

HUN 混 Chaos, blend; the primordial state of *dao* where heaven and earth are blended to form a perfect unity beyond human comprehension.

HUNTUN 混屯 Primordial state of *dao,* personified as Emperor Huntun of the center in *Zhuangzi*.

HUO 火 The fire element.

JIN 金 The metal element.

JING 精 Essence; the microcosmic representation of *dao* as undifferentiated potential.

JING 經 The warp of a fabric, the meridians, the classic texts; denotes the framework which holds a thing together whether it be a cloth, the functional integrity of a human being, or a body of knowledge.

JINGGONG 精宮 Acupuncture point Bladder-52 (47), "palace of essence."

JINGSHEN 精神 Synonymous with *shenjing*.

JINMEN 金門 "Golden gate," the interface between being and nonbeing; an alternate name for acupuncture point Conception Vessel-1.

KARMA (JIEMA) 羯磨 From the Sanskrit *kri*, "to do"; literally, "deed"; signifies all that we bring to this life from past lives and ancestors.

KE 克 Destruction; the *ke* cycle.

KONG 恐 Fear; the emotion associated with the water officials.

KONGQI 空氣 *Qi* gained from respiration.

KUN 坤 *Yijing* hexagram 2, "earth."

KUN 困 Constraint; depicts a tree growing within a sealed box.

KUNLUN MOUNTAIN 崑崙 In early Chinese myth, a mountain thought to be the center of the earth. The earthly representation of the pillar that joins heaven and earth. The home of Xi Wang Mu.

LAOZI (LAO TZU) 老子 Daoist philosopher ascribed as the author of the *Dao De Jing*. The name means literally "old infant."

LE 樂 Music, joy; the emotion associated with the fire officials.

LI 豊 Sacrificial vessel.

LI 禮 Virtue associated with the fire element; propriety.

LI 離 *Yijing* hexagram 30, "fire."

LI 利 Profit, advantage; worldly gain.

LI 立 To establish.

LIN 林 Two trees together; a forest.

LING 靈 *Yin* aspect of heart spirit that complements *shen*. The character *ling* depicts two female shaman performing a ritual to summon rain from heaven. The human potency to fulfill destiny and thereby be effective in influencing heaven and evoking changes in the world.

LINGBAO 靈寶 Bipartite term signifying the notion of *dao* as a treasure existing in both human and heaven. *Ling* is the heavenly aspect and *bao* is the earthly aspect identified with *jing*. Pure potential.

LINGFU 靈府 Spirit storehouse; the heart.

LINGTAI 靈台 Spiritual tower; the heart; the name of acupuncture point Governor-10.

LINGSHU (The Spiritual Pivot) 靈樞 Medical text compiled during the Warring States period (480–222 B.C.E.).

LIU YIMING 劉一明 Daoist scholar who wrote from the late 1700s to the early 1800s. Liu explained the esoteric language of the great Daoist alchemical texts. His work is of deep significance in understanding the spiritual and psychological aspects of Chinese physiology and the inner tradition of healing in Chinese medicine.

LO 絡 Silk, to connect, denotes the meridians when paired with the character *jing*.

LUAN 亂 In early Daoism, the chaos that results in the world after the human fall from original nature and the ensuing institution of society and culture.

LUNHUI 輪迴 Reincarnation. Transmigration of the spirit.

MAI 脈 Meridian, vessel.

MAILI 脈理 The pulse.

MENCIUS, MENGZI (C. 372–289 B.C.E.) 孟子 Confucian philosopher who authored the text that bears his name.

MI 米 Rice.

MIN 皿 A vase.

MING 命 Destiny. One's life mandate in the form of a contract with heaven.

MING 名 Personal name. That which distinguishes one's self from others and sows the seed for the loss of original nature.

MING 明 Illumination. Comprised of the characters for sun and moon, it denotes either the delusion of the material world or enlightenment, respectively.

MING 冥 Darkness, obscurity. In religious Daoism and Buddhism, refers to the underworld.

MINGMEN 命門 "Gate of destiny." The furnace that infuses our complements of primordial *yin* and *yang,* early and later heaven, and *shen* and *jing,* thus maintaining the integrity of these interactions which empower health and evolution.

MINGMING 命名 To distinguish; literally, to give a thing a destiny by naming it.

MINGXUE 名學 Logic; literally, the study of names.

MU 木 Wood.

MU 母 Mother.

MU ZI TOU SHOU ZHUO 目自頭首辶 The *dao* as "the way one comes to see and understand oneself."

NANJING (The Classic of Difficult Issues) 難經 Medical text dating to the first century C.E.

NEI 內 Internal, inner.

NEI BIAN 內篇 Inner volume. Signifies a work that focuses on the inner aspects of a subject such as spiritual transformation in the discipline of internal alchemy.

NEI JING SU WEN (The Yellow Emperor's Classic of Internal Medicine) (c. 200 B.C.E.) 內經素問 The oldest and most respected of the Chinese medical classics.

NU 怒 Anger; the emotion associated with the wood officials.

PANGU 盤古 Mythological giant who stood on earth and supported heaven. Mythological ancestor of the human race.

PO 魄 *Shen* associated with the lung official. Governs the human descent in life. Upon death, the *po* leaves the body through the anus to decay in the earth. It consists of the seven emotions: fear, fright, anger, joy, worry, sadness, and grief. The *po* allows for the construction of the body out of spirit (contrast with *hun*).

PO 剝 *Yijing* hexagram 23, "splitting apart." Termed by Liu Yiming "the door of death."

QI 氣 The motivating force that supports all of life's functional and physical manifestations.

QI 泣 To weep silent tears.

QIHAI 氣海 Sea of *qi*. Depending on the text, several "seas of *qi*" are said to be located throughout the body. Often synonymous with the dantian. A reserve of *qi*.

QING 青 The blue-green color associated with new growth in spring.

QINGMING 青冥 "Blue-green darkness"; the *Bai Wen Bian* uses this term to refer to the color of the penetrating fire in the *dantian*.

QIZHI 氣質 The acquired temperament according to Liu Yiming.

QUAN 泉 A spring gushing out from the ground. Part of the character *yuan*, meaning "source."

REN 仁 Virtue associated with the wood element; benevolence.

RENBUZHI 人不智 Those who do not know; ignorance. Contrast with *daoxin*.

RENDAO 人道 Human way, the ways of humanity. The tendency of human beings to lose original nature.

RI 日 The sun.

SANMAI 散脈 *Qi* wild; a pulse quality denoting the separation of *yin* and *yang*.

SHE 社 Altar to the spirit of the earth. On the left is the character for spirit; on the right is the character for earth.

SHEN 神 *Yang* aspect of heart spirit that complements *ling*. The spirit associated with the heart official. The character *shen* gives the notion of heaven extending itself toward humanity. In the microcosm, the *shen* is that aspect of self that we extend in order to discover and manifest potential (*jing* and *ling*). The impulse (lightning in the macrocosm and spiritual activity in the microcosm) that activates potential.

SHEN 申 Terrestrial branch associated with the metal element.

SHENG 生 Life.

SHENGQI 生氣 Anger.

SHENGREN 聖人 Sage.

SHENHUA 神話 Literally, "spirit talk"; Myth.

SHENJING 神精 Interpenetration of *shen* with *jing* and the empowerment that springs forth.

SHENJING 神經 Literally, "lines that transmit spirit"; The nervous system.

SHENMEN 神門 Name of acupuncture point Heart-7, "spirit gate."

SHENMING 神明 Bright spiritual influence that radiates from heaven.

SHEN NONG BEN CAO (The Treatise of the Spiritual Farmer) 神農本草 China's first text on herbal medicine (c. second century C.E.) attributed to the mythological figure Shen-nong.

SHI 爪 Radical 113; the moon, the stars, and the sun.

SHI JING (The Book of Poetry) 詩經 Confucian classic; collection of poetry written c. 722 B.C.E.

SHISHEN 識神 The "distinguishing spirit"; the discriminating aspect of mind that leads us away from true nature.

SHU 恕 Virtue associated with the earth element; reciprocity. According to Legge (1971, p. 469), "Making our own feelings the rule for our dealing with others."

SHU 數 Literally, "numbers"; fate.

SHU 儵 Literally, "uncertainty." The emperor of the south sea in the myth of Huntun.

SHUI 水 The water element.

SHU JING (The Book of Documents) (date unknown) 書經 One of the Confucian classics.

SHUN 順 To go along or follow; to align one's self with events.

SI 思 Sympathy; the emotion associated with the earth officials.

SI 四 The number four.

SI 死 Death.

TANG 堂 Palace.

TIAN 天 Heaven; corresponds to the highest aspect of being toward which the human spirit ascends.

TIANMING 天命 Destiny, as appointed by heaven; heavenly ordinance.

TAIQUAN 太泉 Alternate name for Lung-9, which denotes the origin of a stream.

TAIYUAN 太淵 Name of acupuncture point Lung-9; refers to the void or abyss between heaven and earth.

TING 聽 To listen.

TONG 通 To be in communication with, to interpenetrate.

TONG SHENMING 通神明 Spiritual brightness; to be in communication with the bright spiritual influence radiating from heaven within (one's heart spirit) and without (the spiritual influence radiating from the moon, stars, and sun).

TOU 頭 The head. The right half of the character *dao*.

Tu 土 The earth element.

WAI 外 External, outer.

WAI BIAN 外篇 Outer volume. Focuses on the external application of a discipline, such as turning lead into gold in external alchemy.

WAIMING 外命 Alternate name for acupuncture point Kidney-7, meaning literally "beyond destiny."

WANG 王 King.

WEI 為 Being.

WEIQI 衛氣 Defensive *qi*.

WO 我 Self.

WU 巫 Female shaman.

WU 五 The number five.

WUJI 無幾 Without limit.

WUJI 無極 Pole of emptiness; the central axis of being.

WUMING 無名 Nameless; not having a personal sense of self as denoted by one's name. A characteristic of the sage and of *dao*.

WUSHENGWUXIU: Neither sound nor smell; devoid of senses.

WUWEI 無為 Nonbeing, inaction, alignment with *dao*.

WUXING 五行 The five transformations or "elements."

XI 覡 Male shaman.

XIAN 仙 Daoist immortal. Sage.

XIANG 相 An official. Mutual.

XIANGKEXU 相克序 The control cycle of the five elements.

XIANGSHENGXU 相生序 The creation cycle of the five elements; literally, the "mutual production cycle."

XIANTIAN 先天 Early heaven. All influences acquired in life prior to the first breath. Includes the notion of *karma* and the modern concept of genetics.

XIN 心 Heart, mind. In health, these two are present as one and empower spontaneity and intuition.

XIN 信 Virtue associated with the earth element; faith, trust. A person standing by his or her word; integrity.

XING 形 Form.

XING 性 Inborn nature.

XING 星 Star.

XI WANG MU 西王母 Daoist immortal. The Queen Mother of the West who presides over birth and death.

XU 虛 Emptiness, void. 墟 Burialground.

XUAN 玄 Dark, mysterious; a characteristic of *dao*.

XUAN WANG (826–781 B.C.E.) 宣王 Emperor of the Zhou dynasty, author of a poem in the *Book of Odes*.

XUANGUAN 玄關 Dark gate, a name for the mysterious pass; the interface between being and nonbeing. Refers also to Daoism, the philosophy that provides an entrance to the primordial aspects of being.

XUE 血 Blood, whose highest function is to empower us to choose vulnerability from a position of strength.

XUEMAI 血脈 Blood vessel.

XUEQI 血氣 Blood and *qi*.

XUJI 虛極 Pole of emptiness; the central axis around which cosmological transformation occurs.

XUKONG 虛空 The void.

XUNZI (HSUN TZU) (born 312 B.C.E.) 荀子 Confucian author who wrote the text bearing his name.

YANG 陽 The active principle, complementary in nature to *yin*. The impulse that acts on potential.

YANGMING 陽明 The functional relationship between the stomach and large intestine officials.

YANGQI 陽氣 According to the alchemy of Liu Yiming, the enlivening influence of early heaven.

YI 一 The number one.

YI 義 The virtue associated with the metal element; righteousness, justice.

YI 意 The *shen* associated with the spleen official; ideation.

YIJING (I Ching) (The Book of Changes) (Zhou dynasty, c. 770 B.C.E.) 易經 One of the Confucian classics. A text that helps guide the reader's intuition to comprehend the dynamic movements of *qi*, which are the foundation of material reality.

YIN 陰 The passive principle, complementary in nature to *yang*. The potential basis for all of life's manifestations.

YIN 音 A sound.

YING 營 An encampment, an army camp.

YING 盈 To be nourished by the fruits of one's labors.

YINGQI 營氣 The highest essence gleaned from respiration and alimentation that constitutes the nourishing aspect and blood.

YINQI 陰氣 According to the alchemy of Liu Yiming, the mundane conditioning influences acquired during later heaven.

YOU 憂 Grief; the emotion associated with the metal officials.

YOUMING 有名 Named; to have a personal name and thus to have lost one's original nature. To direct one's will externally for worldly gain.

YU 禹 Mythological founder and emperor of China's first dynasty, the Xia (2205–1766 B.C.E.). Son of Gun.

YU 愈 To heal.

YU 遇 To meet.

YU 俞 To transmit. A class of acupuncture points.

YUAN 原 Source, origin.

YUAN 淵 Abyss, the void.

YUAN 元 Primordial.

YUAN 遠 Far, distant.

YUANQI 元氣 Primordial (original) *qi*. Our inherited endowment of *yin* and *yang*.

YUANYANG 元陽 Our primordial complement of *yang* associated with the function of the right kidney.

YUANYIN 元陰 Our primordial complement of *yin* associated with the function of the left kidney.

YUANSHI 元始 The primordial beginning; zero.

YUE 月 The moon.

YUE 曰 Speak.

ZANG 臓 Hidden; the *yin* organs (臟).

ZHANG BODUAN Daoist philosopher and alchemist (Yuan dynasty).

ZHEN 真 Upright, correct, authentic; that which is true.

ZHENQI 真氣 That *qi* which supports the human to stand upright between heaven and earth and thus fulfill destiny. That *qi* which reflects the pristine quality of authentic *dao*.

ZHENXING 真性 True nature.

ZHI 治 To treat, to heal, "to set in order," as Emperor Yu did with the floods.

ZHI 智 The virtue associated with the water element; wisdom.

ZHI 質 Substance.

ZHI 志 Human will. The *shen* associated with the kidney official.

ZHIQI 志氣 Willpower.

ZHISHI 志室 Acupuncture point Bladder-52 (47), "room of will."

ZHUANGZI (369?–286? B.C.E.) 莊子 Daoist philosopher to whom the text of the same name is ascribed. Literally may be translated as "serious child." Of interest owing to the great humor displayed in his writing.

ZHUO 辶 Radical 162; walking. The left half of the character *dao*.

ZHUXI (1130–1200 C.E.) 朱喜 Confucian philosopher.

ZIRAN 自然 The natural spontaneity of primordial *dao*; that which emerges in ultimate health.

ZONG 宗 Ancestor. An ancestral hall, the building from which emanates the influence of the deceased ancestors over their posterity.

ZONGQI 宗氣 Ancestral *qi*. That which governs all rhythmic movements in the microcosm such as the heartbeat and the respiratory rhythm.

ZU 祖 Ancestor, origin, beginning.

ZU 足 Foot.

GLOSSARY OF ENGLISH TERMS

ACUPUNCTURE Art of inserting fine needles into the body at specific locations to influence the function of specific aspects of being.

AGGRESSIVE ENERGY Pernicious *qi* that perpetuates dysfunctional relationships between the officials across the *ke* cycle.

ALCHEMY Process of infusing two or more aspects of being into a unity that has been elevated in status to its individual components. The outer aspect of alchemy involves combining various metals in the quest to produce gold. The inner aspect involves the interpenetration of our acquired and primordial influences in a way that leads to the fulfillment of destiny. Therefore we gain immortality by cultivating a virtue perfectly expressed and of everlasting merit.

BLOOD The combination of innate and acquired influences that nourish the embodiment of virtue.

COLD In Chinese medicine, one of the seven "external devils" or environmental pathogens. Any internal state characterized by the dysfunctional display of cold. The nature of cold is to contract and slow functional processes within any aspect of being. Hence slow digestion or thought may be considered indicative of pathological cold. Cold is generally associated with the water element.

CONCEPTION VESSEL One of the eight extra meridians that governs the overall quality and function of *yin*.

DAMP In Chinese medicine, one of the seven "external devils" or environmental pathogens. Internal damp represents the transformation into burden of that which should have nourished us in life. Dampness tends to result from, or potentiate, dysfunction of the earth element.

DRY In Chinese medicine, one of the seven "external devils" or environmental pathogens. Internally, dryness arises from *yin* deficiency and is generally associated with the metal element.

EIGHT EXTRAORDINARY MERIDIANS In addition to the twelve meridians associated with the officials are eight meridians called the "eight extraordinary meridians." These meridians are more primordial in nature and emerge embryologically before the twelve principal meridians. The eight extraordinary meridians may be thought of as oceans, whereas the principal meridians are rivers. The eight extra meridians are Conception Vessel, Governor Vessel, Penetrating Vessel, Belt Vessel, *Yin* Linking Channel, *Yang* Linking Channel, *Yin* Heel Channel, and *Yang* Heel Channel.

EXIT/ENTRY POINTS The exit point of a meridian is where *qi* exits to enter the following meridian's entry point according to the dynamic flow of the Chinese clock. Functional blocks between these points can be detected on the pulse and denote specific qualities of separation between a person's heart and mind.

FIVE-ELEMENTS THEORY The five-element system views nature as comprised of five broad qualities of *qi*, namely, water, wood, fire, earth, and metal. These five elements exist together in a dynamic system of interdependent forces, each balanced by the others. The five-element system is a qualitative standard of reference that may be used to assess the functional relationships inherent in any dynamic process.

FUNCTION The dynamic quality of relationship that exists between two or more things.

GOVERNOR VESSEL One of the eight extra meridians that governs the overall quality and function of *yang*.

HEAT In Chinese medicine one of the seven "external devils" or environmental pathogens. Any internal state characterized by the dysfunctional display of heat. The nature of heat is to expand and accelerate functional processes within any aspect of being. Hence a rapid heart rate or speech may be considered indicative of pathological heat. Heat is generally associated with the fire element.

HERBALISM Art of prescribing herbs in order to influence the function of specific aspects of being.

HOMEOSTASIS Self-regulated state in which the functional dynamics of a system maintain harmony.

HORARY POINT Each meridian contains an element point that accesses the same elemental energy as the meridian itself. For instance, the lung official is associated with the metal element and therefore Lung-8, the metal point associated with the lung official, is the horary point. The accompanying table lists all of the horary points. Horary points are especially effective during the high point of their meridian according to the Chinese clock. During this time, a horary point may be used in order to give an extra tonification or sedation to the associated meridian. Horary points are also particularly effective during the seasonal high point associated with the given meridian as shown in the table here.

Horary Points

HORARY POINTS		HIGH TIME	SEASONAL HIGH POINT
Water	Bl-66	3–5 P.M.	Winter Solstice, December 21
	Ki-10	5–7 P.M.	
Wood	Gb-41	11 P.M.–1 A.M.	Spring Equinox, March 21
	Lv-1	1–3 A.M.	
Fire	Ht-8	11 A.M.–1 P.M.	Summer Solstice, June 21
	SI-5	1–3 P.M.	
	HP-8	7–9 P.M.	
	TH-6	9–11 P.M.	
Earth	St-36	7–9 A.M.	Late Summer, August 21
	Sp-3	9–11 A.M.	
Metal	Lu-8	3–5 A.M.	Fall Equinox, September 21
	LI-1	5–7 A.M.	

HUSBAND/WIFE IMBALANCE Dysfunctional state as determined by pulse diagnosis in which *yin* and *yang* are at a terminal point of separation. Illness has reached a point at which serious pathology is near if the condition is not rectified.

INHERITED ENDOWMENT *Jing, yuanqi,* and *shen.*

MACROCOSM The totality of *dao* as it exists externally to each human being.

MERIDIAN Theoretical construct that denotes a strong functional relationship between a series of acupuncture points. For example, nine points may be discerned that are especially associated with the function of the heart official. Drawing a line through these points creates the heart meridian.

MICROCOSM Totality of *dao* as it exists within each human being.

NEEDLE In the practice of acupuncture, to insert a fine needle in an acupuncture point.

OFFICIAL Sum total of an organ's sphere of influence in every aspect of being.

PRIMORDIAL INFLUENCES Used in this text to signify the influence of those aspects of the inherited endowment that are closest in nature to *dao,* the *jing* and *yuanqi.*

PULSE DIAGNOSIS Craft of discerning the functional state of a patient's being through palpation of specific points along the radial artery at the wrist bilaterally.

SEDATION In acupuncture, the technique of diminishing the functional influence of a specific aspect of being.

SOURCE POINTS Each of the meridians includes a "source" (character *yuan)* point. Source points have the unique characteristic of being able to access the virtue of every point on a given meridian but in a more general and less specific way. My feeling is that the source points on the *yin* meridians connect the function of the associated official to the *dao* as the ultimate source of primordial *qi.* The source points on the *yang* meridians connect the function of the associated official to the *dao* as the ultimate source of acquired *qi.*

SPIRITUAL Those aspects of self that transcend physical being.

TONIFICATION In acupuncture, the technique of strengthening the functional influence of a specific aspect of being.

WIND In Chinese medicine one of the seven "external devils" or environmental pathogens. Any internal state characterized by chaos. Wind is generally associated with the wood element.

WINDOW OF HEAVEN POINTS (*Tianchuang*: 天窗) Located on the upper chest, neck, and face, these acupuncture points have a strong effect in promoting unity of the heart and mind. As confluent points of the divergent meridians they may help bring to the surface emotional material that has been too painful to consciously assimilate.

YIN/YANG THEORY System that allows us to assess the relative qualities of *yin* and *yang* as they serve as the foundation for the manifestation of existence.

REFERENCES

ALLINSON, R. E. (ed.). (1989). *Understanding the Chinese Mind: The Philosophical Roots*. Hong Kong; New York: Oxford University Press.

ANDERSON, P. (1989). *The Method of Holding the Three Ones: A Taoist Manual of Meditation of the Fourth Century* A.D. London: Curzon Press.

ANTHONY, C. K. (1981). *The Philosophy of the* I Ching. Stow, Mass.: Anthony Publishing.

AYSCOUGH, F. (1930). "Notes on the symbolism of the purple forbidden city." *Journal of the North China Branch of the Royal Asiatic Society* 52: 51–78.

BEIJING COLLEGE OF TRADITIONAL CHINESE MEDICINE. (1980). *Essentials of Chinese Acupuncture*. Beijing: Foreign Languages Press.

BENSKY, D., AND BAROLET, R. (1990). *Chinese Herbal Medicine: Formulas and Strategies*. Seattle: Eastland Press.

BENSKY, D., AND GAMBLE, A. (1986). *Chinese Herbal Medicine: Materia Medica*. Seattle: Eastland Press.

BIRCH, S. (1994, Spring). "An historical study of radial pulse six position diagnosis: Naming the unnameable." *Journal of Acupuncture Society of New York* 1, nos. 3 and 4:19–32.

BISHOP, C. W. (1933). "The worship of earth in ancient China." *Journal of the North China Branch of the Royal Asiatic Society* 64: 24–43.

BLOOM, I. (1985). "On the matter of the mind: The metaphysical basis of the expanded self." In *Individualism and Holism: Studies in Confucian and Taoist Values,* edited by D. J. Munro, pp. 293–327. Ann Arbor: Center for Chinese Studies, University of Michigan.

BOHM, D. (1971). "Quantum theory as an indication of the new order in physics. Part A: The development of new orders as shown through the history of physics." *Foundations of Physics,* Vol. 1, pp. 359–381.

———. (1973). "Quantum theory as an indication of the new order in physics. Part B: Implicate and explicate order in physical law." *Foundations of Physics,* Vol. 3, pp. 139–168.

BONNEFOY, Y. (1991). *Asian Mythologies.* Chicago: University of Chicago Press.

CAPRA, F. (1975). *The Tao of Physics.* Berkeley, Calif.: Shambhala.

CHAMBERLAIN, S. (1980, Summer). *"Shen* and *ling." Journal of Traditional Acupuncture,* pp. 16–19.

CHAN, WING-TSIT. (1973). *A Source Book in Chinese Philosophy.* Princeton, N.J.: Princeton University Press.

CHEN, E. M. (1973). "The meaning of *te* in the *Tao Te Ching:* An examination of the concept of nature in Chinese Taoism." *Philosophy East and West* 23: 457–470.

———. (1989). *The Tao Te Ching.* New York: Paragon House.

CH'EN, CH'I-YUN (trans.). (1980). *Hsun Yueh and the Mind of Late Han China.* Princeton, N.J.: Princeton University Press.

CHENG XINNONG. (1990). *Chinese Acupuncture and Moxibustion.* Beijing: Foreign Language Press.

CHRISTIE, A. (1975). *Chinese Mythology.* New York: Hamlyn.

CLEARY, T. (1986a). *The Inner Teachings of Taoism.* Boston: Shambhala.

———. (1986b). *The Taoist I-Ching.* Boston: Shambhala.

———. (1989). *The Book of Balance and Harmony.* San Francisco, Calif.: North Point Press.

COHEN, P. (1979). *Selected Works of Peter A. Broodberg.* Berkeley: University of California Press.

CONNELLY, D. (1994). *Traditional Acupuncture: The Law of the Five Elements.* Columbia, Md.: Traditional Acupuncture Institute.

DALE, R. A. (1993). "The demystification of Chinese pulse diagnosis: An overview of the validations, holograms, and systemics for learning the principles and techniques." *American Journal of Acupuncture* 21, no. 1: 63–80.

DE BARY, T., CHAN, W. T., AND WATSON, B. (1960). *Sources of Chinese Tradition*, Vol. 1. New York: Columbia University Press.

DELANEY, C., LEONARD, D., AND KISCH, L. (1989). *The Acupuncture Point Book*. Makawao, Hawaii: Roast Duck Productions.

DORE, H. (1987). *Chinese Customs*, trans. by M. Kennelly. Singapore: Graham Brash.

DUMONT, T. (1972). *Mental Therapeutics*. Chicago: Yoga Publication Society.

EBERHARD, W. (1986). *A Dictionary of Chinese Symbols: Hidden Symbols in Chinese Life and Thought*. London; New York: Routledge and Kegan Paul.

ECKMAN, P. (1987). *The Book of Changes in Traditional Oriental Medicine*. Columbia, Md.: Traditional Acupuncture Institute.

EINSTEIN, A., AND INFELD, L. (1938). *The Evolution of Physics*. New York: Simon & Schuster.

ELLIS, A., WISEMAN, N., AND BOSS, K. (1989). *Grasping the Wind*. Brookline, Mass.: Paradigm.

ENO, R. (1990). *The Confucian Creation of Heaven*. Albany: State University of New York Press.

ESSENTIALS OF CHINESE ACUPUNCTURE. (1980). Beijing: Foreign Language Press.

FINGARETTE, H. (1972). *Confucius—The Secular as Sacred*. New York: Harper & Row.

FISCHER, E. S. (1930). "A journey to the Tung Ling and a visit to the desecrated Eastern mausolea of the Ta Tsing dynasty in 1929." *Journal of the North China Branch of the Royal Asiatic Society* 61: 20–39.

FOUNDATION FOR INNER PEACE. (1975). *A Course in Miracles*. Huntington Station, N.Y.: Author.

FUNG YU-LAN. (1983). *A History of Chinese Philosophy*, Vols. 1 and 2. Princeton, N.J.: Princeton University Press.

GARDNER, D. K. (trans.). (1990). *Learning to Be a Sage*. Berkeley: University of California Press.

GEBSER, J. (1984). *The Ever-Present Origin*. Athens: Ohio University Press.

GIRARDOT, N. J. (1983). *Myth and Meaning in Early Taoism*. Berkeley: University of California Press.

GRAHAM, A. C. (trans.). (1990). *The Book of Lieh-tzu: A Classic of*

Tao. New York: Columbia University Press.

GRANET, M. (1930). *Chinese Civilization.* New York: Knopf.

GWEI-DJEN, L., AND NEEDHAM, J. (1980). *Celestial Lancets: A History and Rationale of Acupuncture and Moxabuxtion.* Cambridge; New York: Cambridge University Press.

————. (1983). *Science and Civilisation in China: Chemistry and Chemical Technology,* Vol. 5. Cambridge: Cambridge University Press.

HAMMER, L. (1990). *Dragon Rises, Red Bird Flies.* Barrytown, N.Y.: Station Hill Press.

————. (1993a). "Contemporary pulse diagnosis—part I: New perspectives on reviving an ancient art." *American Journal of Acupuncture* 21, no. 2: 123–139.

————. (1993b). "Contemporary pulse diagnosis—part II: Pulse taking method." *American Journal of Acupuncture* 21, no. 3: 219–235.

HAMMER, L. (in press). *Contemporary Chinese Pulse Diagnosis.* Seattle: Eastland Press.

HENDERSON, J. B. (1984). *The Development and Decline of Chinese Cosmology.* New York: Columbia University Press.

HENRICKS, R. G. (trans.). (1989). *Lao-Tzu Te-Tao Ching.* New York: Ballantine Books.

HICKS, S. (1985). *Catalogue of Acupuncture Point Translations.* Columbia, Md.: Traditional Acupuncture Institute.

HOMANN, R. (trans.). (1976). *Pai Wen Pien or The Hundred Questions: A Dialogue Between Two Taoists on the Macrocosmic and Microcosmic System of Correspondence.* Leiden: E. J. Brill.

HUMPHREYS, C. (1984). *A Popular Dictionary of Buddhism.* London: Curzon Press.

JARRETT, L. S. (1985, Autumn). "The holographic paradigm and acupuncture." *Journal of Traditional Acupuncture* 8, no. 2: 36–41.

————. (1992a, April). "Myth and meaning in Chinese medicine." *Traditional Acupuncture Society Journal,* no. 11: 45–48.

————. (1992b, October). "The returned spirit (*gui ling*) of traditional Chinese medicine." *Traditional Acupuncture Society Journal,* no. 12: 19–31.

————. (1992c). "The role of human will (*zhi*), and the spirit of Bladder-52." *American Journal of Acupuncture* 20, no. 4: 349–358.

————. (1993a). "Constitutional type and the internal tradition of Chinese medicine—Part I: The ever present cause." *American Journal of Acupuncture* 21, no. 1: 19–32.

————. (1993b). "Constitutional type and the internal tradition of Chinese medicine—Part II: The ontogeny of life." *American Journal of Acupuncture* 21, no. 2: 141–158.

————. (1994a). "The loss and return of original nature: The law of husband/wife." *American Journal of Acupuncture* 22, no. 1: 29–45.

————. (1994b, Fall). "The use of entry and exit points in traditional acupuncture." *Journal of the National Academy of Acupuncture and Oriental Medicine* 1, no. 1: 19–30.

————. (1995a). "Chinese medicine and the betrayal of intimacy: The theory and treatment of abuse, incest, rape and divorce with acupuncture and herbs—Part I." *American Journal of Acupuncture* 23, no. 1: 35–51.

————. (1995b). "Chinese medicine and the betrayal of intimacy: The theory and treatment of abuse, incest, rape and divorce with acupuncture and herbs—Part II." *American Journal of Acupuncture* 23, no. 2: 123–151.

————. (1995c). "Chinese medicine and the betrayal of intimacy: The theory and treatment of abuse, incest, rape and divorce with acupuncture and herbs—Part III: Case study." *American Journal of Acupuncture* 23, no. 3: 241–267.

————. (1996). *"Niu Huang Qing Xin Wan."* Internet: http://www.spiritpathpress.com/articles.html.

KAPTCHUK, T. J. (1983). *The Web That Has No Weaver.* Chicago: Congdon & Weed.

KI, S., AND YUNKYO, L. (1985). *The Canon of Acupuncture: Huang Ti Nei Ching Ling Shu.* Seoul, Korea: Korea Acupuncture Society.

KOHN, L. (1992). *Early Chinese Mysticism: Philosophy and Soteriology in the Taoist Tradition.* Princeton, N.J.: Princeton University Press.

————. (1993). *The Taoist Experience.* Albany: State University of New York Press.

KUANG-MING, WU. (1989). "Chinese aesthetics." In *Understanding the Chinese Mind: The Philosophical Roots,* edited by R. E. Allinson, pp. 236–264. New York: Oxford University Press.

LAGERWEY, J. (1987). *Taoist Ritual in Chinese Society and History.* New York: Macmillan.

LARRE, C., AND ROCHAT DE LA VALLEE, E. (1985). *The Secret Treatise of the Spiritual Orchard.* East Grinstead, U.K.: International Register of Oriental Medicine.

————. (1989). *The Lung.* Paris: Institut Ricci.

————. (1995). *Rooted in Spirit: The Heart of Chinese Medicine.* Barrytown, N.Y.: Station Hill Press.

LARRE, C., SCHATZ, J., AND ROCHAT DE LA VALLEE, E. (1986). *Survey of Traditional Chinese Medicine.* Columbia, Md.: Traditional Acupuncture Institute.

LAU, D. C. (trans.). (1970). *Mencius.* Harmondsworth, U.K.: Penguin Books.

LEGEZA, L. (1975). *Tao Magic: The Secret Language of Diagrams and Calligraphy.* New York: Thames and Hudson.

LEGGE, J. (trans.). (1970). *The Works of Mencius.* New York: Dover.

————. (1971). *Confucius: Confucian Analects, The Great Learning and the Doctrine of the Mean.* New York: Dover.

LIEBENTHAL, W. (1952, January). "The immortality of the soul in Chinese thought." *Monumenta Nipponica* 8, no. 8: 327–397.

LIN, P. J. (1977). *A Translation of Lao Tzu's Tao Te Ching and Wang Pi's Commentary.* Ann Arbor: Center for Chinese Studies, University of Michigan.

LIN, YUTANG (1942). *The Wisdom of Lao Tzu.* New York: Modern Library.

LOW, R. (1985). *The Secondary Vessels of Acupuncture.* New York: Thorsons.

LU, H. C. (trans.). (1978). *A Complete Translation of: The Yellow Emperor's Classic of Internal Medicine and the Difficult Classic.* Vancouver, B.C.: Academy of Oriental Heritage.

MAJOR, J. S. (1973). *Topography and Cosmology in Early Han Thought: Chapter Four of Huai-Nan-Tzu.* Cambridge, Mass.: Harvard University Press. Yen Ching Institute.

MANN, F. (1974). *The Treatment of Disease by Acupuncture.* London: William Heinemann Medical Books.

MATHEWS, R. H. (1931). *Mathews' Chinese-English Dictionary.* Cambridge, Mass.: Harvard University Press.

MING, OU. (1982). *Chinese-English Glossary of Common Terms in Traditional Chinese Medicine.* Hong Kong: Joint Publishing.

MORGAN, E. (1920). "Destiny, fate." *Journal of the North China Branch of the Royal Asiatic Society* 51: 25.

MUNRO, D. J. (ed.). (1985). *Individualism and Holism: Studies in Confucian and Taoist Values.* Ann Arbor: Center for Chinese Studies, University of Michigan.

O'CONNOR, J., AND BENSKY, D. (trans. and eds.). (1987). *Acupuncture: A Comprehensive Text.* Seattle: Eastland Press.

OMURA, Y. (1982). *Acupuncture Medicine.* Tokyo: Japan Publications.

PALUDAN, A. (1991). *The Chinese Spirit Road: The Classical Tradition of Stone Tomb Statuary.* New Haven, Conn.: Yale University Press.

PORKERT, M. (1982). *The Theoretical Foundations of Chinese Medicine.* Cambridge, Mass.: MIT Press.

―――――. (1983). "The essentials of Chinese diagnostics." *Acta Medicinae Sinensis.* Zurich, Switzerland: Chinese Medicine Publications.

PRIBRAM, K. (1982). "What the fuss is all about." In *The Holographic Paradigm and Other Paradoxes,* edited by K. Wilber, p. 34. Boulder, Colo.: Shambhala.

RAWSON, P., AND LEGEZA, L. (1973). *The Chinese Philosophy of Time and Change: Tao.* New York: Thames and Hudson.

RITSEMA, R., AND KARCHER, S. (1994). *I Ching: The Classic Chinese Oracle of Change.* Rockport, Mass.: Element Books.

SASO, M. (1990). *Blue Dragon, White Tiger: Taoist Rites of Passage.* Washington, D.C.: The Taoist Center; Honolulu: University of Hawaii Press.

SHEN NUNG BEN TSAO. (1982). Beijing: Chung I Ku chih Chu Bian She.

SOOTHILL, W. E., AND HODOUS, L. (1995). *A Dictionary of Chinese Buddhist Terms.* Surrey, U.K.: Curzon Press.

SUN TZU. (1973). *The Art of War.* Hong Kong: Grand Cultural Service Company.

T'ANG, CHUN-I. (1962, January). "The *t'ien ming* [heavenly ordinance] in pre-Ch'in China—I." *Philosophy and Culture: East and West* 11: 195–218.

―――――. (1962, April). "The *t'ien ming* [heavenly ordinance] in pre-Ch'in China—II." *Philosophy and Culture: East and West* 12: 29–49.

TU, WEI-MING. (1985). "Subjectivity in Liu Tsung-chou." In *Individualism and Holism: Studies in Confucian and Taoist Values,* edited by D. Munro, pp. 215–238. Ann Arbor: Center for Chinese Studies, University of Michigan.

UNSCHULD, P. U. (1985). *Medicine in China: A History of Ideas.* Berkeley: University of California Press.

―――――. (1986). *Nan-Ching: The Classic of Difficult Issues.* Berkeley: University of California Press.

―――――. (1988). *Introductory Readings in Classical Chinese Medicine.* Boston: Kluwer Academic.

VAN OVER, R. (1973). *Taoist Tales.* New York: Meridian.

VEITH, I. (1949). The *Yellow Emperor's Classic of Internal Medicine.* Berkeley: University of California Press.

WARE, J. R. (1966). *Alchemy, Medicine, and Religion in the China of*

A.D. *320*. Mineola, N.Y.: Dover.

WATSON, B. (trans.). (1964a). *Chuang Tzu: Basic Writings*. New York: Columbia University Press.

————. (1964b). *Han Fei Tzu, Basic Writings*. New York: Columbia University Press.

————. (1968). *The Complete Works of Chuang Tzu*. New York: Columbia University Press.

WIEGER, L. (1965). *Chinese Characters*. New York: Paragon Book Reprint.

WILDER, G. D., AND INGRAM, J. H. (1974). *Analysis of Chinese Characters*. New York: Dover.

WILHELM, R. (1962). *The Secret of the Golden Flower*. New York: Harcourt, Brace & World.

————. (1968). *The I-Ching or Book of Changes*. Princeton, N.J.: Princeton University Press.

WILLIAMS, C. A. S. (1974). *Chinese Symbolism and Art Motifs*. Rutland, Vt.: Charles E. Tuttle.

WORSLEY, J. R. (1979). *The Meridians of Ch'i Energy: Point Reference Guide*. Columbia, Md.: Traditional Acupuncture Institute.

WU, JING-NUAN (trans.). (1991). *Yi Jing*. Washington, D.C.: The Taoist Center.

————. (1993). *Ling Shu, or The Spiritual Pivot*. Washington, D.C.: The Taoist Center.

PINYIN INDEX

ENGLISH INDEX

The way to transcend karma lies in the proper use of the mind and will. The oneness of all life is a truth that can be fully realized only when false notions of a separate self, whose destiny can be considered apart from the whole, are forever annihilated.

– Li Junfan

LONNY S. JARRETT, M. AC., has been a student of Chinese medicine since 1980. He is a graduate of the Traditional Acupuncture Institute and a fellow of the National Academy of Acupuncture and Oriental Medicine. He holds a master's degree in neurobiology and a fourth degree black belt in Tae Kwon Do. Lonny teaches and publishes extensively on inner traditions of Chinese medicine and pulse diagnosis. He maintains his clinical practice in Stockbridge, Massachusetts. A current teaching schedule as well as many of his articles are available on his Web page at http://www.spiritpathpress.com.